Vascular Liver Disease

Laurie D. DeLeve
Guadalupe Garcia-Tsao
Editors

Vascular Liver Disease

Mechanisms and Management

Springer

Editors
Laurie D. DeLeve
Division of Gastrointestinal
and Liver Diseases
University of Southern California
Keck School of Medicine
Los Angeles, CA 90033, USA
deleve@usc.edu

Guadalupe Garcia-Tsao
Section of Digestive Diseases
Yale University School of Medicine
New Haven, CT 06520, USA
guadalupe.garcia-tsao@yale.edu

ISBN 978-1-4419-8326-8 e-ISBN 978-1-4419-8327-5
DOI 10.1007/978-1-4419-8327-5
Springer New York Dordrecht Heidelberg London

Library of Congress Control Number: 2011922497

Printed on acid-free paper

Springer is part of Springer Science+Business Media (www.springer.com)

Dedicated to our familes and friends, mentors and colleagues.

Preface

Functions of the liver are highly dependent on its vascular connections to the "outside world" (the gut and the splanchnic circulation) and the "inside world" (the heart and the systemic circulation). These connections not only allow the liver to process nutrients and store vitamins that are absorbed from the gut, but also permit removal of bacteria that come from the gut before they reach the systemic circulation. The liver detoxifies and metabolizes endogenous toxins (e.g., ammonia) and, importantly, exogenous substances such as alcohol and most medications that arrive to the liver via the systemic or splanchnic circulations. Additionally, the liver synthesizes substances such as albumin and clotting factors that are secreted into the systemic circulation and produces bile acids that are secreted through the biliary ducts into the gut, facilitating fat absorption.

It follows that abnormalities that directly or indirectly affect the hepatic vasculature will lead to significant disease. These abnormalities can be microscopic, at the level of the hepatic sinusoids, or can affect the larger afferent or efferent vessels. This book approaches all of these disease entities and includes the mechanisms and management of intrahepatic vascular disease, including the most common cause of intra- and extrahepatic vascular disease of the liver, cirrhosis, and also reviews the mechanisms and management of less common diseases of the liver vasculature such as sinusoidal obstruction syndrome (previously known as veno-occlusive disease), portal vein thrombosis, the Budd-Chiari syndrome, and congenital vascular malformations. The very fact that these entities are rare increases the challenge to physicians and physician scientists; the low incidence complicates the accrual of patients for clinical research and reduces physician experience in managing patients with these disorders.

Although many textbooks have been written on the consequences of cirrhosis on the liver vasculature, this is the only textbook that focuses on the liver vasculature as a separate entity. The authors are authorities in their field, from six different countries – one-third of the chapters are from authors outside of the United States (United States, Australia, Italy, Switzerland, Spain, and France).

The book is organized in three sections. The first section examines the pathophysiology of circulatory liver diseases. It examines the cellular and biochemical changes of the hepatic microcirculation in aging (Chap. 2), with fibrosis (Chaps. 2 and 4), and toxic injury (Chap. 2) and discusses general and liver-specific mechanisms involved in hemostasis and thrombosis (Chap. 1). Pathogenic factors underlying circulatory injury in liver transplantation (Chap. 5) and the mechanisms leading to portal hypertension (Chaps. 6 and 7) are also discussed. This section will be of particular interest to basic scientists and clinical investigators interested in the liver circulation, and to gastroenterologists, hepatologists, and hepatobiliary surgeons who would like to read about new developments in the field.

Section 2 provides in-depth information on the clinical approach to vascular liver diseases. Chapters 8 and 9 provide descriptions and images of the histology and radiological appearance of vascular liver disease, as well as discussions of the utility of liver biopsy and imaging modalities in diagnosis. The remaining five chapters discuss diagnosis and medical treatment of various vascular liver diseases.

Finally, the three chapters in Sect. 3 discuss the interventional radiology and surgical approaches to portal hypertension (Chaps. 15 and 16, respectively) and the indications for liver transplantation in patients with vascular liver disease (Chap. 17). Sections 2 and 3 will be of particular interest to gastroenterologists and hepatologists, to hepatobiliary surgeons and transplant surgeons, and to interventional radiologists with a particular interest in the liver, who will use this as a reference in patient management.

Los Angeles, CA Laurie D. DeLeve
New Haven, CT Guadalupe Garcia-Tsao

Contents

Contributors

Juan G. Abraldes
Hepatic Hemodynamic Laboratory, Liver Unit, Hospital Clinic-Idibaps, University of Barcelona and Centro de Investigación Biomédica de Enfermedades Hepáticas y Digestivas (Ciberehd), Barcelona, Spain

Eliano Bonaccorsi-Riani
Department of Abdominal and Transplantation Surgery, St. Luc Université Catholique de Louvain (UCL), Avenue Hippocrates 10, Brussels, Belgium

Jaime Bosch
Hepatic Hemodynamic Laboratory, Liver Unit, Hospital Clinic-Idibaps, University of Barcelona and Centro de Investigación Biomédica de Enfermedades Hepáticas y Digestivas (Ciberehd), Barcelona, Spain

Christophe Bureau
Hepato-Gastro-Enterologie, University of Toulouse, CHU Toulouse-Purpan Place du Dr Baylac, Toulouse, 31059, France

Pierre-Alain Clavien
Department of Surgery, University Hospital of Zurich, Ramistrase 100, CH-8091 Zurich, Switzerland

Victoria C. Cogger
Centre for Education and Research on Ageing, Sydney Medical School and ANZAC Research Institute, Sydney, NSW, Australia

Laurie D. DeLeve
Division of Gastrointestinal and Liver Diseases, University of Southern California, Keck School of Medicine, 2011 Zonal Avenue- HMR 603, Los Angeles, CA 90033, USA

Philipp Dutkowski
Department of Surgery, The Swiss HPB (Hepato-Pancreatico-Biliary) and Transplantation Center, University Hospital of Zurich, Zurich, Switzerland

Ashraf Mohammad El-Badry
Department of Surgery, The Swiss HPB (Hepato-Pancreatico-Biliary) and Transplantation Center, University Hospital of Zurich, Zurich, Switzerland

Robin Fraser
Department of Pathology, University of Otago, Christchurch, New Zealand

Juan Carlos García-Pagán
Hepatic Hemodynamic Laboratory, Liver Unit, Hospital Clinic
Barcelona-CIBERehd-IDIBAPS-Institut Clinic de Malalties Digestives
I Metaboliques, Villarroel 170 street, Barcelona 08036, Spain

Guadalupe Garcia-Tsao
Section of Digestive Diseases, Yale University School of Medicine,
333 Cedar Street, LMP 1080, New Haven, CT 06520, USA;
Section of Digestive Diseases, VA Connecticut Health Care System,
West Haven, CT, USA

Pierre Goffette
Department of Medical Imaging, St. Luc Université Catholique de
Louvain (UCL), Brussels, Belgium

Roberto J. Groszmann
Department of Medicine-Digestive Diseases, Yale University School
of Medicine, PO Box 208019, New Haven, CT 06520-8019, USA

J. Michael Henderson
Department of General Surgery, The Cleveland Clinic Foundation,
9500 Euclid Avenue/E32, Cleveland, OH 44195-000, USA

Dhanpat Jain
Department of Pathology, Yale University School of Medicine,
New Haven, CT USA

David G. Le Couteur
Centre for Education and Research on Ageing, The University of Sydney
and Concord R.G. Hospital, Sydney, NSW, Australia

Jan P. Lerut
Department of Abdominal and Transplantation Surgery, Starzl Abdominal
Transplant Unit, St. Luc Université Hospitals Universite catholique de
Louvain (UCL), Avenue Hippocrates 10, Brussels, Belgium

Joseph K. Lim
Section of Digestive Diseases, Yale University School of Medicine,
New Haven, CT 06520, USA;
Section of Gastroenterology, VA Connecticut Health Care System,
West Haven, CT, USA

Robert S. McCuskey
Department of Cell Biology and Anatomy, University of Arizona,
Tucson, AZ, USA

George B. McDonald
Gastroenterology/Hepatology Section (D2-190), Fred Hutchinson
Cancer Research Center and University of Washington School of Medicine,
1100 Fairview Avenue North, Seattle, WA 98109-1024, USA

Donald G. Mitchell
Department of Radiology, Thomas Jefferson University Hospital, Philadelphia, PA 19102, USA

Philippe Otal
Radiologie, University of Toulouse, CHU-Toulouse-Rangueil, 1 Ave J Poulhes, Toulouse 31059, France

Massimo Pinzani
Dipartimento di Medicina Interna, Center for Research, High Education and Transfer DENOThe, Università degli Studi di Firenze, Viale G.B. Morgagni, 85, 50134 Firenze, Italy

Simon C. Robson
Beth Israel Deaconess Medical Center, 330 Brookline Avenue, E/CLS-612, Boston, MA 02215, USA

Christopher G. Roth
Department of Radiology, Thomas Jefferson University Hospital, Philadelphia, PA 19102, USA

Susana Seijo-Rios
Hepatic Hemodynamic Laboratory, Liver Unit, Hospital Clinic Barcelona-CIBERehd-IDIBAPS-Institut Clinic de Malalties Digestives 1 Metaboliques, Villarroel 170 street, Barcelona 08036, Spain

Bård Smedsrød
Vascular Biology Research Group, Department of Medical Biology, University of Tromsø, Tromsø, Norway

Dmitri Svistounov
Vascular Biology Research Group, Department of Medical Biology, University of Tromsø, Tromsø, Norway

Puneeta Tandon
Hepatic Hemodynamic Laboratory, Liver Unit, Hospital Clinic Barcelona-CIBERehd-IDIBAPS-Institut Clinic de Malalties Digestives 1 Metaboliques, Villarroel 170 street, Barcelona 08036, Spain

Dominique-Charles Valla
Hépatologie, Hopital Beaujon, APHP; Université Denis, Diderot-Paris 7; and INSERM U773, 100 Bvd Leclerc, 92118 Clichy, France

Jean-Pierre Vinel
Hepato-Gastro-Enterologie, University of Toulouse, CHU Toulouse-Purpan, Place du Dr Baylac, Toulouse 31059, France

Alessandra Warren
ANZAC Research Institute and Center for Education and Research on Ageing, The University of Sydney, Sydney, NSW, Australia

A. Brian West
Department of Pathology, Yale University School of Medicine, New Haven, CT, USA

Alexander Zipprich
First Department of Internal Medicine, Martin-Luther-University Halle-Wittenberg, Halle/Saale, Germany

Svetlana N. Zykova
Department of Pathology, University Hospital of Northern Norway, Tromsø, Norway;
Centre for Education and Research on Ageing, Sydney Medical School and ANZAC Research Institute, Sydney, NSW, Australia

Part I

Mechanisms

Liver Endothelial Cells: Hemostasis, Thrombosis, and Hepatic Vascular Diseases

1

Simon C. Robson

Abstract

The liver is the source of blood plasma coagulation proteins and hepatic vascular elements are unique from the inflow or outflow macrovessels to the hepatic sinusoidal endothelium. The hemostatic process may be considered a defense mechanism that maintains normal blood vessel homeostasis and thereby preserves the integrity of the circulation. This chapter will cover mechanisms of hemostasis, summarize regulation of coagulation pathways, and indicate how thrombosis may develop in the diseased hepatic vasculature.

Patients with liver disease can exhibit coagulation factor synthetic dysfunction, thrombocytopenia, excessive fibrinolysis, and associated features of portal hypertension that might provoke massive bleeding. Procoagulative abnormalities in liver diseases also exacerbate disordered sinusoidal remodeling, provoke abnormal angiogenesis, and contribute to venous thrombosis and further vascular compromise. Clearly, dysregulation of hemostasis and coagulation may result in a hemorrhagic tendency and may also provoke thrombosis. However, coagulation and hemostatic disorders are difficult to monitor or treat effectively; these processes greatly contribute to the morbidity and mortality seen in progressive liver disease.

Disordered hemostasis in acute and chronic liver diseases remains an important clinical problem that is still poorly understood and where ongoing research is critically needed.

Keywords

Liver • Endothelium • Platelet • Coagulation • Thrombosis • Hemostasis • CD39

Introduction

The liver is a vital organ with a diverse range of functions, including crucial metabolic pathways, protein synthesis, detoxification, and bile secretion, among others. These functions are absolutely necessary for survival and are chiefly performed by the parenchymal cells or hepatocytes.

S.C. Robson (✉)
Beth Israel Deaconess Medical Center,
330 Brookline Avenue, E/CLS-612,
Boston, MA 02215, USA
e-mail: srobson@bidmc.harvard.edu

L.D. DeLeve and G. Garcia-Tsao (eds.), *Vascular Liver Disease: Mechanisms and Management*,
DOI 10.1007/978-1-4419-8327-5_1,

The life-preserving functions and properties of the liver appear wholly dependent upon distinct elements of organization of the hepatic vasculature. It has been proposed that the endothelium (a single layer of cells lining the inner surface of these blood vessels and comprising the sinusoids) organizes components of the vasculature in an organ-specific manner and thereby determines the functional relationships between blood constituents and perfused tissues, including those within the liver [1–4]. The hepatic vasculature is unique at all levels – from the inflow and outflow macrovessels to the details of the microvasculature and hepatic sinusoids. As discussed in Chaps. 7, 8, and 11, liver disease leads to important changes in vascular function and blood flow (hepatic arterial, portal, and hepatic venous systems), which result in portal hypertension and its associated complications.

This chapter will introduce and discuss mechanisms of hemostasis and thrombosis and apply these to the hepatic circulation. The hemostatic process may be considered a defense mechanism to maintain normal blood vessel homeostasis and preserve the integrity of the closed high- and low-pressure circulatory systems [5–7]. This process becomes disordered in several pathological states. The common liver diseases have at their core major perturbations in coagulation as a consequence of synthetic dysfunction and portal hypertension [8, 9]. There are wide swings in hemostasis manifesting in overt bleeding tendencies with hemorrhage, or as hyperfibrinolysis, and then a predisposition towards hypercoagulability [8, 10–12]. These divergent manifestations may also be seen simultaneously or concurrently in acute liver injury and/or cirrhosis suggesting major perturbations and differential compartmentalization of thromboregulatory mechanisms in these disease states. Such hemostatic abnormalities can also be ascribed, at least in part, to endothelial cell (EC) dysfunction and the disordered blood flow to the liver with portosystemic shunting. Hence, variceal hemorrhage may often coexist with the development of thrombosis of major veins and microvasculature of the diseased liver [8, 9, 13].

We will describe the role of the endothelial dysfunction in hepatic pathophysiology and indicate how these cells might contribute to the divergent manifestations of coagulopathy and thrombotic vascular diseases of liver [8–12]. We will also briefly address endothelial heterogeneity and focus on its importance in regard to hemostasis and hepatic function under both physiological and pathologic states [2, 3].

Finally, alterations in the hemostatic response and coagulopathy may also be pathogenetic abinitio and further provoke injury, architectural changes, and parenchymal extinction in the diseased liver with sinusoidal vascular and accessory cell activation, microvascular thrombosis, and obliteration [10–12, 14–17]. There is increasing evidence that coagulation factors and platelet mediators not only regulate hemostasis and innate immunity, but may also impact adaptive immunity by specifically driving chronic inflammatory cells resulting in fibrogenesis [18].

Coagulation and hemostatic disorders are difficult to monitor and treat effectively. As an introduction to other chapters, we will speculate as to how differential hemostatic responses might dictate onset of thrombosis in any hypercoagulable state to occur specifically in large venous vessels (as in portal or hepatic vein thrombosis, described in Chaps. 12 and 13, or in the microvasculature). Lastly, we discuss disorders of hemostasis and endothelial dysfunction and review their relevance with respect to vascular complications of transplantation.

Vascular Anatomy of the Liver

Blood vessels develop by a process of vasculogenesis followed by angiogenesis, with induction of endothelial and other vascular cell phenotypes. Blood vessels may be considered as tubular structures comprised of the endothelial inner lining with smooth muscle and other cells. These may form single layers as in capillaries that are comprised of typical endothelium and pericytes. With increasing size, several layers are then organized within a complex cell matrix, as is seen in arterioles or venules. These larger structures are divided by elastic laminae to form the tunica intima and media that have variable thicknesses dictated according to the vessel size and internal pressure. The outer connective tissue sheath of a larger blood vessel is termed the tunica adventitia. The vasa vasorum refers to the network of capillaries supplying the outer media in larger vessels [19].

The major elements of the circulation of the liver comprise the hepatic artery and portal vein that perfuse the liver with around 20% of cardiac output; drainage is via the hepatic veins, but the liver can also serve to some extent as a passive reservoir. In contrast, in most other vascular beds and in vital organs such as the heart and kidneys, perfusion would be only arterial.

With respect to the microanatomic arrangements, liver cells are largely supplied by the hepatic sinusoids, which are tortuous structures analogous to capillaries. Blood flow into the sinusoids is derived from two "inflow" sources (see Fig. 1.1). Inflow into the sinusoids by hepatic arteries carries oxygenated blood, whereas the portal vein branches provide venous blood at lower pressure and with lower oxygen tension albeit containing nutrients, immunologically active mediators, hormones, growth factors, and immune cells from the intestines, pancreas, and spleen [20, 21].

Blood circulates through the sinusoids culminating in the central vein of each anatomical lobule of the liver (see Fig. 1.1) [4, 19, 22]. The central veins join to form larger veins, which drain the liver ultimately via the hepatic veins into the inferior vena cava. The liver cells produce bile that is kept separate from the blood and is collected in canaliculi that join to form bile ducts. Interestingly, such bile ducts are supplied only by hepatic artery branches and therefore bear the brunt of hepatic arterial disorders including arterial inflammatory processes such as that seen in reperfusion injury and oxidative stress reactions (Fig. 1.1).

Hemostasis and Coagulation Pathways

Hemostasis must remain inactive under basal conditions, but ready to immediately close off defects, shut off blood loss, and thereby minimize

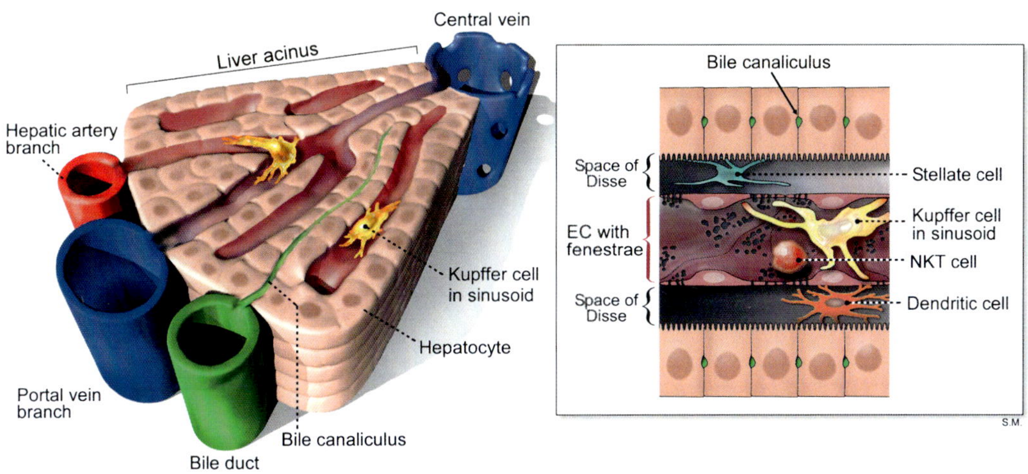

Fig. 1.1 Microanatomy of hepatic sinusoids. As detailed in the text, portal vein and hepatic artery branches culminate in portal tracts, which contain a "triad" including a biliary duct branch. Terminal portal veins generate septal branches that empty into the sinusoids. Blood circulates via the sections of the anatomical lobule to the central vein. Hepatic artery branches that course parallel to the portal vein radicles terminate in a periductular plexus and in the sinusoids supplying periportal regions of acinus zone 1. Functional areas 1–3 of the acinus are associated with decreasing oxygen tensions towards the central vein. Sinusoids are lined by distinct LSEC as described in text (and see adjacent area). Kupffer cells reside adjacent to the space of Disse, which contains extracellular matrix proteins and hepatic stellate cells. Dendritic and NKT lymphoid cells (in transit) have the capacity to pass through the space of Disse. Figure courtesy of Steve Moskowitz, Advanced Medical Graphics, Boston, MA. Concept adapted from: Adams and Eksteen [21]

tissue injury. The pathophysiology of coagulation pathways and platelet-activating mechanisms in hemostasis are integral to an understanding of thrombosis and pathological processes in the vasculature, including the hepatic sinusoids and large vessels of the liver [8, 9, 13, 23].

Coagulation Cascades

The initiating event of blood coagulation is the exposure of abluminal tissue factor (TF; potentially also within circulating microparticles) to circulating factor VII(a) (see Fig. 1.2a). Any disruption in the endothelial barrier between abluminal TF-expressing cells and circulating blood or activation of ECs and endogenous expression of TF might be considered as initiating events in blood coagulation.

TF-Factor VIIa is known to activate two clotting factors: factor IX and factor X. Factor IX (complexed with factor VIII and stabilized by von Willebrand Factor (vWF)) activates a positive feedback loop to activate more factor X. Activated factor Xa together with factor V activates thrombin (from prothrombin or factor II), which has the potential at low concentrations to activate platelets to potentiate clotting (see below).

In addition, thrombin accelerates most components of the clotting process with positive feedback loops, activating more factor V, factor VIII, and factor XI (increasing activated factor IXa) (see Fig. 1.2b). Thrombin also activates factor XIII, which covalently links fibrin molecules in a transglutaminase reaction to form an insoluble mesh (see Fig. 1.2b).

In summary, the TF-Factor VIIa complex initiates a chain reaction by activating other zymogen coagulation factors in the blood and amplifying feedback loops to enhance clotting activity [6]. This cascade of activated zymogens and positive feedback loops propagates fibrin formation to fully impede local hemorrhage. The "intrinsic pathway" involving factor XII-dependent activation of factor XI adds to the positive feedback of the whole coagulation pathway (Fig. 1.2a, b). Noteworthy is that occlusive pathological thrombotic processes are not seen in mice null for factor XII and deficiency in factor XII does not cause hemostatic defects [24].

Hemostasis and Platelet Function

This hemostatic process is initiated by damage to the endothelium with exposure of circulating platelets to subendothelial surfaces and low levels of thrombin arising from the initiation phase serine proteases of the coagulation cascade. There appear to be two separate and independent pathways for platelet activation: these involve vascular collagen-dependent activation and thrombin-dependent pathways [6, 25]. Vascular-associated vWF also plays a major role in hemostasis by mediating platelet activation [26, 27]. Vascular injury exposes circulating platelets to collagen-bound vWF, which binds via the glycoprotein receptor GP1bα and integrins such as GPIIbIIIa (which can also interact with fibrin(ogen)) to initiate rolling (Fig. 1.3a). This process in turn activates other platelets by release of serotonin, thromboxane A2, and adenosine triphosphate and diphosphate (ATP and ADP) [28, 29]. Recruitment of other platelets to the thrombus is made possible by activation of GPIIbIIIa, which exhibits increased affinity for fibrinogen and vWF after a process of "inside out" integrin signaling (Fig. 1.3b), potentially augmented by the actions of protein disulfide isomerase [6, 7]. Platelet stabilization is further achieved through the action of CD40, growth-arrest-specific gene 6, ephrin-Eph, and others [6].

Low levels of thrombin initially generated in the coagulation cascade cleave protease-activated receptors (PAR1 in humans) to also initiate platelet activation [25]. Simultaneous activation of the coagulation cascade and platelets is proposed to synergize to further propagate thrombus formation [5].

The hemostatic process can be further facilitated by expression of functionally active TF by cell-derived microparticles. It is of interest that such thrombus formation promoted by circulating microparticles can develop without implicating

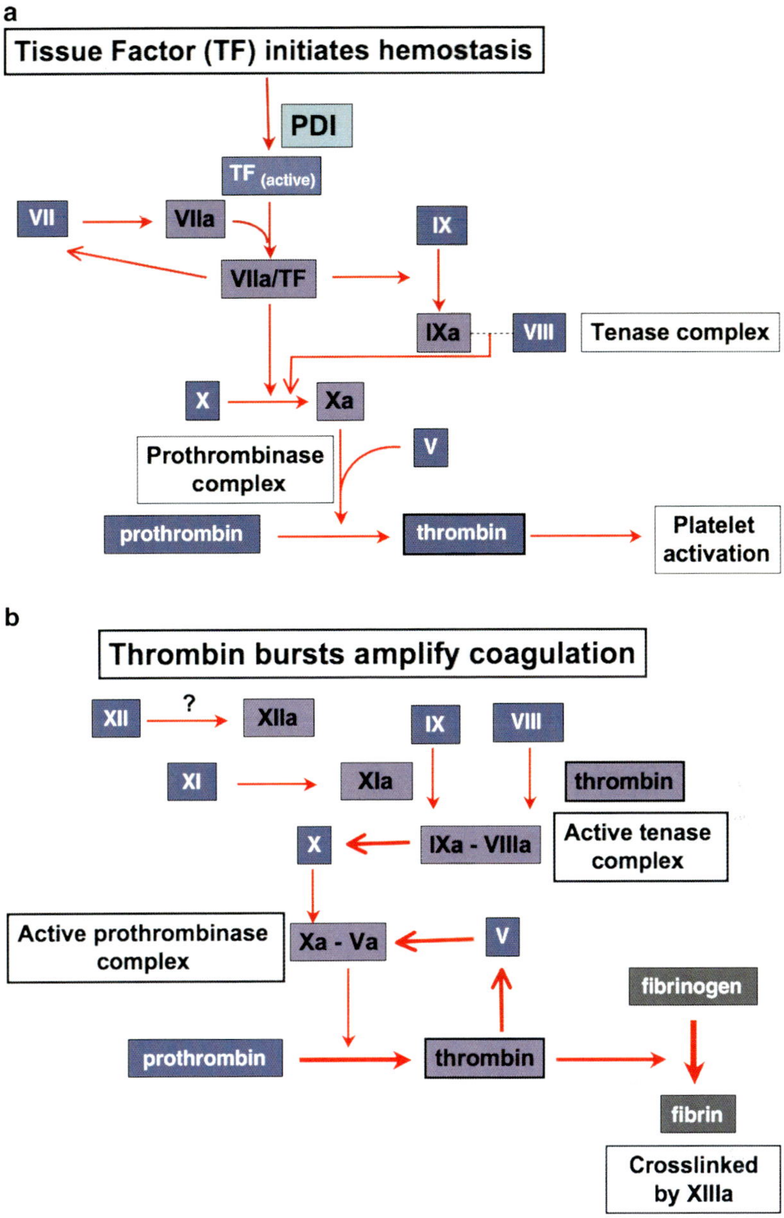

Fig. 1.2 Phases of coagulation cascade. (**a**) Initiation: the process of coagulation comprises an *initiation phase* with platelet activation triggered by low levels thrombin generated by TF-VII(a) with factors Xa, VIII, and V. The complex formed between TF and circulating factor VIIa has the capacity to further activate factor VII, together with factors IX and X. A form of TF that is initially inactive (or "encrypted") can be derived from circulating cells or their derived microparticles and transformed via activated isomerization of a mixed disulfide and a free thiol to an intramolecular disulfide at sites of thrombus formation, as mediated by PDI (protein disulphide isomerase) [31]. In turn, factor IXa binds to nonactivated factor VIII to form a "tenase complex" that can activate factor X (albeit inefficiently) to form factor Xa. Factor Xa, generated by the TF–factor VIIa complex or the factor IXa–factor VIII complex, binds factor V on membrane surfaces. This complex converts small amounts of prothrombin to thrombin to activate platelets. (**b**) Amplification: this phase of initiation is followed by a series of positive feedback loops in a so-called *amplification phase* to generate higher levels of thrombin that can now also induce fibrin formation to form fibrin as a component of the hemostatic plug. During amplification loops, the thrombin generated feeds back and can cause activation of factors VIII and V, together with the dual mode of activation of factor XI, leading to higher levels of thrombin generation in bursts that converts large amounts of fibrinogen to fibrin, then in turn cross-linked by FXIII. Control is at the level of natural anticoagulants antithrombin, tissue factor pathway inhibitor, thrombomodulin, and the protein C and S system (not shown here; see text for details). Figure design assisted by Dr. Joel Wedd, Beth Israel Deaconess Medical Center, Boston MA

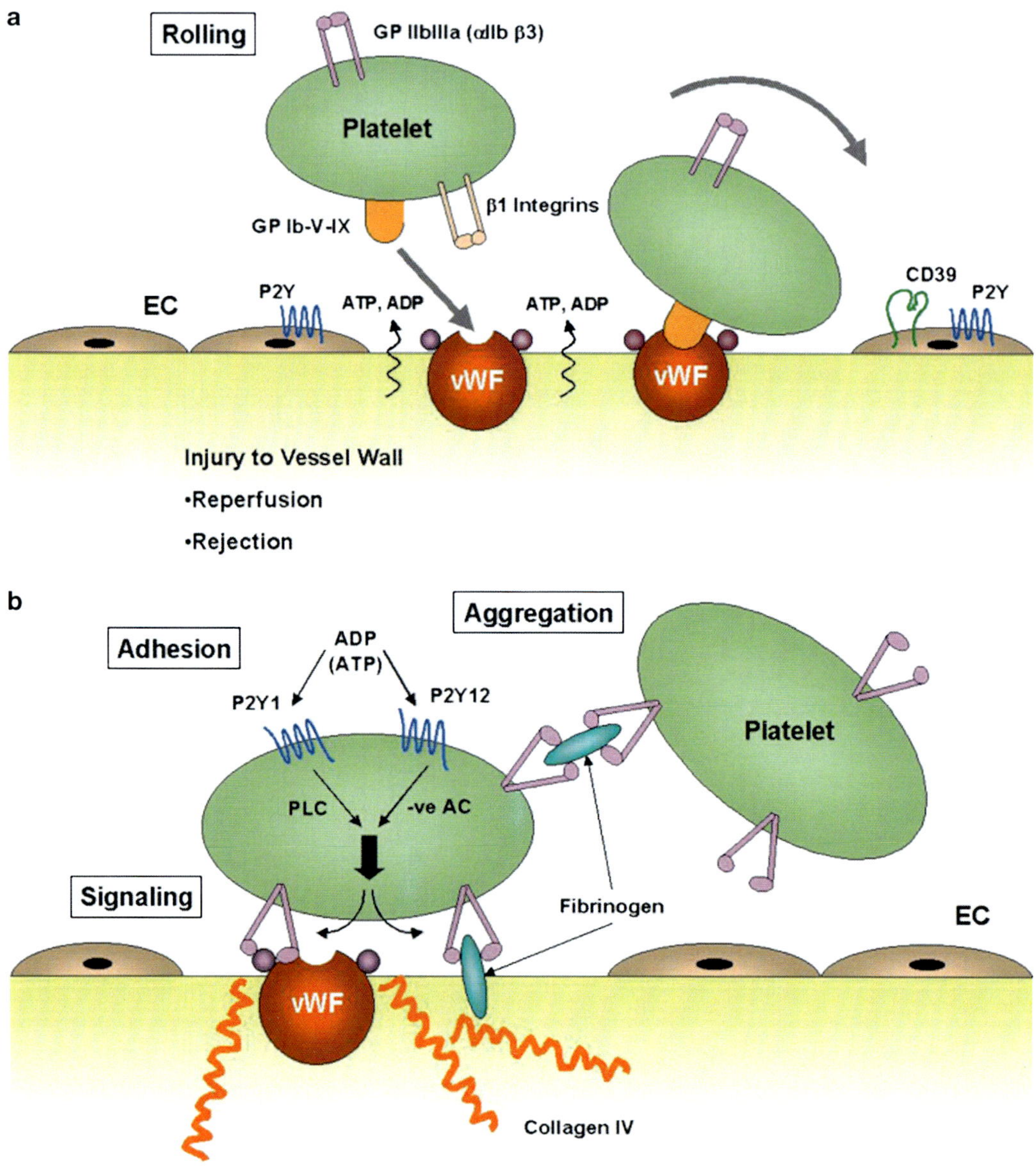

Fig. 1.3 Thrombin-independent mechanisms of platelet activation. The process of coagulation comprises an initiation phase with platelet activation triggered by low levels of thrombin generated by TF-VII(a) with factors Xa, VIII, and V (panel 2A above). Platelets are also primarily triggered by subendothelial collagen and vWF, as shown here. (**a**) Rolling: nonactivated platelets make contact, via integrins and the GPIb complex, with subendothelial vWF and collagen exposed at sites of injury. (**b**) Activation: platelet adhesion and aggregation occur that are induced by the local release of ADP, a purinergic signaling mediator operative at P2Y1 and P2Y12 receptors. These G-protein coupled receptors are linked to phospholipase C and adenylate cyclases, respectively. Activation of GPIIbIIIa fibrinogen receptors follows and leads to fibrin(ogen) interactions that cause hemostatic platelet plug. See text for details

direct endothelial damage [6, 7]. An interesting theoretical consideration is that a form of TF that is initially inactive (or "encrypted") can be derived from circulating cells or their derived microparticles and transformed via activated isomerization of a mixed disulfide and a free thiol to an intramolecular disulfide at sites of thrombus formation [30]. Thrombogenesis is blocked when the extracellular protein disulfide isomerase is inhibited [30], perhaps preventing the activation of critical functions in platelet receptors and TF [6, 31].

Thromboregulation

The hemostatic process described above is sensitive to thromboregulation and is highly responsive to these inhibitory signals. Without negative regulation, pathological coagulation would cause clotting far in excess of what is needed to provide hemostasis and cause thrombosis. Therefore, several mechanisms are in place to slow, stop, and reverse clot formation [29, 32].

Natural anticoagulants include antithrombin, which inactivates thrombin and the active forms of factors X, IX, XI, and XII. Protein C and Protein S, which when complexed together, inactivate factor V and factor VIII (see Fig. 1.2). Protein S is a cofactor to protein C, which is activated by thrombin binding to thrombomodulin and undergoing changes in catalytic specificity.

Initially, thrombomodulin binds thrombin as this becomes more plentiful during active coagulation. With thrombomodulin bound, thrombin is less able to cleave fibrinogen, affect factor V, and activate platelets. This complex then activates protein C, a process aided by binding to the EC protein C receptor. The activated protein C directly affects the coagulation cascade by destroying the activated forms of factor V and factor VIII. Protein S acts as a cofactor in this process. The thrombomodulin–protein C interaction significantly slows the effects of thrombin in the clotting cascade. Thrombomodulin protein also has anti-inflammatory properties directly tied to protein C activation [33, 34].

Platelet regulatory properties are governed by other important mechanisms that include the release of prostacyclin [35], the generation of nitric oxide [36], a purinergic/pyriminergic signaling system (see below) [32, 37, 38], and heparan sulfate expression within the associated cellular glycocalyx [39]. These vascular-based systems operate together with the localized expression of natural anticoagulants such as tissue factor pathway inhibitor or thrombomodulin and fibrinolytic mechanisms involving tissue plasminogen activator [40].

Fibrinolysis

Lastly, there is a process of fibrinolysis, integral to regulated hemostasis and thrombosis that results in clot solubilization, which is largely accomplished by the plasminogen system. Plasminogen is activated to plasmin by plasminogen activators, chief of which is tissue Plasminogen Activator (t-PA). Plasmin degrades factor VIII, factor V, vWF, and factor XIII to impede coagulation and also solubilizes fibrin to generate degradation products such as D-dimer, a marker for fibrin turnover and inflammation. In addition, t-PA is inhibited by plasminogen activator inhibitor type-1 (PAI-1), which is produced by ECs.

Purinergic Signaling in Hemostasis

Extracellular nucleotides (e.g., ATP, ADP, UTP, and UDP) are released by leukocytes, platelets, and ECs in the blood, where they provide extracellular signals crucial in hemostasis [41]. These mediators bind the multiple type-2 purinergic/pyrimidinergic (P2Y1-14 and P2X1-7) receptors on platelets, endothelium and the vascular smooth muscle, and leukocytes [42]. Extracellular nucleotide stimulation of purinergic/pyrimidinergic-(P2) receptors is associated with activation of platelets, leukocytes, and ECs and may culminate in vascular thrombosis and inflammation in vivo [6]. The 15 defined and characterized P2 receptors of the P2Y and P2X families have different specificities and trigger short-term (acute) processes affecting cellular metabolism, nitric oxide (NO) release, adhesion, activation, and migration together with other more protracted developmental responses, such as cell proliferation, differentiation, and apoptosis [43–45].

ATP and ADP regulate hemostasis through the activation of platelet P2 receptors, most notably P2Y12 and P2Y1 (Figs. 1.3 and 1.4). P2X1 is rapidly desensitized and likely important under very high shear stress. ADP is a major platelet-recruiting

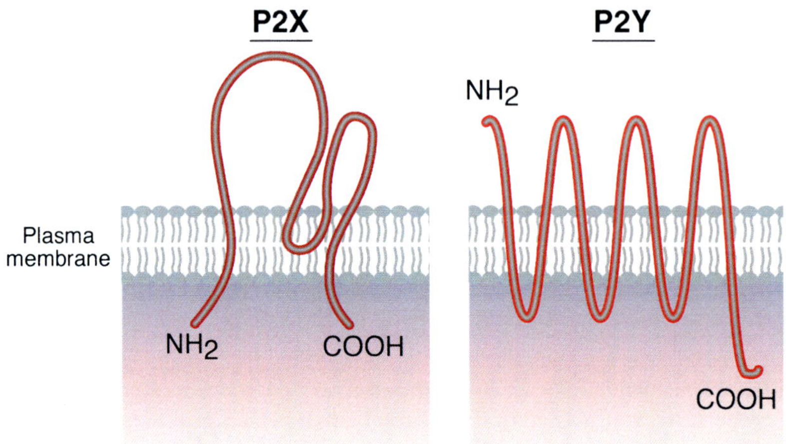

Fig. 1.4 Two families of membrane-bound P2-type receptors that recognize extracellular nucleotides. Representative elements of the two families of nucleotide type-P2 receptors are depicted here. P2X are "rapid" ligand-gated ion channels permeable for Na^+, K^+, and also Ca^{2+} (subtypes P2X1-7). P2Y are the "slow" metabotropic receptors (P2Y1-14) and are 7-transmembrane G_q- or G_i-protein linked receptors. See text for details. Figure courtesy of Steve Moskowitz, Advanced Medical Graphics, Boston, MA

Table 1.1 Vascular ectonucleotidases: hepatic NTPDases of CD39 family [37, 55, 99]

Protein designation	Previous or other nomenclature and localization	Gene name		Chromosome location		Accession number
		Human	Mouse	Human	Mouse	
NTPDase1	CD39, ATPDase, ecto-apyrase	*ENTPD1*		10q24		U87967
	Endothelium and vascular smooth muscle cells	*Entpd1*		19C3		NM009848
	Activated LSEC					
NTPDase2	CD39L1, ecto-ATPase	*ENTPD2*		9q34		AF144748
	Adventitial myofibroblastic cells and pericytes; also portal nerves	*Entpd2*		2A3		AY376711
NTPDase3	CD39L3, HB6	*ENTPD3*		3p21.3		AF034840
	Endothelium albeit at low levels	*Entpd3*		9F4		AY376710
NTPDase8	Liver canalicular ecto-ATPase, hATPDase	*ENTPD8*		9q34		AY430414
	Variable expression noted on centrally located LSEC	*Entpd8*		2A3		AY364442

factor originating from platelet dense granules during activation, whereas ATP derived from the same sources has been considered a competitive antagonist of ADP for platelet P2Y receptors and a putative agonist for P2X1 receptors [41, 46, 47]. ATP (and UTP) also stimulates endothelial P2Y1 and P2Y2 receptors to release prostacyclin (PGI2) and nitric oxide (NO), two vasodilators and inhibitors of platelet aggregation [48–52]. This latter protective action of ATP may limit the extent of intravascular platelet aggregation and help localize thrombus formation to areas of vascular damage [50, 53, 54].

The above P2 receptor-mediated effects are closely modulated by ecto-enzymes termed ecto-nucleotidases (e.g., ecto-ADPases, ecto-ATPases) that bind and then hydrolyze extracellular nucleotides, ultimately to their respective nucleosides (that in turn activate a series of adenosine or P1 receptors) [45, 55]. The dominant ecto-enzymes or ectonucleotidases of the vasculature are now more fully characterized as ecto-nucleoside triphosphate diphosphohydrolases or E-NTPDases of the CD39 family (Table 1.1). This important biological property expressed by the endothelium, and associated cells, is responsible for the regulation of extracellular levels of nucleotides [37, 56–59]. CD39 is the dominant ectonucleotidase in the vasculature and is responsible for phosphohydrolysis of ADP (and ATP) thereby generating AMP and ultimately adenosine. This action reduces platelet activation in the area of clot via reduced interaction with P2Y1 and P2Y12. At areas of vascular injury, localized vascular CD39 bioactivity is lost which tends to promote platelet activation locally [58].

The concepts above have developed from studies involving protein chemistry, platelet aggregometry, and vascular cell biological approaches. Recent work has tested their validity by studying thrombus formation in live mice using intravital microscopy of mesenteric and cremasteric vessels by Drs. Furie and Furie with others [6, 7, 60, 61]. As alluded to before [6], TF can exist in a latent (or "encrypted") form that lacks coagulant activity or in an active form that initiates blood coagulation. Furthermore in such systems, it is proposed that exposed collagen primarily triggers the accumulation and activation of platelets, whereas TF initiates the generation of thrombin that not only converts fibrinogen to fibrin, but also activates platelets [6, 7]. Still how these two pathways might contribute to platelet activation is uncertain, and participation of each is likely to depend upon the anatomical site and/or disease process. In addition, such studies have not been possible in the liver circulation to date.

One recent development of note given the ready access of platelets to the hepatic sinusoids has been the observation that platelets may interact directly with liver sinusoidal endothelial cell (LSEC) and consequently with hepatocytes [62, 63]. These interactions are mediated by the Ashwell receptor, which is a major carbohydrate binding protein lectin, expressed by hepatocytes. This hepatic asialoglycoprotein receptor rapidly clears glycan ligands, e.g., galactose and *N*-acetylgalactosamine. These are typically seen on soluble glycoproteins, but are also expressed by thromboregulatory components such as vWF and the GPIb receptor on platelets (Fig. 1.3a, b). Such interactions likely evolved to eliminate platelets that bear receptors desialylated by bacterial neuraminidase or altered by "cold stress" and senescence [62, 63] that could be aberrantly activated at a peripheral site and cause tissue injury. How these mechanisms of platelet sequestration relate to the well-established glycosylation abnormalities of coagulation factors seen in chronic liver disease and hepatocellular carcinoma with hyperfucosylation and increased side chain branching is unknown [64–67].

Secondary Manifestations of Liver Disease with Disordered Hemostasis and Hemorrhage

The functioning of the hemostatic system is closely linked to liver dysfunction in that hepatocytes produce most of the factors of the coagulation and fibrinolytic systems [65, 66, 68, 69]. Liver disease results in abnormal and decreased synthesis of vitamin-K-dependent and -independent clotting factors, platelet production abnormalities, anemia, and hypersplenism with associated platelet consumption. These coagulation factor quantitative and qualitative abnormalities are associated with excessive consumption and uncontrolled fibrinolysis. These underpin, at least in part, the bleeding diathesis seen in patients with liver disease [70–72].

Acute and chronic liver diseases therefore impact all hemostatic mechanisms and a detailed discussion of these is beyond the scope of this chapter. However, it is of interest that patients with extrahepatic portal hypertension with normal liver function and histology also exhibit coagulation abnormalities and thrombocytopenia [13]. This has been ascribed to a low-grade disseminated intravascular coagulopathy and consumptive features associated with portosystemic shunting as noted in cirrhosis together with platelet sequestration secondary to hypersplenism, as mentioned above [66, 68, 69].

Bleeding complications in patients with liver disease are unpredictable, with the majority of hemorrhagic episodes occurring secondary to portal hypertension and gastroesophageal varices. Standard laboratory tests for coagulation abnormalities are typically performed in patients with liver disease, but are not wholly predictive of bleeding risk as in those patients who have coagulation factor deficiencies and normal liver function [72]. Likewise, large randomized, controlled clinical trials are needed to better define the role of coagulation factor administration and recombinant activated factor VII in the prophylaxis and treatment of hemorrhage, other than variceal (see Chap. 11), noted in liver disease [71]. Although further work is required to dissect out the mechanisms and the clinical settings where it might be useful, activated factor XII might be of potential therapeutic import [24].

Finally, thrombopoietin has been shown to be the major regulator of megakaryocytopoiesis and platelet formation. Boosting platelet levels with the use of eltrombopag, a thrombopoietic drug operative at the thrombopoietin receptor or c-mpl, has been useful in the setting of chronic hepatitis C therapy. It has not been established whether treating thrombocytopenia per se will improve the associated coagulopathy seen in chronic liver disease [70].

Vascular and Sinusoidal Endothelial Heterogeneity

We will focus on the heterogeneity of hepatic vascular EC and LSEC and consider their respective roles in the regulation of coagulation. These seem dependent upon natural anticoagulatory factors as well as complement regulatory mechanisms that result in thromboregulation within the hepatic vasculature and within sinusoids. Morphological and functional aspects of hepatic vascular elements in disease states are covered further elsewhere in this textbook.

The prototypic vascular endothelium provides a barrier that separates blood cells and plasma factors from highly reactive elements of the deeper layer of the vessel wall and maintains blood fluidity and flow by inhibiting coagulation and platelet activation and promoting fibrinolysis [40]. Although ECs in the hepatic vasculature are in general comprised of a thin layer cytoplasm to permit fluid, electrolyte, and low Mr. solute exchange, their structures are also typically continuous to facilitate the retention of blood cells, oncotic factors, and high Mr. proteins. Such elements are further enhanced at several sites. For example, pores and microvascular transport systems are lacking in the vasculature of the nervous system where there is a pronounced "blood–brain barrier" that is functionally traversed only by the intermediary glial cells [73].

There are unique remodeling properties attributed to the hepatic and portal venous endothelium. These vascular beds are characterized by fairly rapid turnover under conditions of stress with replacement in transplanted organs by host-derived circulating pluripotent progenitor cells (endothelial precursor cells) of the recipient, capable of differentiating into venous EC [74–76]. This ability of the liver graft to repopulate the venous endothelium appears far more pronounced than the equivalent levels in cardiac allografts, as shown by Quaini et al. [77].

The hepatic sinusoids have fenestrated LSEC that exhibit unique dynamism and functionality. In this and other specialized vascular beds, notably in bone marrow and the spleen, the endothelial monolayer is discontinuous with large fenestrations and the basement membrane rudimentary to permit filtration of high Mr. solutes (chylomicrons, immune complexes) or even platelets (see Fig. 1.1) [78, 79].

LSEC also secrete cytokines and growth factors important in hepatocellular regeneration, angiogenesis, and liver remodeling [80].

Although vascular EC share common features and functions, it is clear from the above that there are significant features of functional, structural, and anatomic heterogeneity of these cells within the liver. It is clear that the unique hemodynamics, circumstances, and pressures in the portal or hepatic venous system contrast markedly with those associated with the arterial systems and the hepatic sinusoids. Hence, studies conducted in vitro on "typical" macrovascular EC may not be comparable to those conducted in the context of blood flow and in the unique microenvironment of the organ-specific vascular bed.

There are also a whole host of other considerations that impact endothelium and potentially the hepatic vascular EC and LSEC: these include epigenetic modifications, exposure to environmental factors, nutrients, and toxins as well as conditions that range from pregnancy, preeclampsia, surgery, trauma, and sepsis [19, 22, 81].

Acute insults to the endothelium result in a form of vascular injury characterized by interstitial edema and hemorrhage with associated vascular thrombosis. The rapidity of such a process (minutes to hours) precludes any absolute requirements for transcriptional up-regulation and synthesis of proinflammatory factors by vascular cells; this form of EC stimulation has been termed type I activation [82]. The second major process of EC activation has been termed type II, as the mechanisms are protein synthesis-dependent [82]. Further perturbation of the quiescent vascular antithrombotic surface is linked to the production of procoagulants. Other features of the activated endothelium are dependent upon the new expression of adhesion molecules such as E-selectin, vascular cell adhesion molecule (VCAM-1), and intercellular adhesion molecule (ICAM-1) with secretion of chemoattractant chemokines IL-8 and monocyte chemoattractant protein (MCP-1) [83]. The transcription factor NF-kappaB appears to play a pivotal role in the up-regulation of transcription of "inflammatory genes" during EC activation; many of the genes associated with this process have one or more NF-kappaB binding sites within their promoters [84]. Thrombin, which is present in many situations, activates EC in an NF-kappaB-dependent manner; thrombin and TNF act synergistically in this regard [85]. Reactive oxygen species are generated in many situations and would activate NF-kappaB thereby leading to type II EC activation [86].

Despite these considerations of phenotypic changes with activation and other caveats, the successful cell culture of several types of EC has provided further evidence for remarkable differences in the specific biochemical functioning and antigenic determinants of these cells [80, 87]. In addition to these organ-specific EC antigens, there are site-specific EC antigens and an interesting differential ability of EC to act as antigen-presenting cells in vitro that have implications for disease, as well as in transplantation and rejection processes (see later) [88, 89].

Vascular Signaling Pathways in Hemostasis, Liver Disease, and Portal Hypertension

Endothelial dysfunction in liver cirrhosis has been ascribed to impaired endothelial-dependent relaxation that contributes to increased intrahepatic vascular resistance, promoting portal hypertension [16] (see Chap. 7). Increased production of vasodilator molecules, e.g., nitric oxide (NO), contributes to increased endothelium-dependent relaxation within the systemic and splanchnic arterial circulations [90] (see Chap. 8).

Over the past decade, extracellular nucleotides and derivatives have been increasingly recognized as important mediators of vascular inflammation and thrombosis with varying impacts in different experimental systems and in models of human disease [55]. Extracellular nucleotides/nucleosides are also recognized as influencing liver metabolism and function, vasomotor responses, platelet activation, thrombosis, and inflammatory processes [91–94].

Studies demonstrated that regulatory steps have evolved in purinergic responses at the level of nucleotide release, receptor expression and/or desensitization, and the phosphohydrolysis of the nucleotide mediators to the specific derivatives. Each of these steps is involved in mediating specificity of purinergic/pyrimidinergic signaling: (1) the derivation or source of the extracellular nucleotides [41, 42, 92]; (2) the expression of specific receptors for these molecular transmitters (or the nucleotide and nucleoside derivatives) [95–98] (Molecular Recognition Section of National Institutes of Health http://mgddk1.niddk. nih. gov: 8000/nomenclature.html) (see Fig. 1.4); and (3) the existence of ectonucleotidases that dictate the cellular responses by hydrolyzing the nucleotides (to nucleosides) [37, 55, 99].

Several mechanisms account for the presence of nucleotides or nucleosides in plasma [100]. As alluded to above, these include aggregating platelets, degranulating macrophages, excitatory neurons, injured cells, and cells undergoing mechanical or oxidative stress resulting in lysis, selective permeabilization of cellular membranes, and exocytosis of secretory vesicles, such as from platelet dense bodies [41, 46]. It is important to note here that many processes of arterial vascular injury are associated with the release of adenine nucleotides that exert a variety of inflammatory effects on the endothelium, platelets, and leukocytes (reviewed in [41, 92]).

In contrast, ATP released from ECs during changes in flow (shear stress) or following exposure to hypoxic conditions activates P2Y receptors expressed by these cells and by vascular smooth muscle cells in an autocrine and paracrine manner to release nitric oxide, resulting in vessel relaxation as a purinergic event. Any nucleotide released will be ultimately hydrolyzed to adenosine and will result in vasodilatation via the effects of vascular smooth muscle adenosine P1 receptors. P2X receptors also appear on vascular cells and are thought to be associated with changes in cell adhesion and permeability (see Fig. 1.4) [45].

P1 (adenosine) can be differentiated from P2 (ATP/ADP) receptors by direct pharmacological and molecular means. To date, four subtypes of P1 receptors have been cloned, namely A1, A2A, A2B, and A3 with substantial interspecies differences [95–98]. The adenosine receptors are classified according to their affinities for adenosine and variant coupling to adenylate cyclase [98].

The endothelial membrane-expressed CD39/NTPDase-1 is the major ectonucleotidase in the vasculature of the liver (Table 1.1) [101]. The ecto-enzyme CD39/NTPDase1 can be shown to efficiently bind and hydrolyze extracellular ADP (and ATP) to AMP; the product AMP does activate select P1 receptors, but is preferentially hydrolyzed to adenosine by the ubiquitous CD73 and ecto-5′-nucleotidases. This phosphohydrolytic reaction limits the platelet activation response that is dependent upon the autocrine and paracrine release of ADP with activation of specific purinergic receptors [56, 58, 102]. In contrast, CD39L1/NTPDase2, a preferential nucleoside triphosphatase, activates platelets by converting the competitive antagonist (ATP) of platelet ADP receptors to the specific agonist (ADP) of the P2Y1 and P2Y12 receptors (Table 1.1).

In keeping with these biochemical properties, CD39 is mainly expressed by EC and vascular smooth muscle where it serves as a thromboregulatory factor within the liver. CD39 is rapidly upregulated by LSEC with cell activation or post-partial hepatectomy (see Supplemental Fig. 1 in Beldi et al. 2008; Ref. 140).

In contrast, CD39L1 is associated with the adventitial surfaces of muscularized vessels, microvascular pericytes, and stromal cells and could potentially serve as a hemostatic factor [103]. There are other hepatic NTPDases as summarized in Table 1.1.

Various biological functions of these P2 and adenosine receptors, together with NTPDases, could be influenced by differential expression in various vascular beds, certain unique biochemical characteristics and the effects of their relevant substrate nucleotides, or products on various subtypes of receptors expressed in the local environment. It has been proposed that in concert with the nearly 20 described P2 or P1 or adenosine receptors, combinations of NTPDases have the capacity to terminate signaling, alter specificities of the response, or even generate signaling molecules (e.g., ADP) from precursors (e.g., ATP) [55]. However, little is currently known of the structural or functional associations of NTPDases, with one another or with P2 receptors. It is proposed that under certain conditions, hepatic and other NTPDases may protect the integrity of any future response by preventing receptor desensitization reactions [101, 104]. In contrast, coexpression of ectonucleotidases may be essential for the survival of cells that express P2X7 receptors, as these receptors do not readily autoregulate by desensitization [105] responses and can induce apoptosis [106].

In testing these mechanisms in vivo, we have noted that genetic deletion of CD39 results in deleterious outcomes in the setting of portal hypertension and hepatic ischemia reperfusion that are associated with significant microcirculatory derangements and major intestinal hemorrhage [107]. These develop as a consequence of decreased generation of adenosine in the hepatosplanchnic circulation [108].

Hepatic Sinusoidal Responses and Coagulation Multicellular Composition of Hepatic Sinusoids

This section addresses the unique compositions of the cells of the sinusoids and how these may be impacted by hemostatic mediators. As mentioned above, LSEC are unique among vascular EC, as they lack a developed basement membrane. Indeed, pores called fenestrae exist throughout the endothelium, allowing diffusion of macromolecules and complexes (see Fig. 1.1) (see Chap. 2). It is highly likely that the different EC and LSEC phenotypes have developed progressive specialization as a consequence of cues from surrounding tissues and cells in the sinusoids, as proposed by Spemann and Mangold for local angioblast development (Table 1.2) [109].

Hepatic sinusoids are formed by at least four different cell types, each with different phenotypic characteristics, functions, and topography [110, 111]. The LSEC facilitate the generation of extracellular fluid that resembles plasma within the space of Disse [112]. The fenestrae are grouped together in "sieve plates," and without a basal lamina, small particles are free to diffuse into the perisinusoidal space and into contact with hepatocytes (see Fig. 1.1). With this adaptation, the LSE acts as a filter between the sinusoidal lumen and the space of Disse adjacent to the hepatic parenchymal cells (hepatocytes) which process the nutrients taken from the portal blood. The substrates, products, and constituents of hepatocyte metabolism can be filtered both ways through the fenestrated sinusoidal endothelium.

The dynamic fenestrae are affected by multiple local factors like the presence of toxins and vasoactive substances such as NO. The ECs lining the sinusoid are responsible for endocytosis of particles that reach them through the portal circulation. In addition, they release multiple factors, many of which are notably involved in the inflammatory response. IL-1, IL-6, interferon, and ICAM-1 are among the signaling messengers released. These cells are also integral in a purine/pyrimidinergic signaling pathway that may be directly related to vascular autoregulation, thrombosis, and inflammation [107].

Kupffer cells are tissue macrophages with an intrasinusoidal location and a pronounced phagocytic capacity. These cells function to remove cellular breakdown products, microbes, and other particles from the sinusoidal area. In performing this function, these cells release cytokines, free radicals, lysosomal enzymes, and platelet-activating factors. Their possible role in thrombosis and injured or activated platelet sequestration remains speculative [62, 113].

Stellate cells are astrocyte-like cells present in the perisinusoidal space of Disse, which are thought to represent the main hepatic source of extracellular matrix components. Stellate cells are actually perisinusoidal and may help to control blood flow in the sinusoidal space and interact closely with other cells in autocrine and paracrine manners that show responsiveness to metabolic needs imposed by liver growth and repair by impacting extracellular matrix content [17, 114]. These cells are clearly impacted by hemostatic mediators, as discussed later [14, 17, 23].

Table 1.2 Vascular development, vasculogenesis, angiogenesis, and changes in endothelial cell pluripotential capacity

	Pluripotential capacity
Vasculogenesis	
Hemangioblast → Angioblast → Endothelium → Vascular prototype	
Angiogenesis	
vs. liver sinusoidal endothelial phenotype	
vs. renal glomerular endothelium etc.	
Increasing differentiation	
Ultimate specialization	

Endothelial cell and vascular development involves a process characterized by further differentiation and specialization that occurs at the expense of pluripotentiality (see [153, 154] from where table adapted)

"Pit cells" are granular lymphocyte lineages that exhibit natural killer T cell (NKT) activity and attach to the sinusoid wall [115]. These and other intrahepatic lymphocytes have distinctive phenotypes and unique functions. Such cells include both conventional CD4+ and CD8+ alpha beta T cell receptor (TCR)+ T cells, B cells, natural killer (NK) cells as well as other lymphoid cells (natural killer T (NKT) cells, gamma delta TCR+ T cells, CD4− CD8− T cells), which may well influence inflammatory and immune reactions in the liver sinusoids [20].

Capillarization, Thrombosis, and Parenchymal Extinction

At least in part, it is feasible that sinusoidal endothelial and the accessory cells have a certain degree of plasticity and behave as adaptive "input–output" devices. Signals arise from the extracellular milieu and may include biochemical signals triggered by extracellular nucleotides (or nucleosides) and thrombin (amongst other coagulation factors) (Fig. 1.5) [17, 18, 107, 116]. Triggering of these responses results in biomechanical responses transduced by adhesion receptors following P2-mediated or protease-activated receptor (PAR)-mediated signals, such as the affinity changes in integrins [8, 14, 117, 118]. These manifest as alterations in cellular phenotype, such as with activation responses, and include a number of structural and functional changes implicated in diverse pathophysiological processes including vascular inflammation and thrombotic disease (see Fig. 1.5) [18, 107, 116].

Coagulation factors and platelet mediators clearly impact innate and adaptive immunity and modulate cells in the liver to fundamentally alter the microvasculature of the liver. Extracellular nucleotides and thrombin, as examples, further exacerbate disordered sinusoidal remodeling, capillarization, and abnormal angiogenesis provoking fibrosis and vascular distortion. These

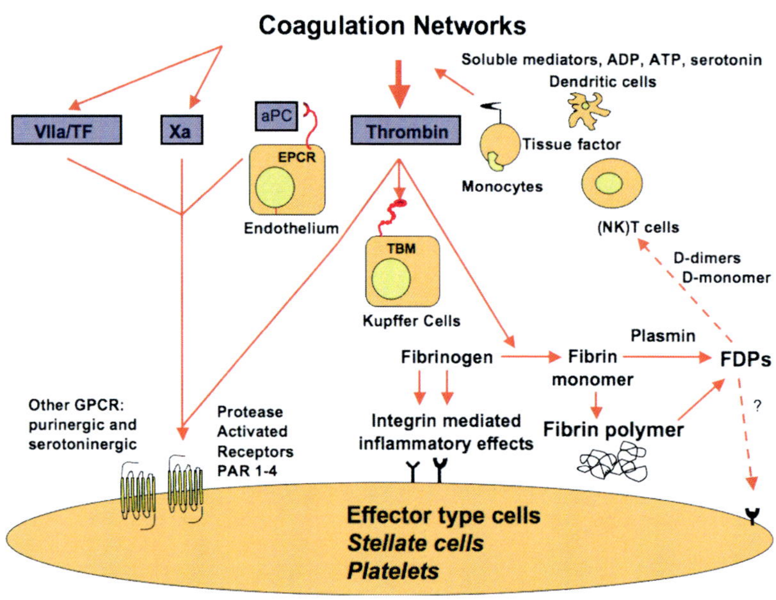

Fig. 1.5 Activated coagulation factors in the liver trigger multicellular inflammatory responses. Hemostasis is triggered by coagulation factors and controlled by natural anticoagulants, as detailed in text and Fig. 1.2 (and also from [18]). However, these proteases also have multiple other effects, some of which are independent of fibrin generation. These latter develop via specific interactions with specific cell membrane-expressed "protease activated receptors" expressed on platelets, endothelium, and sinusoidal cells. See: [17, 18, 116] for more details. Other G-protein coupled receptors recognizing platelet-derived mediators, e.g., serotonin and ADP, interact in signaling pathways [107, 138, 139]. Fibrin is also generated and is subject to proteolysis via plasmin to yield fibrin degradation products that also feedback to influence immune responsiveness in liver diseases [13, 151]

processes destroy the normal sinusoid structures and contribute to the morbidity and mortality seen in progressive liver disease and in complications of hepatic transplantation [9, 14].

Hypercoagulable events occur in cirrhosis patients despite the predisposition to bleeding [8]. Thrombotic events may be clinically evident, such as in portal vein thrombosis or pulmonary embolism, but may also contribute to portopulmonary hypertension as well as thrombosis of extracorporeal circuits in dialysis or liver assist devices [9]. Thromboses of medium and large venous vessels are an additional serious complication in cirrhosis and are important in causing progression of disease.

Portal venous lesions in cirrhosis have generally been attributed to thrombosis, but the pathogenesis of the hepatic vein lesions has not been investigated to the same extent in cirrhosis and mechanisms remain unknown. In cardiac cirrhosis, initial sinusoidal thrombosis occasionally propagates and causes both secondary hepatic and portal thrombosis with ischemia, parenchymal extinction, and fibrosis [11, 12]. In chronic hepatitis C infection, factor V Leiden mutation, protein C deficiency, and increased expression of factor VIII are all associated with rapid progression to cirrhosis [14].

These studies suggest a role for coagulation cascade activity in hepatic fibrogenesis with pathogenic mechanisms downstream of thrombin and other coagulation factor activation. Thrombosis is therefore an increasingly recognized complication of liver disease and systemic hypercoagulability may contribute to the development of vascular thrombosis, parenchymal extinction, and the associated hepatic fibrosis [10–12, 119].

Microvascular vs. Macrovascular Endothelial Mediated Diseases

Why a defined hypercoagulable state elicits thrombogenesis at a specific site in either the venous or arterial system of the liver is an important question that is still unanswered [2, 120, 121]. Advances in the understanding of hemostatic mechanisms and platelet thromboregulation unfortunately do not provide clear insights into this problem. There is increasing evidence that the coagulation process can be promoted by prothrombotic microparticles that sequester at sites of vascular thrombosis [6, 7]. Important thromboregulatory factors, e.g., CD39, can be also incorporated into these cell-derived membrane elements [122].

It is known that toxic and direct insults to the LSEC may result in sinusoidal obstruction syndrome, hepatic peliosis, and nodular regenerative hyperplasia. These conditions have been typically associated with LSEC associated drug injury or herbal toxicity (e.g., azathioprine, 6-mercaptopurine, oral contraceptives, anabolic steroids, and Senecio type alkaloids). The primary injury is followed by a series of biologic processes that lead to circulatory compromise of centrilobular hepatocytes, sinusoidal fibrosis, and obstruction with portal hypertension [123]. In elegant animal models, bone marrow-derived CD133+ progenitors can be shown to repopulate the sites of LSEC denudation and injury with therapeutic benefit [124, 125].

The major etiological factors and conditions that predispose to and are associated with large vessel thrombosis viz. of portal vein and hepatic veins are discussed elsewhere in this textbook. In such primary circulatory liver diseases and the relevant animal models, portal hypertension and/or hemostatic changes usually precede liver dysfunction [13, 108, 123–127].

Transplantation

Reperfusion injury and acute and chronic rejection are dictated by endothelial and vascular responses [107, 128, 129]. Vascular inflammation is also modulated by resident and circulating lymphoid regulatory and NKT cells [107, 130, 131]. These aspects are addressed in detail in Chap. 6 [132, 133], and elsewhere.

Reperfusion Injury, Endothelial Cytoprotection, and Regeneration

Organ ischemia and the sequelae of reperfusion injury are a major cause of morbidity and mortality in hepatobiliary surgery and liver transplantation

[132, 133]. Systemic inflammatory responses to ischemia reperfusion injury are characterized by vascular EC and neutrophil activation with cytokine and free oxygen radical release. Profound ischemia reperfusion injury may result in primary graft failure as a consequence of severe LSEC injury [132, 134, 135]. The biliary system largely exhibits delayed consequences of vascular injury with stricturing and anastomotic breakdown. This is because the hepatic arterial inflow is directed to the bile ducts (see Fig. 1.1) that are markedly and selectively affected by acute arterial processes, such as seen in reperfusion injury [134].

Vascular-mediated protection of the graft or injured liver is dependent upon normal functioning of hepatic endothelium [76, 80, 136]. Typically, EC activation seen during ischemic insults is associated with apoptosis responses, procoagulant induction, and loss of protective thromboregulatory factors such as tissue factor pathway inhibitor, thrombomodulin, and vascular NTPDase activity [58, 128, 137].

EC turnover is critically important during liver regeneration that is required for restoration of parenchymal cell mass postsurgery and resection. The process of liver regeneration is further facilitated by vascular endothelial growth factor responses and hemostatic mediators and factors derived from platelets and vascular cells [23, 80, 138, 139].

Immunological Injury

One of the important features of acute cellular rejection recognized by the Banff Working Group on Liver Allograft Pathology is that of endothelial injury and central vein damage [140, 141]. The arterial lesions of chronic rejection are termed transplant arteriosclerosis or vasculopathy. These obliterative lesions are associated with major neointimal proliferation that comprises alpha-actin vascular smooth muscle cells [142, 143]. Chronic rejection of these allografts manifests as a progressive vascular obliterative disease with specific ischemic injury to the biliary system in the liver graft known as the "vanishing bile duct syndrome" [142, 143].

Some long-term human recipients of liver allografts and some animal species (pigs and rats) show little requirement for immunosuppression to maintain their grafts [144]. Immunological properties of LSEC have been described which might contribute to this phenomenon. These cells function uniquely among vascular EC as antigen-presenting cells *without cytokine prestimulation* and have the capacity to present antigen in a mode that facilitates regulatory tolerance [145]. Recipients of a liver and the donor-specific heart or kidney can further exhibit allospecific tolerance mediated at least in part by sinusoidal cells. In this instance, the liver induces specific tolerance for another distant but allo-identical graft. High levels of release from the liver into the blood of allogeneic (donor type) MHC Class 1 proteins from sinusoidal cells and hepatocytes could blind host immune cells. Alternatively, passenger immune cells (lymphocytes and dendritic) from the donor liver could migrate into the host creating a level of microchimerism [144].

LSEC also express cell adhesion molecules either constitutively (for example, CD54 (intercellular adhesion molecule-1 or ICAM-1), CD102 (ICAM-2), and CD58) or following stimulation (an example would be vascular cell adhesion molecule-1 (VCAM-1)). The expression of these adhesion molecules by LSEC results in the liver selectively trapping postactivated CD8+ T cells, thus explaining the role of the liver as a "T cell sink" [145, 146]. Finally, intrahepatic entrapment and deletion by LSEC of the activated host T cells, as a consequence of the lack of costimulatory signals, could also block alloreactivity [145, 146].

In the context of the vascular endothelial heterogeneity within livers, kidneys, and hearts, there are likely to be differential EC responses [4]. As mentioned above, the unique features of LSEC have implications for the remarkable ability of the liver to induce tolerogenicity to alloantigen and to be relatively resistant to both acute and chronic rejection [144, 146].

The enhanced ability of the liver to form chimeric type hepatic veins, with a dominant proportion of the endothelium being from the host, might have implications for long-term graft survival [75, 76, 136]. There are substantial data to indicate that these cells are of recipient origin that have migrated to sites of vascular injury and may be important in maintenance of initial vascular integrity [147]. Despite this, the liver is not entirely spared from damaging host-versus-graft rejection responses targeting both portal and hepatic venous branches [148]. The liver is also a site for graft versus-host (GVH) disease after hematopoietic cell transplantation [112, 146].

Conclusions

In summary, hemostasis research and the understanding of platelet responses have advanced significantly over the past decade. However, disordered hemostasis in acute and chronic liver diseases remains poorly understood and remains a serious problem. Coagulation and hemostatic disorders are difficult to monitor and treat effectively with current agents. They contribute to the morbidity and mortality seen in progressive liver disease, decompensation, and in complications of transplantation [8, 9, 13–16, 107, 129, 149].

Coagulation and platelet abnormalities in hepatic decompensation not only provoke hemorrhage, but further exacerbate disordered sinusoidal remodeling, abnormal angiogenesis, venous thrombosis, and vascular distortion mediated by fibrosis [118, 150].

Acknowledgments I apologize in advance if, because of space and time constraints, I have not adequately referenced the work of others and have instead cited review articles.

I am grateful, as always, to Dr. Bruce Furie for important discussions and enlightenment in hemostasis and thrombosis.

Grant support from NIH.

References

1. Aird WC. Endothelial cell dynamics and complexity theory. Crit Care Med. 2002;30(5 Suppl S):S180–5.
2. Aird WC. Vascular bed-specific hemostasis: role of endothelium in pathogenesis. Crit Care Med. 2001; 29(7 Suppl S):S28–34.
3. Gross PL, Aird WC. The endothelium and thrombosis [Review]. Semin Thromb Hemost. 2000;26(5):463–78.
4. Aird WC. Endothelial cell heterogeneity. Crit Care Med. 2003;31(4 Suppl S):S221–30.
5. Furie B, Furie BC. Thrombus formation in vivo. J Clin Invest. 2005;115(12):3355–62.
6. Furie B. Pathogenesis of thrombosis. Hematology Am Soc Hematol Educ Program. 2009:255–8.
7. Furie B, Furie BC. Mechanisms of thrombus formation. N Engl J Med. 2008;359(9):938–49.
8. Roberts LN, Patel RK, Arya R. Haemostasis and thrombosis in liver disease. Br J Haematol. 2010;148: 507–21.
9. Northup PG, Sundaram V, Fallon MB, et al. Hypercoagulation and thrombophilia in liver disease. J Thromb Haemost. 2008;6(1):2–9.
10. Shimamatsu K, Wanless IR. Role of ischemia in causing apoptosis, atrophy, and nodular hyperplasia in human liver. Hepatology. 1997;26(2):343–50.
11. Wanless IR, Wong F, Blendis LM, Greig P, Heathcote EJ, Levy G. Hepatic and portal vein thrombosis in cirrhosis: possible role in development of parenchymal extinction and portal hypertension. Hepatology. 1995;21(5):1238–47.
12. Wanless IR, Liu JJ, Butany J. Role of thrombosis in the pathogenesis of congestive hepatic fibrosis (cardiac cirrhosis). Hepatology. 1995;21(5):1232–7.
13. Robson SC, Kahn D, Kruskal J, Bird AR, Kirsch RE. Disordered hemostasis in extrahepatic portal hypertension. Hepatology. 1993;18(4):853–7.
14. Anstee QM, Wright M, Goldin R, Thursz MR. Parenchymal extinction: coagulation and hepatic fibrogenesis. Clin Liver Dis. 2009;13(1):117–26.
15. Bosch J. Vascular deterioration in cirrhosis: the big picture. J Clin Gastroenterol. 2007;41 Suppl 3:S247–53.
16. Iwakiri Y, Groszmann RJ. Vascular endothelial dysfunction in cirrhosis. J Hepatol. 2007;46(5):927–34.
17. Friedman SL. Hepatic stellate cells: protean, multifunctional, and enigmatic cells of the liver. Physiol Rev. 2008;88(1):125–72.
18. Shrivastava S, McVey JH, Dorling A. The interface between coagulation and immunity. Am J Transplant. 2007;7(3):499–506.
19. Aird WC. Phenotypic heterogeneity of the endothelium: II. Representative vascular beds. Circ Res. 2007;100(2):174–90.
20. Nemeth E, Baird AW, O'Farrelly C. Microanatomy of the liver immune system. Semin Immunopathol. 2009;31(3):333–43.
21. Adams DH, Eksteen B. Aberrant homing of mucosal T cells and extra-intestinal manifestations of inflammatory bowel disease. Nat Rev Immunol. 2006;6(3): 244–51.
22. Aird WC. Phenotypic heterogeneity of the endothelium: I. Structure, function, and mechanisms. Circ Res. 2007;100(2):158–73.
23. Calvaruso V, Maimone S, Gatt A, et al. Coagulation and fibrosis in chronic liver disease. Gut. 2008;57(12):1722–7.
24. Kleinschnitz C, Stoll G, Bendszus M, et al. Targeting coagulation factor XII provides protection

from pathological thrombosis in cerebral ischemia without interfering with hemostasis. J Exp Med. 2006;203(3):513–8.
25. Coughlin SR. Protease-activated receptors in hemostasis, thrombosis and vascular biology. J Thromb Haemost. 2005;3(8):1800–14.
26. Varga-Szabo D, Pleines I, Nieswandt B. Cell adhesion mechanisms in platelets. Arterioscler Thromb Vasc Biol. 2008;28(3):403–12.
27. Ruggeri ZM. The role of von Willebrand factor in thrombus formation. Thromb Res. 2007;120 Suppl 1:S5–9.
28. Marcus AJ. Platelet function (third of three parts). N Engl J Med. 1969;280(24):1330–5.
29. Marcus AJ, Safier LB, Broekman MJ, et al. Thrombosis and inflammation as multicellular processes: significance of cell-cell interactions. Thromb Haemost. 1995;74(1):213–7.
30. Reinhardt C, von Bruhl ML, Manukyan D, et al. Protein disulfide isomerase acts as an injury response signal that enhances fibrin generation via tissue factor activation. J Clin Invest. 2008;118(3):1110–22.
31. Cho J, Furie BC, Coughlin SR, Furie B. A critical role for extracellular protein disulfide isomerase during thrombus formation in mice. J Clin Invest. 2008;118(3):1123–31.
32. Marcus AJ, Safier LB, Kaminski WE, et al. Principles of thromboregulation: control of platelet reactivity in vascular disease. Adv Prostaglandin Thromboxane Leukot Res. 1995;23:413–8.
33. Esmon CT, Fukudome K, Mather T, et al. Inflammation, sepsis, and coagulation. Haematologica. 1999;84(3):254–9.
34. Castellino FJ, Ploplis VA. The protein C pathway and pathologic processes. J Thromb Haemost. 2009;7 Suppl 1:140–5.
35. Sinzinger H, Virgolini I, Gazso A, Ogrady J. Review – eicosanoids in atherosclerosis. Exp Pathol. 1991;43(2):2–19.
36. Cooke JP, Dzau VJ. Nitric oxide synthase – role in the genesis of vascular disease [Review]. Annu Rev Med. 1997;48(489):489–509.
37. Robson SC, Wu Y, Sun X, Knosalla C, Dwyer K, Enjyoji K. Ectonucleotidases of CD39 family modulate vascular inflammation and thrombosis in transplantation. Semin Thromb Hemost. 2005;31(2):217–33.
38. Atkinson B, Dwyer K, Enjyoji K, Robson SC. Ectonucleotidases of the CD39/NTPDase family modulate platelet activation and thrombus formation: potential as therapeutic targets. Blood Cells Mol Dis. 2006;10:10.
39. Ihrcke NS, Wrenshall LE, Lindman BJ, Platt JL. Role of heparan sulfate in immune system-blood vessel interactions. Immunol Today. 1993;14(500):500–5.
40. Ross R. Cell biology of atherosclerosis. [Review]. Annu Rev Physiol. 1995;57(791):791–804.
41. Luthje J. metabolism and function of extracellular adenine nucleotides in the blood [published erratum appears in Klin Wochenschr 1989 May 15;67(10):558]. [Review]. Klinische Wochenschrift. 1989;67(6):317–27.
42. Abbracchio MP, Burnstock G. Purinoceptors – are there families of P2X and P2Y purinoceptors [Review]. Pharmacol Ther. 1994;64(3):445–75.
43. Harden TK, Lazarowski ER, Boucher RC. Release, metabolism and interconversion of adenine and uridine nucleotides: implications for G protein-coupled P2 receptor agonist selectivity. Trends Pharmacol Sci. 1997;18(2):43–6.
44. Weisman GA, Erb L, Garrad RC, et al. P2Y nucleotide receptors in the immune system: Signaling by a P2Y(2) receptor in U937 monocytes. Drug Dev Res. 1998;45(3–4):222–8.
45. Burnstock G, Knight G. Cellular distribution and functions of P2 receptor subtypes in different systems. Int Rev Cytol. 2004;240:31–304.
46. Fijnheer R, Boomgaard MN, van den Eertwegh AJ, et al. Stored platelets release nucleotides as inhibitors of platelet function. Thromb Haemost. 1992;68(5):595–9.
47. Hechler B, Vigne P, Leon C, Breittmayer JP, Gachet C, Frelin C. Atp derivatives are antagonists of the P2y(1) receptor – similarities to the platelet Adp receptor. Mol Pharmacol. 1998;53(4):727–33.
48. Yang S, Cheek DJ, Westfall DP, Buxton IL. Purinergic axis in cardiac blood vessels. Agonist-mediated release of ATP from cardiac endothelial cells. Circ Res. 1994;74(3):401–7.
49. Fisette PL, Denlinger LC, Proctor RA, Bertics PJ. Modulatoin of marcrophage function by P2Y-purinergic receptors [Review]. Drug Dev Res. 1996; 39(3–4):377–87.
50. Marcus AJ, Safier LB. Thromboregulation: multicellular modulation of platelet reactivity in hemostasis and thrombosis. [Review]. FASEB J. 1993;7(6):516–22.
51. Juul B, Plesner L, Aalkjaer C. Effects of ATP and related nucleotides on the tone of isolated rat mesenteric resistance arteries. J Pharmacol Exp Ther. 1993;264(3):1234–40.
52. Motte S, Communi D, Pirotton S, Boeynaems JM. Involvement of multiple receptors in the actions of extracellular ATP: the example of vascular endothelial cells. [Review]. Int J Biochem Cell Biol. 1995; 27(1):1–7.
53. Cote YP, Picher M, St JP, Beliveau R, Potier M, Beaudoin AR. Identification and localization of ATP-diphosphohydrolase (apyrase) in bovine aorta: relevance to vascular tone and platelet aggregation. Biochim Biophys Acta. 1991;1078(2):187–91.
54. Cote YP, Filep JG, Battistini B, Gauvreau J, Sirois P, Beaudoin AR. Characterization of ATP-diphosphohydrolase activities in the intima and media of the bovine aorta: evidence for a regulatory role in platelet activation in vitro. Biochim Biophys Acta. 1992;1139(1–2):133–42.
55. Robson SC, Enjyoji K, Goepfert C, et al. Modulation of extracellular nucleotide-mediated signaling by CD39/nucleoside triphosphate diphosphohydrolase-1. Drug Dev Res. 2001;53(2–3):193–207.

56. Marcus AJ, Safier LB, Hajjar KA, et al. Inhibition of platelet function by an aspirin-insensitive endothelial cell ADPase. Thromboregulation by endothelial cells. J Clin Investig. 1991;88(5):1690–6.
57. Kaczmarek E, Koziak K, Sevigny J, et al. Identification and characterization of Cd39 vascular ATP diphosphohydrolase. J Biol Chem. 1996;271(51):33116–22.
58. Robson SC, Kaczmarek E, Siegel JB, et al. Loss of ATP diphosphohydrolase activity with endothelial cell activation. J Exp Med. 1997;185(1):153–63.
59. Marcus AJ, Broekman MJ, Drosopoulos JH, et al. Metabolic control of excessive extracellular nucleotide accumulation by CD39/ecto-nucleotidase-1: implications for ischemic vascular diseases. J Pharmacol Exp Ther. 2003;305(1):9–16.
60. Enjyoji K, Sevigny J, Lin Y, et al. Targeted disruption of Cd39/ATP diphosphohydrolase results in disordered hemostasis and thromboregulation. Nat Med. 1999;5(9):1010–7.
61. Wagner DD, Frenette PS. The vessel wall and its interactions. Blood. 2008;111:5271–81.
62. Rumjantseva V, Grewal PK, Wandall HH, et al. Dual roles for hepatic lectin receptors in the clearance of chilled platelets. Nat Med. 2009;15(11):1273–80.
63. Grewal PK, Uchiyama S, Ditto D, et al. The Ashwell receptor mitigates the lethal coagulopathy of sepsis. Nat Med. 2008;14(6):648–55.
64. Karpatkin S, Finlay TH, Ballesteros AL, Karpatkin M. Effect of warfarin on prothrombin synthesis and secretion in human Hep G2 cells. Blood. 1987;70(3):773–8.
65. Kerr R. New insights into haemostasis in liver failure. Blood Coagul Fibrinolysis. 2003;14 Suppl 1:S43–5.
66. Straub PW. Diffuse intravascular coagulation in liver disease? Semin Thromb Hemost Summer. 1977;4(1):29–39.
67. Blomme B, Van Steenkiste C, Callewaert N, Van Vlierberghe H. Alteration of protein glycosylation in liver diseases. J Hepatol. 2009;50(3):592–603.
68. Bloom AL. Intravascular coagulation and the liver. Br J Haematol. 1975;30(1):1–7.
69. Losowsky MS. Impaired coagulation in the bleeding of chronic liver disease. J R Coll Physicians Lond. 1973;8(1):79–86.
70. Giannini EG, Savarino V. Thrombocytopenia in liver disease. Curr Opin Hematol. 2008;15(5):473–80.
71. Franchini M, Montagnana M, Targher G, Zaffanello M, Lippi G. The use of recombinant factor VIIa in liver diseases. Blood Coagul Fibrinolysis. 2008;19(5):341–8.
72. Thachil J. Relevance of clotting tests in liver disease. Postgrad Med J. 2008;84(990):177–81.
73. Luscinskas FW, Ma S, Nusrat A, Parkos CA, Shaw SK. Leukocyte transendothelial migration: a junctional affairs [Review]. Semin Immunol. 2002;14(2):105–13.
74. Hove WR, van Hoek B, Bajema IM, Ringers J, van Krieken JH, Lagaaij EL. Extensive chimerism in liver transplants: vascular endothelium, bile duct epithelium, and hepatocytes. Liver Transpl. 2003;9(6):552–6.
75. Gao ZH, Williams GM. Vascular endothelial-cell turnover: a new factor in the vascular microenvironment of the liver.[comment]. Trends Immunol. 2001;22(8):421–2.
76. Gao Z, McAlister VC, Williams GM. Repopulation of liver endothelium by bone-marrow-derived cells. Lancet. 2001;357(9260):932–3.
77. Quaini F, Urbanek K, Beltrami AP, et al. Chimerism of the transplanted heart.[comment]. N Engl J Med. 2002;346(1):5–15.
78. Burt AD, Le BB, Balabaud C, Bioulac SP. Morphologic investigation of sinusoidal cells. [Review]. Semin Liver Dis. 1993;13(1):21–38.
79. McCuskey RS, Reilly FD. Hepatic microvasculature: dynamic structure and its regulation. [Review]. Semin Liver Dis. 1993;13(1):1–12.
80. LeCouter J, Moritz DR, Li B, et al. Angiogenesis-independent endothelial protection of liver: role of VEGFR-1.[comment]. Science. 2003;299(5608):890–3.
81. Minami T, Aird WC. Endothelial cell gene regulation. Trends Cardiovasc Med. 2005;15(5):174–84.
82. Cotran RS, Pober JS. Endothelial activation and inflammation. Prog Immunol. 1989;8:747.
83. Hancock WW. Delayed xenograft rejection. World J Surg. 1997;21(9):917–23.
84. Baeuerle PA, Baltimore D. Activation of DNA-binding activity in an apparently cytoplasmic precursor of the NF-kappaB transcription factor. Cell. 1988;53(211):211–7.
85. Anrather D, Millan MT, Palmetshofer A, et al. Thrombin activates nuclear factor-kappa-B and potentiates endothelial cell activation by TNF. J Immunol. 1997;159(11):5620–8.
86. Ferran C, Millan MT, Csizmadia V, et al. Inhibition of NF-kappaB by pyrrolidine dithiocarbamate blocks endothelial cell activation. Biochem Biophys Res Commun. 1995;214(1):212–23.
87. Takagi H, King GL, Robinson GS, Ferrara N, Aiello LP. Adenosine mediates hypoxic induction of vascular endothelial growth factor in retinal pericytes and endothelial cells. Investig Ophthalmol Vis Sci. 1996;37(11):2165–76.
88. Murray AG, Khodadoust MM, Pober JS, Bothwell ALM. Porcine aortic endothelial cells activate human T cells: direct presentation of MHC antigens and co-stimulation by ligands for human CD2 and CD28. Immunity. 1994;1:57–63.
89. Savage CO, Hughes CC, McIntyre BW, Picard JK, Pober JS. Human CD4+ T cells proliferate to HLA-DR+ allogeneic vascular endothelium. Identification of accessory interactions. Transplantation. 1993;56(1):128–34.
90. Wiest R, Groszmann RJ. Nitric oxide and portal hypertension: its role in the regulation of intrahepatic and splanchnic vascular resistance. Semin Liver Dis. 1999;19(4):411–26.
91. Boeynaems J-M, Pearson JD. P2 purinoreceptors on vascular endothelial cells: physiological significance

and transduction mechanisms. TIPS (Trends Pharnmacol Sci). 1990;11:34–7.
92. Dubyak GR, Elmoatassim C. Signal transduction via P2-purinergic receptors for extracellular ATP and other nucleotides [Review]. Am J Physiol. 1993;265(3 Part 1):C577–606.
93. Brake A, Schumacher M, Julius D. ATP receptors in sickness, pain and death. Chem Biol. 1996;3(4): 229–32.
94. Franceschi C, Abbracchio MP, Barbieri D, et al. Purines and cell death. Drug Dev Res. 1996;39(3–4):442–9.
95. Fredholm BB, Abbracchio MP, Burnstock G, et al. Nomenclature and classification of purinoreceptors. Pharmacol Rev. 1994;46:143–52.
96. Buell G, Collo G, Rassendren F. P2X receptors – an emerging channel family [Review]. Eur J Neurosci. 1996;8(10):2221–8.
97. Roman RM, Fitz JG. Emerging roles of purinergic signaling in gastrointestinal epithelial secretion and hepatobiliary function. Gastroenterology. 1999;116: 964–79.
98. Palmer TM, Stiles GL. Adenosine receptors. Neuropharmacology. 1995;34:683–94.
99. Plesner L. Ecto-ATPases: identities and functions. Int Rev Cytol. 1995;158:141–214.
100. Traut TW. Physiological concentrations of purines and pyrimidines [Review]. Mol Cell Biochem. 1994;140(1):1–22.
101. Robson SC. Endothelial cell phenotypes associated with organ transplantation. In: William C. Aird, editor. Endothelial cells in health and disease. Taylor and Francis. Boca Raton, FL. USA: 2005. pp. 439–476.
102. Robson SC, Sevigny J, Imai M, Enjyoji K. Thromboregulatory potential of endothelial CD39/ nucleoside triphosphate diphosphohydrolase: modulation of purinergic signalling in platelets. Emerg Ther Targets. 2000;4:155–71.
103. Sevigny J, Sundberg C, Braun N, et al. Differential catalytic properties and vascular topography of murine nucleoside triphosphate diphosphohydrolase 1 (NTPDase1) and NTPDase2 have implications for thromboregulation. Blood. 2002;99(8):2801–9.
104. Vigne P, Breittmayer JP, Frelin C. Analysis of the influence of nucleotidases on the apparent activity of exogenous ATP and ADP at P2Y(1) receptors. Br J Pharmacol. 1998;125(4):675–80.
105. Simon T, Verstuyft C, Mary-Krause M, et al. Genetic determinants of response to clopidogrel and cardiovascular events. N Engl J Med. 2009;360(4):363–75.
106. Von Albertini M, Palmetshofer A, Kaczmarek E, et al. Extracellular ATP and ADP activate transcription factor NF-kappa-B and induce endothelial cell apoptosis. Biochem Biophys Res Commun. 1998; 248(3):822–9.
107. Beldi G, Enjyoji K, Wu Y, et al. The role of purinergic signaling in the liver and in transplantation: effects of extracellular nucleotides on hepatic graft vascular injury, rejection and metabolism. Front Biosci. 2008;13:2588–603.
108. Sun X, Cardenas A, Wu Y, Enjyoji K, Robson SC. Vascular stasis, intestinal hemorrhage, and heightened vascular permeability complicate acute portal hypertension in cd39-null mice. Am J Physiol Gastrointest Liver Physiol. 2009;297(2):G306–11.
109. Spemann H, Mangold H. Induction of embryonic primordia by implantation of organizers from a different species. 1923. Int J Dev Biol. 2001;45(1): 13–38.
110. Barbera-Guillem E, Vidal-Vanaclocha F. Sinusoidal structure of the liver. Revis Biol Celular. 1988; 16(1–34):54–68.
111. Bouwens L, De Bleser P, Vanderkerken K, Geerts B, Wisse E. Liver cell heterogeneity: functions of non-parenchymal cells. Enzyme. 1992;46(1–3):155–68.
112. Knolle PA, Limmer A. Neighborhood politics: the immunoregulatory function of organ-resident liver endothelial cells.[comment]. Trends Immunol. 2001;22(8):432–7.
113. Hoffmeister KM, Felbinger TW, Falet H, et al. The clearance mechanism of chilled blood platelets. Cell. 2003;112(1):87–97.
114. Reeves HL, Friedman SL. Activation of hepatic stellate cells – a key issue in liver fibrosis. Front Biosci. 2002;7:d808–26.
115. Wisse E, Luo D, Vermijlen D, Kanellopoulou C, De Zanger R, Braet F. On the function of pit cells, the liver-specific natural killer cells. Semin Liver Dis. 1997;17(4):265–86.
116. Chen D, Dorling A. Critical roles for thrombin in acute and chronic inflammation. J Thromb Haemost. 2009;7 Suppl 1:122–6.
117. Borensztajn K, von der Thusen JH, Peppelenbosch MP, Spek CA. The coagulation factor Xa/protease activated receptor-2 axis in the progression of liver fibrosis: a multifaceted paradigm. J Cell Mol Med. 2010;14:143–53.
118. Fiorucci S, Antonelli E, Distrutti E, et al. PAR1 antagonism protects against experimental liver fibrosis. Role of proteinase receptors in stellate cell activation. Hepatology. 2004;39(2):365–75.
119. Tanaka M, Wanless IR. Pathology of the liver in budd-chiari-syndrome – portal vein thrombosis and the histogenesis of veno-centric cirrhosis, veno-portal cirrhosis, and large regenerative nodules. Hepatology. 1998;27(2):488–96.
120. Valla DC. Portal vein thrombosis and prothrombotic disorders. J Gastroenterol Hepatol. 1999;14(11): 1051–2.
121. Darwish Murad S, Plessier A, Hernandez-Guerra M, et al. Etiology, management, and outcome of the Budd-Chiari syndrome. Ann Intern Med. 2009; 151(3):167–75.
122. Banz Y, Beldi G, Wu Y, Atkinson B, Usheva A, Robson SC. CD39 is incorporated into plasma microparticles where it maintains functional properties and impacts endothelial activation. Br J Haematol. 2008;142(4):627–37.
123. DeLeve LD, Shulman HM, McDonald GB. Toxic injury to hepatic sinusoids: sinusoidal obstruction

syndrome (veno-occlusive disease). Semin Liver Dis. 2002;22(1):27–42.
124. Harb R, Xie G, Lutzko C, et al. Bone marrow progenitor cells repair rat hepatic sinusoidal endothelial cells after liver injury. Gastroenterology. 2009; 137(2):704–12.
125. DeLeve LD, Valla DC, Garcia-Tsao G. Vascular disorders of the liver. Hepatology. 2009;49(5):1729–64.
126. DeLeve LD. Vascular liver diseases. Curr Gastroenterol Rep. 2003;5(1):63–70.
127. Robson SC, Jaskiewicz K, Engelbrecht G, Kahn D, Hickman R, Kirsch RE. Haemostatic and immunological sequelae of portacaval shunt in rats. Liver. 1995;15(6):293–9.
128. Robson SC, Candinas D, Hancock WW, Wrighton C, Winkler H, Bach FH. Role of endothelial cells in transplantation [Review]. Int Arch Allergy Immunol. 1995;106(4):305–22.
129. Dwyer K, Deaglio S, Crikis S, et al. Salutary roles of CD39 in transplantation. Transplant Rev. 2007;21: 54–63.
130. Lappas CM, Day YJ, Marshall MA, Engelhard VH, Linden J. Adenosine A2A receptor activation reduces hepatic ischemia reperfusion injury by inhibiting CD1d-dependent NKT cell activation. J Exp Med. 2006;203(12):2639–48.
131. Beldi G, Banz Y, Kroemer A, et al. Deletion of CD39 on natural killer cells attenuates hepatic ischemia/reperfusion injury in mice. Hepatology. 2010;51(5):1702–11.
132. Clavien PA. Sinusoidal endothelial cell injury during hepatic preservation and reperfusion. Hepatology. 1998;28(2):281–5.
133. de Rougemont O, Lehmann K, Clavien PA. Preconditioning, organ preservation, and postconditioning to prevent ischemia-reperfusion injury to the liver. Liver Transpl. 2009;15(10):1172–82.
134. Serracino-Inglott F, Habib NA, Mathie RT. Hepatic ischemia-reperfusion injury [Review]. Am J Surg. 2001;181(2):160–6.
135. Bilzer M, Gerbes AL. Preservation injury of the liver: mechanisms and novel therapeutic strategies [Review]. J Hepatol. 2000;32(3):508–15.
136. Baccarani U, Donini A, Risaliti A, Bresadola F. Replacement of liver venous endothelium. Lancet. 2001;357(9274):2137.
137. Kopp CW, Robson SC, Siegel JB, et al. Regulation of monocyte tissue factor activity by allogeneic and xenogeneic endothelial cells. Thromb Haemost. 1998;79(3):529–38.
138. Lesurtel M, Graf R, Aleil B, et al. Platelet-derived serotonin mediates liver regeneration. Science. 2006;312(5770):104–7.
139. Beldi G, Wu Y, Sun X, et al. Regulated catalysis of extracellular nucleotides by vascular CD39/ENTPD1 is required for liver regeneration. Gastroenterology. 2008;135(5):1751–60.
140. Demetris AJ, Adeyi O, Bellamy CO, et al. Liver biopsy interpretation for causes of late liver allograft dysfunction. Hepatology. 2006;44(2):489–501.
141. Demetris AJ, Ruppert K, Dvorchik I, et al. Real-time monitoring of acute liver-allograft rejection using the Banff schema. Transplantation. 2002;74(9):1290–6.
142. Libby P, Pober JS. Chronic rejection. Immunity. 2001;14(4):387–97.
143. Demetris AJ, Murase N, Lee RG, et al. Chronic rejection. A general overview of histopathology and pathophysiology with emphasis on liver, heart and intestinal allografts. Ann Transplant. 1997;2(2):27–44.
144. Starzl TE. The "privileged" liver and hepatic tolerogenicity. Liver Transplant. 2001;7(10):918–20.
145. Crispe IN, Dao T, Klugewitz K, Mehal WZ, Metz DP. The liver as a site of T-cell apoptosis: graveyard, or killing field? Immunol Rev. 2000;174:47–62.
146. Mackay IR. Hepatoimmunology: a perspective. Immunol Cell Biol. 2002;80(1):36–44.
147. Hillebrands JL, Klatter FA, van den Hurk BM, Popa ER, Nieuwenhuis P, Rozing J. Origin of neointimal endothelium and alpha-actin-positive smooth muscle cells in transplant arteriosclerosis.[comment]. J Clin Investig. 2001;107(11):1411–22.
148. Dhillon AP, Burroughs AK, Hudson M, Shah N, Rolles K, Scheuer PJ. Hepatic venular stenosis after orthotopic liver transplantation. Hepatology. 1994; 19(1):106–11.
149. Treiber G, Csepregi A, Malfertheiner P. The pathophysiology of portal hypertension. Dig Dis. 2005;23(1):6–10.
150. Pinzani M, Marra F. Cytokine receptors and signaling in hepatic stellate cells. Semin Liver Dis. 2001;21(3):397–416.
151. Robson SC, Saunders R, Purves LR, Dejager C, Corrigall A, Kirsch RE. Fibrin and fibrinogen degradation products with an intact D-domain C-terminal gamma-chain inhibit an early step in accessory cell-dependent lymphocyte mitogenesis. Blood. 1993;81(11):3006–14.
152. Poole TJ, Coffin JD. Vasculogenesis and angiogenesis: two distinct morphogenetic mechanisms establish embryonic vascular pattern. J Exp Zool. 1989;251(2):224–31.
153. Coffin JD, Poole TJ. Embryonic vascular development: immunohistochemical identification of the origin and subsequent morphogenesis of the major vessel primordia in quail embryos. Development. 1988;102(4):735–48.

Vascular Liver Disease and the Liver Sinusoidal Endothelial Cell

2

Laurie D. DeLeve

Abstract

The hepatic sinusoidal endothelial cell is highly differentiated, with unique morphology and function. It provides a porous barrier that facilitates access of the hepatocyte to oxygen and small molecules in the microcirculation. Other specialized functions include clearance of colloids and macromolecules, promotion of hepatic stellate cell quiescence, and induction of immune tolerance. The hepatic sinusoidal endothelial cell may be injured by a variety of toxins, ischemia–reperfusion, and even bacteria, leading to vascular liver diseases such as sinusoidal obstruction syndrome, nodular regenerative hyperplasia, and peliosis hepatis.

Keywords

Liver • Liver circulation • Endothelial cells • Hepatic veno-occlusive disease • Nodular regenerative hyperplasia

Introduction

The liver sinusoidal endothelial cell (LSEC) has a number of important functions, as will be addressed below. To summarize these functions, LSECs: (1) provide a porous barrier that facilitates oxygenation of hepatocytes and enhances hepatocyte exposure to macromolecules in the portal circulation; (2) clear colloids and macromolecules from the circulation; (3) act as a gatekeeper against hepatic stellate cell (HSC) activation; and (4) provide a microcirculation.

Wisse was first able to demonstrate that the endothelial cells lining the hepatic sinusoids were distinct from Kupffer cells using electron microscopic studies of the perfusion-fixed liver [1, 2]. The next major step forward in LSEC research was the description of a method to isolate a pure population of LSEC using elutriation [3, 4]. Isolation by elutriation requires specialized equipment, which has limited the number of laboratories working in this field. Subsequent development of a method using density gradient centrifugation with selective adherence has provided an alternative method for rapid and inexpensive isolation of LSEC [5]. In recent years, several methods have been described for LSEC isolation using immunomagnetic separation. Immunomagnetic separation yields a very small fraction of the number of cells isolated by either of the two earlier methods, with the inherent risk

L.D. DeLeve (✉)
Division of Gastrointestinal and Liver Diseases, University of Southern California, Keck School of Medicine, 2011 Zonal Avenue- HMR 603, Los Angeles, CA 90033, USA
e-mail: deleve@usc.edu

L.D. DeLeve and G. Garcia-Tsao (eds.), *Vascular Liver Disease: Mechanisms and Management*,
DOI 10.1007/978-1-4419-8327-5_2,

that subpopulations are being isolated. Most of the immunomagnetic protocols have not yet validated that the cells being isolated have both ultrastructural features and functional characteristics specific to LSEC. With proper validation, the use of immunomagnetic separation should facilitate more widespread study of LSEC.

SEC Phenotype

Two specific phenotypic features can be used to definitively identify LSEC. By electron microscopy [1, 2], LSEC have nondiaphragmed fenestrae organized in clusters termed sieve plates. Functionally, endocytosis of labeled formaldehyde-treated serum albumin or collagen alpha chains can be used to identify LSEC (see Sect. Function and Dysfunction). Although there are a number of surface markers present on LSEC (Table 2.1), few if any are specific for LSEC within the liver.

Morphology

Endothelial Cell Fenestration

The permeability of endothelial barriers is dependent on the structure of the cell itself and the underlying basement membrane. Endothelial cells are divided into continuous or discontinuous cells. Continuous endothelial cells have continuous cytoplasm and fusion of the luminal and abluminal plasma membrane only occurs at cell junctions. The subset of discontinuous endothelium that has larger gaps or pores is referred to as fenestrated cells. Fenestrae traverse the cytoplasm and connect the luminal and abluminal cytoplasmic membrane. Fenestrae can be closed with a diaphragm or completely open. With the exception of the LSEC and renal glomerular endothelial cell, fenestrated endothelial cells in the mammal are diaphragmed. The LSEC and the glomerular endothelial cell differ from each other in that the LSEC does not have an organized basement membrane and the glomerular endothelial cell does. Thus, the LSEC has a unique morphology in that it is the only mammalian cell with both open fenestrae and the lack of an organized basement membrane. The LSEC is therefore the most permeable of all mammalian endothelial cells. The fenestrae in LSEC are grouped together in clusters, termed sieve plates (Fig. 2.1).

The LSEC morphology varies across the sinusoid. LSEC in the periportal region are smaller than perivenular LSEC. Compared to perivenular LSEC, periportal LSEC have fewer fenestrae per sieve plate and fenestrae that are slighter larger in size, but overall porosity (percentage of the cell surface occupied by fenestrae) of periportal LSEC is lower than of perivenular LSEC.

Table 2.1 Selected markers present on LSEC

CD31 or PECAM-1	Classic endothelial cell marker present on cell surface, facilitates transendothelial migration of leukocytes [6]. Absent from cell surface of LSEC, but present in cytoplasm [7]
CD45	Leukocyte common antigen. Present on 85–90% of LSEC isolated by elutriation [8]
CD33	A myeloblast antigen, also present on the LSEC surface [8]
CD4	Present on T cells, monocytes, macrophages, dendritic cells, and LSEC [9]
ICAM-1	Ligand for LFA-1 on leukocytes [9]
CD36	Thrombospondin-1 receptor [9]
Fcγ(gamma) receptor IIb_2	Predominant receptor on LSEC for the Fc receptor of immunoglobulin G, endocytoses immune complexes. Present on dendritic cells
Stabilin-2	Main scavenger receptor on LSEC, thought within the liver to be unique for LSEC [10–12]
Integrin $\alpha(\text{alpha})_1\beta(\text{beta})_1$	Preferentially binds collagen IV [13]
Integrin $\alpha(\text{alpha})_5\beta(\text{beta})_1$	Binds fibronectin [13]

Other antigens reported on LSEC include LYVE-1, MCAM (CD46), MHC class I and class II molecules, CD80, CD86, CD40

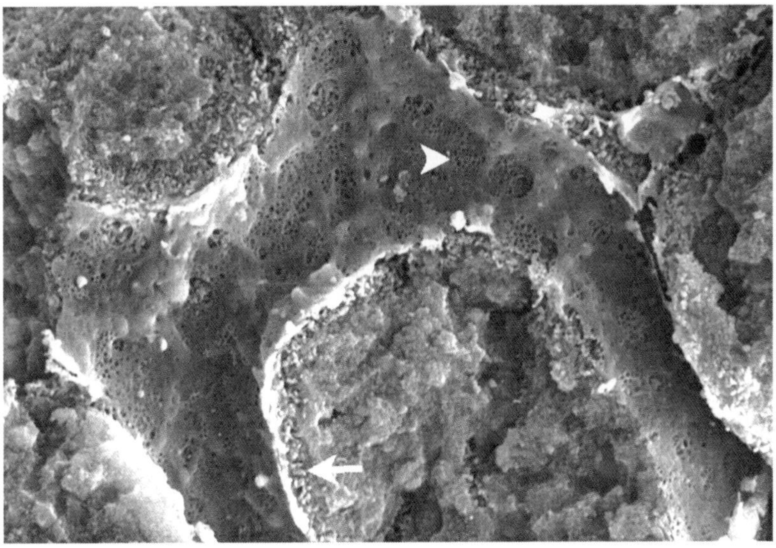

Fig. 2.1 Hepatic sinusoid. Scanning electron microscopy picture of hepatic sinusoid. *Arrowhead* indicates a sieve plate in the LSEC. *Arrow* indicates hepatocyte villi in the space of Disse

Other Sinusoidal Endothelial Cells

Sinusoids are tortuous terminal blood vessels with a discontinuous endothelial lining and either a discontinuous basement membrane or the lack of an organized basement membrane. In addition to the liver, both the spleen and bone marrow have sinusoids. Both the spleen and bone marrow have interendothelial slits that open up to allow migration of cells through the sinusoids, providing the discontinuity of lining. Splenic sinusoidal endothelial cells have continuous cytoplasm, but a discontinuous basement membrane that forms ring-like structures around the sinusoid [14–16]. The bone marrow has diaphragmed, fenestrated endothelial cells and a discontinuous, irregular basement membrane [17, 18].

Regulation of SEC Phenotype

Fenestrated endothelial cells occur in proximity to epithelial cells with a high constitutive expression of vascular endothelial growth factor (VEGF) [19]. In the liver, the LSEC phenotype is maintained by paracrine secretion of VEGF by hepatocytes and HSCs [7, 20] and a downstream autocrine loop of VEGF-stimulated NO production by eNOS in the LSEC [7].

Function and Dysfunction

Barrier Function

Oxygen Delivery

The liver has a dual blood supply. About 70% of the blood is poorly oxygenated blood from the portal vein and the remaining 30% is well-oxygenated blood from the hepatic artery. The combination of open fenestrae, thin cytoplasm, and lack of an organized basement membrane reduces the distance required for oxygen diffusion and thereby facilitates oxygen delivery to the hepatocyte to compensate for the relatively low pO_2 in sinusoidal blood.

Loss of fenestration, thickening of the cytoplasm, and development of an organized basement membrane is called capillarization [21]. Capillarization precedes fibrosis in chronic liver disease and has been observed in both humans and experimental animals [21–27]. A forme fruste of capillarization, termed pseudocapillarization by LeCouteur and colleagues, occurs with aging in humans and experimental animals (see Chap. 3). In both capillarization and pseudocapillarization, there is evidence of hepatocyte hypoxia. In the cirrhotic liver, oxidative drug metabolism is decreased and can be restored with oxygen supplementation [28–30]. In pseudocapillarization, there is a decline in high-energy phosphate and other metabolites in the hepatocyte, indicative of hepatocyte hypoxia [31]. In the latter case, this occurs without fibrosis or other structural changes that could account for the hypoxia. There are no studies to document whether functions other than oxidative metabolism are impaired by the barrier to oxygenation induced by capillarization.

Passage of Small Molecules

Based on the observation that chylomicron remnants that pass into the space of Disse are smaller than the size of fenestrae, it was postulated many years ago that LSEC fenestration acts as a sieve for chylomicron remnant clearance [1, 32, 33]. This observation gained renewed interest with the recognition of aging-related pseudocapillarization. Chylomicron remnants are thought to play an important role in initiating atherosclerosis [34, 35]. Decreased chylomicron remnant clearance with aging-related LSEC defenestration may contribute to aging-related hyperlipidemia and atherosclerosis [36–38] (see Chap. 3).

In most vascular beds, protein-bound drug is restricted to the circulation and uptake into tissues is restricted to free or unbound drug, but in the liver protein-bound drugs pass into the space of Disse. Consequently, in one pass through the liver free drug in the space of Disse can be cleared by hepatocytes, which allows bound drug to reequilibrate with the free, and the newly formed free drug can be cleared. This allows drug clearance to exceed the free fraction in the liver. The combination of decreased drug clearance and the decline in oxidative drug metabolism (see above) in capillarization and pseudocapillarization is predicted to contribute to the impaired drug disposition in chronic liver disease and the aging liver. However, in both aging and cirrhosis there are also changes in liver blood flow and liver mass, so that it is difficult to determine the relative contribution of changes in LSEC to the decline in drug clearance and drug metabolism.

Scavenger Function of LSEC

LSEC and Kupffer cells play complementary roles in the clearance of waste from portal vein blood. LSEC clear colloids and macromolecules, whereas Kupffer cells phagocytose the larger particulate matter and insoluble waste. As described by Smedsrød et al. [39], there are several factors that make LSEC such effective and important scavengers. The liver, and therefore the LSEC, is the first checkpoint for macromolecules and antigens that enter the portal circulation from the intestine. LSEC clearance is facilitated by the slow and intermittent flow through the sinusoids, the large surface area of LSEC, the numerous positively charged coated pits that aid endocytosis of negatively charged molecules, and the presence of three distinct endocytosis receptors. Finally, LSEC are well suited for disposal of waste products, because of high specific activity of lysosomal enzymes that is as high or even higher than that of Kupffer cells [40].

The three LSEC endocytosis receptors are the collagen-α(alpha)-chain/mannose receptor, the hyaluronan/scavenger receptor, and the Fcγ(gamma) IIb_2 receptor. The collagen-α(alpha)-chain/mannose receptor (CD206) clears circulating collagen alpha chains, i.e., denatured collagen of several types of collagen, and glycoconjugates with terminal mannose, such as lysosomal enzymes, procollagen type I carboxyterminal propeptides, and tissue type plasminogen activator [41, 42]. The hyaluronan/scavenger receptor, SR-H (stabilin-1 and stabilin-2), is the main functional scavenger receptor on the LSEC [10–12]. The hyaluronan/scavenger receptor clears hyaluronan, chondroitin sulphate, formaldehyde-treated serum albumin (FSA, used as a test ligand for scavenger receptor-mediated endocytosis), procollagen type I and III N-terminal peptides, nidogen, acetylated and oxidized low density lipoprotein [43–45], plasma coagulation products, and advanced glycation end-products [46]. The LSEC Fc receptor, Fcγ(gamma) IIb_2 (CD32b or SE-1), clears immune complexes formed with Ig G [47, 48].

Aging-related pseudocapillarization and liver disease-related capillarization both lead to a decline in endocytosis [49, 50]. The pathophysiological consequences of the decline in LSEC scavenger function have not been studied.

Stellate Cell Quiescence

In vitro studies show that LSEC maintain stellate cell quiescence and induce reversion of activated stellate cells to quiescence [51]. When LSEC dedifferentiate to a defenestrated "capillarized" phenotype, this paracrine effect on stellate cells is lost and stellate cell become activated. LSEC capillarization in vivo precedes fibrosis in both human chronic liver disease and in experimental animal models. The in vitro studies suggest that LSEC capillarization not only precedes fibrosis, but also is permissive for fibrosis and that reversal of capillarization could promote resolution of fibrosis. Studies reported in abstract form provide in vivo confirmation that reversal of capillarization promotes reversion of stellate cells to quiescence and reversal of fibrosis [52].

Other LSEC Functions

Two other LSEC functions have not been well studied in chronic liver disease and will only be briefly mentioned.

Immune Function

LSEC may function as an antigen-presenting cell that induces tolerance [53–60]. This effect is consistent with several observations that suggest that the liver can induce tolerance: the success of transplantation of MHC-incompatible livers, induction of immune tolerance to antigens presented in the portal circulation, and the reduction in rejection when the venous drainage of a graft is through the portal vein [61].

Drug Metabolism

Although the specific activity of metabolic enzymes is generally much higher in parenchymal cells, LSEC have both phase I and II enzymes [62, 63]. The ability of LSEC to metabolically activate drugs may contribute to some forms of toxin-induced injury [64–66], particularly given the relatively low glutathione detoxification capacity [67]. There are currently no studies of whether LSEC drug metabolism is altered in chronic liver disease.

Vascular Liver Disease and LSEC (Table 2.2)

Sinusoidal Obstruction Syndrome (SOS)

For decades, SOS was called hepatic veno-occlusive disease. Given that 45% of patients with mild and moderate SOS and 25% of patients with severe SOS after myeloablative regimens do not have involvement of the central venules [68] and that the disease is initiated by damage at the level of the sinusoids (see below), this is a misnomer. This led to the new name, SOS [69], which also serves to distinguish it from liver pathology with veno-occlusive lesions seen in alcoholic liver disease and liver transplantation, sometimes termed hepatic veno-occlusive disease in the literature.

SOS occurs in only two settings. It can be induced by ingestion of pyrrolizidine alkaloids, as first described in South Africa and later described in Jamaica [70–72]. The second setting is due to specific medications alone (see Table 2.3) or medications in combination with irradiation of the liver. The major plant species containing pyrrolizidine alkaloids, *Crotalaria*, *Heliotropium*, and *Senecio*, can be found all around the world. However, pyrrolizidine alkaloid-induced SOS is most commonly seen in undernourished individuals in underdeveloped countries. It can be seen sporadically in individuals that ingest "bush teas" or during local

Table 2.2 Vascular liver injury with LSEC involvement

Sinusoidal obstruction syndrome
Radiation-induced liver disease
Ischemia–reperfusion injury[a]
Heterogeneous liver perfusion
Peliosis hepatitis

[a] See Chap. 5

epidemics, when crops are contaminated by plants containing pyrrolizidine alkaloids. In contrast to the iatrogenic form, pyrrolizidine alkaloid-induced SOS is commonly a more chronic disease. The most common setting for SOS in North America and Western Europe is after myeloablative hematopoietic cell transplantation. It is seen sporadically after chemotherapy unrelated to hematopoietic cell transplantation and with certain immunosuppressive drugs.

Table 2.3 Drugs associated with sinusoidal obstruction syndrome

Actinomycin D
Azathioprine
BCNU [a]
Busulfan [b]
Cyclophosphamide [b]
Cytosine arabinoside
Dacarbazine
Dimethylbusulfan [c]
Gemcitabine [c]
Gemtuzumab-ozogamicin
Mithramycin
Oxaliplatin
6-Thioguanine
Urethane

[a] Only in high doses
[b] Only at high doses and in combination regimens
[c] Rare case reports

Mechanism of Injury (Fig. 2.2)

In vitro studies with drugs and toxins that cause SOS demonstrated that these compounds are selectively more toxic to LSEC, either due to enhanced metabolic activation in the LSEC or due to relatively weak detoxification [64, 66, 73]. SOS has also been studied in a reproducible animal model induced by monocrotaline, a pyrrolizidine alkaloid [74]. This model has the same signs and symptoms as human SOS and follows a more acute course, similar to that seen in humans after high-dose chemotherapy. Monocrotaline is P450 activated to a monocrotaline pyrrole and metabolic activation occurs in both hepatocytes and LSEC. One of the four known adducts of monocrotaline pyrrole is actin [75]. In LSEC, monocrotaline causes depolymerization of F-actin, which in turn leads to increased expression of matrix metalloproteinase-9 (MMP-9) [76], an enzyme that is exocytosed from cytoplasmic granules and then digests extracellular matrix in the space of Disse. The combination of depolymerization of F-actin, an element of the cell skeleton, and digestion of the extracellular matrix tethering of the LSEC leads to rounding up of the LSEC and formation of gaps in the endothelial barrier [77]. With obstruction of sinusoids by swollen LSEC and gaps in the endothelial barrier, the space of Disse becomes

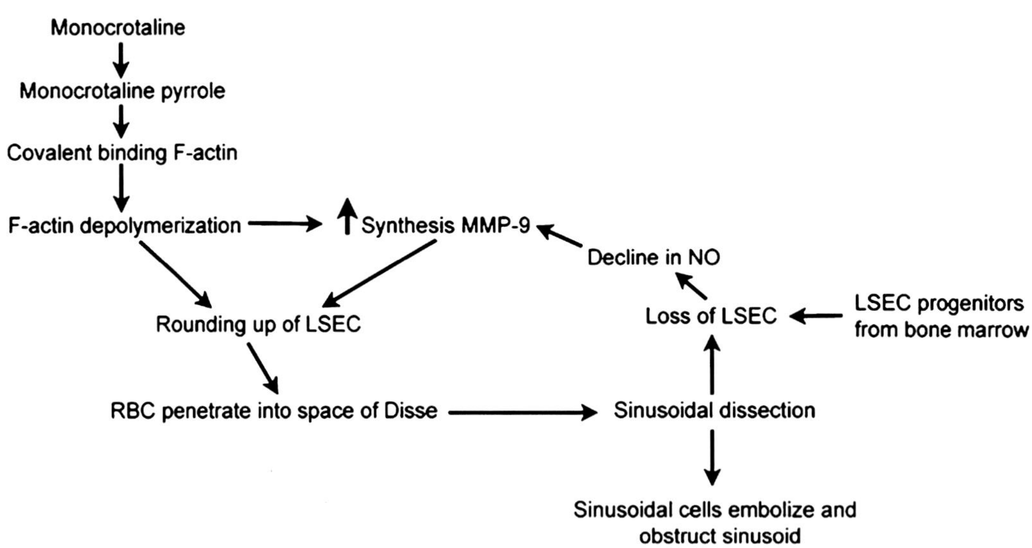

Fig. 2.2 Scheme illustrating mechanism of SOS

the pathway of least resistance. Red cells penetrate between LSEC and eventually blood begins to flow through the space of Disse, dissecting off LSEC and stellate cells. Sinusoidal cells embolize downstream, blocking sinusoidal blood flow. Other changes occur that lead to the perpetuation of the changes described above. At the same time that LSEC round up, the number of Kupffer cells in the liver decreases markedly [74]. Nitric oxide (NO) levels fall in parallel to the decline in Kupffer cells [78]. As the number of viable LSEC declines, there is an additional and parallel drop in NO. NO is known to tonically inhibit MMP synthesis [79–81] and delivery of a liver-specific NO prodrug prevents the increase in MMP-9 synthesis and activity in this model. Monocrotaline depletes LSEC glutathione (GSH) and support of LSEC GSH prevents the development of SOS in the model. GSH inhibits MMP-9 activity [82]. Thus, the decline in NO permits the increased synthesis of MMP-9 and the fall in GSH permits increased MMP-9 activity. All of the events described above are initiating events that occur before there is clear-cut histological evidence of injury and form a feed-forward loop of injury. The more MMP-9 synthesis is upregulated, the more LSEC are lost, the greater the decline in NO, and the less MMP-9 synthesis and activity are inhibited. Inhibition of MMP-9, treatment with a liver-specific NO donor, or support of GSH all prevent development of SOS, demonstrating that the LSEC injury initiates SOS and that protection of the LSEC prevents SOS.

There is a second component to SOS that distinguishes it from other forms of LSEC injury. The normal response to endothelial cell injury is to increase the number of endothelial progenitor cells in the bone marrow and mobilization of these cells to the circulation. In monocrotaline-induced SOS, LSEC progenitors in the bone marrow are reduced by 50% and circulating progenitors are reduced by over 95% [8], demonstrating monocrotaline toxicity to the progenitors. Infusion of LSEC progenitor cells completely prevents SOS. In contrast, when a subtoxic dose of monocrotaline is given to bone marrow-suppressed rats, severe SOS ensues, demonstrating that bone marrow suppression unmasks a subclinical injury. Thus, SOS is due to both LSEC injury and to monocrotaline-induced impairment of repair by bone marrow-derived progenitors. This then explains why SOS occurs almost exclusively after either exposure to pyrrolizidine alkaloids or to chemotherapy regimens that are both toxic to LSEC and that are myeloablative.

In addition to the changes to the LSEC, SOS can also lead to occlusion of the hepatic venules. There is a rough correlation with severity of disease and extension of the injury to the venules [68]. Central vein endothelial cells are damaged and subendothelial edema contributes to the early occlusion of the venules. The impediment to sinusoidal and venular blood flow leads to hepatocyte necrosis. Thus, in early SOS there is congestion, centrilobular hemorrhagic necrosis, extensive centrilobular loss of CD31 positive LSEC, loss of central vein endothelium, and occlusion of the central vein by subintimal edema.

Late SOS is characterized by marked sinusoidal fibrosis and fibrotic occlusion of central veins. LSEC tonically suppress stellate cell activation [51], so that widespread, prolonged loss of LSEC [77] permits stellate cell activation and sinusoidal fibrosis.

Clinical Features of SOS

This section will discuss chemo-irradiation induced SOS: there is much more extensive literature on this than on pyrrolizidine alkaloid-induced SOS and the author assumes that readers of this text are more likely to see chemo-irradiation induced SOS.

Causes of SOS (Table 2.3)

The highest risk for SOS is induced by myeloablative chemotherapy in preparation for hematopoietic cell transplantation (including bone marrow transplantation). Cyclophosphamide by itself does not cause SOS, but two of the highest risk myeloablative regimens contain cyclophosphamide [83]. Busulfan does not cause SOS when given alone, but the busulfan–cyclophosphamide myeloablative regimen is a very high-risk regimen. In contrast, the myeloablative regimen busulfan–fludarabine has a much lower incidence of SOS. Another high-risk regimen is cyclophosphamide combined with total body irradiation (TBI). The doses of TBI used are not in the hepatotoxic range when used alone, but the risk of SOS in the cyclophosphamide–TBI regimen increases with higher doses of TBI [83].

Gemtuzumab-ozogamicin is a humanized monoclonal antibody to CD33, a myeloblast antigen that is linked to the toxin calicheamicin and is used in the treatment of acute myeloid leukemia. Of note, LSEC express CD33 on their surface [8]. As a single agent, gemtuzumab-ozogamicin has a relatively low incidence of SOS. Patients with acute myeloid leukemia may undergo myeloablative hematopoietic cell transplantation and, if the disease relapses, may then be treated with gemtuzumab-ozogamicin, or the converse order of treatments may be used. The incidence of SOS increases markedly when a patient has been exposed to both gemtuzumab-ozogamicin and myeloablative chemotherapy and this risk is greater when the two modalities are given within several months of each other [84–86]. It is not known why there is a persistently increased risk of SOS in the first few months after myeloablative chemo-irradiation or gemtuzumab-ozogamicin, but it is tempting to speculate that this may indicate persistent suppression of the bone marrow LSEC progenitor response.

Treatment of Wilms' tumor with actinomycin D has a significant risk for SOS. The risk is highest when the tumor is in the right kidney, when actinomycin D is given in combination with abdominal irradiation and when a single high dose is given instead of repeated administration of lower doses [87–89]. Among the remaining medications listed in Table 2.3, there are numerous reports of SOS related to standard chemotherapy with dacarbazine, cytosine arabinoside, or oxaliplatin. There are also case series of SOS related to immunosuppression with azathioprine for kidney or liver transplantation and to 6-thioguanine used for inflammatory bowel disease or psoriasis.

Incidence: The incidence of SOS has dropped over the years. This can largely be attributed to the shift towards nonmyeloablative regimens, e.g., fludarabine plus low-dose TBI, which are not hepatotoxic. There are substantial differences in the incidence of SOS across transplant centers, which depends on the regimens used (TBI dose used, use of gemtuzumab-ozogamicin), patient exclusion criteria (preexisting liver disease, prior transplantation), and diagnostic criteria [83]. As McDonald has pointed out in a recent review, although the frequency of SOS varies at different centers, case fatality rate remains relatively constant at 15–20% [83].

Diagnosis: In patients at risk for SOS, the diagnosis can often be made based on the presence of painful hepatomegaly, weight gain, and hyperbilirubinemia, but with careful exclusion of other causes of these signs and symptoms. The diagnosis can be supported in unclear cases by Doppler ultrasound, transjugular liver biopsy, and wedged hepatic venous pressure gradient.

Prognosis: High elevations of ALT, higher portal pressure, and multiorgan failure are predictive of a poor prognosis [83]. For patients who develop SOS due to cyclophosphamide-containing regimens, outcome can be predicted based on bilirubin level and weight gain using published graphs [90].

Prevention: The highest risk patients are those with underlying liver disease, previous myeloablative regimens, and previous evidence of SOS. Regimens that have not been linked to SOS and could be considered in these high-risk patients are the myeloablative regimen fludarabine with targeted busulfan [91, 92] or the nonmyeloablative regimen of fludarabine plus low-dose TBI [93]. If high-risk patients are to be treated with cyclophosphamide–TBI or busulfan–cyclophosphamide, regimens may need to be modified. Lower doses or personalized dosing of cyclophosphamide [94, 95], TBI doses below 12 Gy, or administration of intravenous busulfan after rather than before cyclophosphamide [96] may reduce the risk of SOS. As mentioned earlier, a longer interval between myeloablative regimens and gemtuzumab-ozogamicin decreases the risk for SOS. The risk of SOS from gemtuzumab-ozogamicin is also decreased when a reduced-intensity regimen is used for the hematopoietic cell transplantation, although the risk is still dependent on interval between modalities [97]. Gemtuzumab-ozogamicin has a low incidence of SOS when given alone vs. the higher risk of the combination with 6-thioguanine [97], a drug that also causes SOS when used as a single drug [98–100]. In prospective studies, prophylaxis with heparin, ursodeoxycholic acid, or antithrombin III did not prevent fatal SOS [69]. Various other proposed prophylactic strategies still need to be tested in randomized controlled studies.

Treatment: Treatment of SOS requires pain management and management of fluid overload with diuretics, paracentesis, hemofiltration, or hemodialysis. Defibrotide, a single-stranded polydeoxyribonucleotide, has been used extensively for SOS, but has never been studied in a randomized controlled trial. Liver transplantation should only be considered if the disease that necessitated the chemo-irradiation has a favorable prognosis.

Radiation-Induced Liver Disease (RILD)

RILD occurs in patients who undergo irradiation for primary or metastatic cancer in the liver. Given the radiosensitivity of endothelial cells and the general resemblance to SOS, RILD is assumed to be due to endothelial damage, but it is not known whether this is mainly a venous or a sinusoidal injury. The lesion has not been reproduced in experimental animals.

RILD is a syndrome of anicteric ascites, hepatomegaly, and abnormal liver tests which develops 2 weeks to 4 months after hepatic irradiation in excess of 30–35 Gy. The risk of developing RILD is dependent on the irradiated liver volume and hepatic functional reserve.

Histological features are sinusoidal hemorrhage and congestion, fibrotic veno-occlusive lesions of the central vein but also occasionally of the intermediate size portal veins, and centrilobular atrophy [101–103]. Portal to central bridging fibrosis and persistent fibrotic veno-occlusive lesions of the central veins may be seen months to years later [103]. Ultrastructurally, fibrin has been identified in central venules, but there are no thrombi of fibrin or platelets [102].

The clinical features of RILD are painful hepatomegaly, weight gain, and ascites. Liver tests show normal bilirubin, alkaline phosphatase elevations that are 3–10 times the upper limit of normal, and modest AST and ALT elevations. Most patients recover over 3–5 months, but some progress to chronic liver disease. A small fraction of patients who develop progressive fibrosis with jaundice, refractory ascites, and coagulopathy have a poor prognosis [103].

Although there are similarities between SOS and RILD, these are distinct syndromes. Clinically, SOS is accompanied by hyperbilirubinemia and patients with RILD usually have normal bilirubin levels. The chronic course of RILD resembles the course of pyrrolizidine alkaloid-induced SOS with often greatly delayed onset and a course of months and sometimes years, whereas SOS related to myeloablative regimens occurs within 2–4 weeks of the insult and resolves within weeks to months. On histology, there is centrilobular atrophy but no necrosis in RILD and occasional veno-occlusive lesions can be in the portal veins, whereas the classic lesion of SOS includes centrilobular necrosis and does not involve the portal veins. Ultrastructurally, fibrin is present in the central venules of RILD, but fibrin is absent on ultrastructural studies of SOS.

Heterogeneous Liver Perfusion

Historically, diffuse nodular regenerative hyperplasia, partial nodular transformation, idiopathic noncirrhotic intrahepatic portal hypertension, and incomplete septal cirrhosis were described as distinct forms of liver pathology. However, the current consensus holds that these lesions are a single entity with a common etiology, i.e., uneven perfusion of the liver, that result in a spectrum of pathological lesions and clinical manifestations [104–107]. More than one of these pathological lesions may be found in some patients, supporting the concept that these lesions are a spectrum of responses due to a shared etiology [105]. These lesions of heterogeneous liver perfusion occur, by definition, in the absence of cirrhosis or of chronic liver disease that might cause cirrhosis. The circulatory impairment may be either at the level of the portal vein or the sinusoid, the latter justifying the inclusion of these lesions in this chapter.

It should be stated that it is still an unproven working hypothesis, albeit a widely accepted one, that these lesions are due to heterogeneous perfusion. The hypothesis, first described for nodular regenerative hyperplasia [107], is that impaired regional perfusion of the liver leads to atrophy with apoptotic or atrophic hepatocytes [108] and reactive hyperplasia in adjacent areas with preserved blood flow. The original concept was that impaired perfusion was due to obstructive portal vasculopathy [107] and was subsequently revised to include impaired flow at the level of the sinusoid. A recent study suggests that impairment of flow at the level of the sinusoid may account for a significant proportion of cases [104]. The hypothesis of heterogeneous perfusion is based on histopathological observations, but has never been tested experimentally. Mice with inducible inactivation of Notch1 develop nodular regenerative hyperplasia without vascular obliteration, although ultrastructural studies of the sinusoids were not performed, which would have definitively ruled out abnormalities at the sinusoidal level [109].

Risk factors for lesions with heterogeneous liver perfusion include collagen vascular diseases, clotting disorders, myelo- and lymphoproliferative diseases, immunological disorders, and a variety of drugs and toxins (Table 2.4). For many of the predisposing factors it is apparent how the venous or sinusoidal circulation would be impaired, but for others it is unclear. Inflammation of the hepatic artery in collagen vascular diseases or immune complex diseases may extend to adjacent portal veins [110, 111]. Prothrombotic disorders may cause thrombosis at the level of either the venous or sinusoidal circulation [104]. Azathioprine and myeloablative regimens may damage LSEC [66, 73]. It is noteworthy that there is significant overlap between causes of SOS (see Table 2.3), lesions with heterogeneous liver perfusion (see Table 2.4), and peliosis hepatis (see Table 2.6), supporting the concept that the LSEC may be a common target of some of these risk factors.

Table 2.4 Conditions leading to lesions of heterogeneous liver perfusion

Collagen vascular diseases
Rheumatoid arthritis
Scleroderma
Systemic lupus erythematosus
Polyarteritis nodosa
Glomerulonephritis
Hematological diseases
Polycythemia vera
Essential thrombocythemia
Agnogenic myeloid metaplasia
Chronic myeloid leukemia
Hodgkin's disease
Non-Hodgkin's lymphoma
Multiple myeloma
Primary hypogammaglobulinemia
Immunological disorders
Cryoglobulinemia
Antiphospholipid syndrome
Myasthenia gravis
HIV/AIDS
Drugs and toxins
Anabolic steroids
Azathioprine
Myeloablative conditioning regimens
Oral contraceptives
Oxaliplatin
Thoratrast
Toxic oil syndrome
6-Thioguanine

The common clinical syndrome manifested by these lesions is noncirrhotic portal hypertension. The presentation can vary from asymptomatic disease diagnosed only at autopsy to decompensated liver disease. Symptomatic patients may present with variceal bleeding or splenomegaly. Liver test abnormalities may include changes in prothrombin time, alkaline phosphatase, bilirubin, AST, and ALT [105]. Two large autopsy series found a prevalence of diffuse nodular regenerative hyperplasia of around 2.5% [106, 107]. Given that diffuse nodular regenerative hyperplasia is a relatively uncommon clinical diagnosis, this demonstrates that most cases of diffuse nodular regenerative hyperplasia are

Table 2.5 Lesions due to heterogeneous liver perfusion [105]

Liver lesions	Histology
Diffuse nodular regenerative hyperplasia	Monoacinar nodules consisting of hyperplastic hepatocytes diffusely distributed throughout the liver without a surrounding fibrous septum
Partial nodular transformation	Multiple nodules consisting of hyperplastic hepatocytes, several centimeters in diameter, involving several portal tracts, located in perihilar region
Incomplete septal cirrhosis	Large, diffusely distributed nodules, surrounded by incomplete slender fibrotic septa; septa extend from periportal or perivenular fibrosis; abnormal spacing between portal tracts and between portal tracts and central veins
Idiopathic noncirrhotic intrahepatic portal hypertension	No nodules; portal tracts are fibrotic, thin fibrotic septa may be present, when present, bridging fibrosis is subcapsular; sinusoidal dilatation is common

asymptomatic. Morphology of lesions attributed to heterogeneous perfusion of the liver is described in Table 2.5.

The liver lesions require no therapy, but the predisposing factor may require treatment. Portal hypertension is treated with the conventional approaches. A requirement for liver transplantation has been reported, but is rare.

Peliosis Hepatis

In peliosis hepatis, blood-filled cystic lesions are distributed irregularly throughout the hepatic parenchyma. The peliotic cavities range in size from less than 1 mm to several centimeters. Peliosis is most common in the liver, but also occurs in the spleen, abdominal lymph nodes, and bone marrow.

Table 2.6 lists the hematological disorders, drugs and toxins, and immunological and infectious diseases that predispose to peliosis. Historically, peliosis hepatis was found at autopsy in patients with chronic wasting illnesses, in particular tuberculosis and cancer. In patients with acquired immunodeficiency syndrome (AIDS), infection with *Bartonella henselae* or *Bartonella quintana* may cause peliosis as well as bacillary angiomatosis. One might therefore speculate that, analogous to AIDS, *Bartonella* sp. may play a role in some of the other predisposing factors with associated immunosuppression, such as tuberculosis, cancer, malnutrition, and glucocorticoid therapy.

The initial histological change in peliosis is sinusoidal dilatation and this progresses to formation of cavities without sinusoidal endothelial cells [112, 113]. Later in the course of the disease, the peliotic cavities may reendothelialize. Peliosis due to *Bartonella* species most clearly demonstrates that the lesion is initiated by damage to LSEC. Electron microscopy studies demonstrate the presence of *Bartonella* bacilli in LSEC of peliotic lesions [114] and disruption of the LSEC lining [112]. As described in the section on lesions of heterogeneous liver perfusion, several of the drugs listed in Table 2.6 have also been linked to the other disorders that target LSEC (see Tables 2.3 and 2.4). More strikingly, there are case reports of patients treated with azathioprine who were found to have all three lesions, SOS, diffuse nodular regenerative hyperplasia,

Table 2.6 Conditions associated with peliosis hepatis

Hematological diseases
Myeloproliferative diseases
Lymphoma
Macroglobulinemia
Multiple myeloma
Leukemia
Drugs and toxins
Anabolic steroids
Arsenic
Azathioprine
Oral contraceptives
Oxaliplatin
6-Thioguanine
Thoratrast
Vinyl chloride
Immunological/infectious disorders
AIDS/bartonella infection
Tuberculosis

and peliosis, in their liver. Other predisposing factors listed in Table 2.6 cause peliosis through an as yet undefined mechanism.

Peliosis hepatis is usually asymptomatic, but patients may present with portal hypertension, ascites, cholestasis, or liver failure. Rupture of a peliotic cavity may lead to a hepatic hematoma or an intraperitoneal hemorrhage that may rapidly progress to shock and death. Peliosis may regress if the precipitating cause is withdrawn or resolves.

Conclusions

LSEC have a number of important functions and may be the initiating target of a number of vascular liver diseases. The difficulty in isolating these cells has limited the number of laboratories that have studied LSEC. As more investigators turn their attention to this fascinating cell, we are likely to uncover pathology related to their dysfunction in chronic liver disease and aging and to discover more diseases in which LSEC injury places a role.

References

1. Wisse E. An electron microscopic study of the fenestrated endothelial lining of rat liver sinusoids. J Ultrastruct Res. 1970;31:125–50.
2. Wisse E. An ultrastructural characterization of the endothelial cell in the rat liver sinusoid under normal and various experimental conditions, as a contribution to the distinction between endothelial and Kupffer cells. J Ultrastruct Res. 1972;38:528–62.
3. Knook DL, Blansjaar N, Sleyster EC. Isolation and characterization of Kupffer and endothelial cells from the rat liver. Exp Cell Res. 1977;109:317–29.
4. Knook DL, Sleyster EC. Separation of the Kupffer and endothelial cells of the rat liver by centrifugal elutriation. Exp Cell Res. 1976;99:444–9.
5. Eriksson S, Fraser JRE, Laurent TC, Pertoft H, Smedsrød B. Endothelial cells are a site of uptake and degradation of hyaluronic acid in the liver. Exp Cell Res. 1983;144:223–8.
6. Vaporciyan AA, DeLisser HM, Yan HC, Mendiguren II, Thorn SR, Jones ML, et al. Involvement of platelet-endothelial cell adhesion molecule-1 in neutrophil recruitment in vivo. Science. 1993;262:1580–2.
7. DeLeve LD, Wang X, Hu L, McCuskey MK, McCuskey RS. Rat liver sinusoidal endothelial cell phenotype is under paracrine and autocrine control. Am J Physiol Gastrointest Liver Physiol. 2004;287: G757–63.
8. Harb R, Xie G, Lutzko C, Guo Y, Wang X, Hill C, et al. Bone marrow progenitor cells repair rat hepatic sinusoidal endothelial cells after liver injury. Gastroenterology. 2009;137:704–12.
9. Scoazec JY, Feldmann G. In situ immunophenotyping study of endothelial cells of the human hepatic sinusoid: results and functional implications. Hepatology. 1991;14:789–97.
10. McCourt PA, Smedsrod BH, Melkko J, Johansson S. Characterization of a hyaluronan receptor on rat sinusoidal liver endothelial cells and its functional relationship to scavenger receptors. Hepatology. 1999;30: 1276–86.
11. Hansen B, Longati P, Elvevold K, Nedredal GI, Schledzewski K, Olsen R, et al. Stabilin-1 and stabilin-2 are both directed into the early endocytic pathway in hepatic sinusoidal endothelium via interactions with clathrin/AP-2, independent of ligand binding. Exp Cell Res. 2005;303:160–73.
12. Politz O, Gratchev A, McCourt PAG, Schledzewski K, Guillot P, Johansson S, et al. Stabilin-1 and -2 constitute a novel family of fasciclin-like hyaluronan receptor homologues. Biochem J. 2002;362:155–64.
13. Couvelard A, Scoazec JY, Feldmann G. Expression of cell-cell and cell-matrix adhesion proteins by sinusoidal endothelial cells in the normal and cirrhotic human liver. Am J Pathol. 1993;143:738–52.
14. Weiss L, Chen LT. A scanning electron microscopic study of the spleen. Blood. 1974;43:665–91.
15. Blue J, Weiss L. Electron microscopy of the red pulp of the dog spleen including vascular arrangements, peri-arterial macrophage sheaths, ellipsoids, and the contractive reticular meshwork. Am J Anat. 1981; 161:189–218.
16. Blue J, Weiss L. Vascular pathways in nonsinusal red pulp: an electron microscopic study of the cat spleen. Am J Anat. 1981;161:135–68.
17. De Bruyn PP, Michelson S. Changes in the random distribution of sialic acid at the surface of the myeloid sinusoidal endothelium resulting from the presence of diaphragmed fenestrae. J Cell Biol. 1979;82: 708–14.
18. Inoue S, Osmond DG. Basement membrane of mouse bone marrow sinusoids shows distinctive structure and proteoglycan composition: a high resolution ultrastructural study. Anat Rec. 2001;264:294–304.
19. Risau W. Development and differentiation of endothelium. Kidney Int Suppl. 1998;54:S3–6.
20. Yamane A, Seetharam L, Yamaguchi S, Gotoh N, Takahashi T, Neufeld G, et al. A new communication system between hepatocytes and sinusoidal endothelial cells in liver through vascular endothelial growth factor and Flt tyrosine kinase receptor family (Flt-1 and KDR/Flk-1). Oncogene. 1994;9:2683–90.
21. Schaffner F, Popper H. Capillarization of hepatic sinusoids in man. Gastroenterology. 1963;44:239–42.
22. DeLeve LD, Wang X, Kanel GC, Atkinson RD, McCuskey RS. Prevention of hepatic fibrosis in a murine model of metabolic syndrome with non-alcoholic steatohepatitis. Am J Pathol. 2008;173:993–1001.

23. Dubuisson L, Boussarie L, Bedin C-A, Balabud C, Bioulac-Sage P. Transformation of sinusoids into capillaries in a rat model of selenium-induced nodular regenerative hyperplasia: an immunolight and immunoelectron microscopic study. Hepatology. 1995;21:805–14.
24. Horn T, Christoffersen P, Henriksen JH. Alcoholic liver injury: defenestration in noncirrhotic livers-a scanning electron microscopic study. Hepatology. 1987;7:77–82.
25. Horn T, Junge J, Christoffersen P. Early alcoholic liver injury: changes of the Disse space in acinar zone 3. Liver. 1985;5:301–10.
26. Urashima S, Tsutsumi M, Nakase K, Wang JS, Takada A. Studies on capillarization of the hepatic sinusoids in alcoholic liver disease. Alcohol Alcohol. 1993;S1B: 77–84.
27. Xu B, Broome U, Uzunel M, Nava S, Ge X, Kumagai-Braesch M, et al. Capillarization of hepatic sinusoid by liver endothelial cell-reactive autoantibodies in patients with cirrhosis and chronic hepatitis. Am J Pathol. 2003;163:1275–89.
28. Froomes PRA, Morgan DJ, Smallwood RA, Angus PW. Comparative effects of oxygen supplementation on theophylline and acetaminophen clearance in human cirrhosis. Gastroenterology. 1999;116:915–20.
29. Hickey PL, Angus PW, McLean AJ, Morgan DJ. Oxygen supplementation restores theophylline clearance to normal in cirrhotic rats. Gastroenterology. 1995;108:1504–9.
30. Le Couteur DG, Hickey H, Harvey PJ, Gready J, McLean AJ. Hepatic artery flow and propranolol metabolism in perfused cirrhotic rat liver. J Pharmacol Exp Ther. 1999;289:1553–8.
31. Le Couteur DG, Cogger VC, Markus AM, Harvey PJ, Yin ZL, Annselin AD, et al. Pseudocapillarization and associated energy limitation in the aged rat liver. Hepatology. 2001;33:537–43.
32. Fraser R, Bosanquet AG, Day WA. Filtration of chylomicrons by the liver may influence cholesterol metabolism and atherosclerosis. Atherosclerosis. 1978;29:113–23.
33. Redgrave TG. Formation of cholesteryl ester-rich particulate lipid during metabolism of chylomicrons. J Clin Investig. 1970;49:465–71.
34. Proctor SD, Mamo JC. Retention of fluorescent-labelled chylomicron remnants within the intima of the arterial wall – evidence that plaque cholesterol may be derived from post-prandial lipoproteins.[see comment]. Eur J Clin Investig. 1998;28:497–503.
35. Botham KM, Wheeler-Jones CPD. Introduction to the Biochemical Society Focused Meeting on Diet and Cardiovascular Health: chylomicron remnants and their emerging roles in vascular dysfunction in atherosclerosis. Biochem Soc Trans. 2007;35:437–9.
36. Cogger VC, Warren A, Fraser R, Ngu M, McLean AJ, Le Couteur DG. Hepatic sinusoidal pseudocapillarization with aging in the non-human primate. Exp Gerontol. 2003;38:1101–7.
37. McLean AJ, Cogger VC, Chong GC, Warren A, Markus AM, Dahlstrom JE, et al. Age-related pseudocapillarization of the human liver. J Pathol. 2003;200: 112–7.
38. Warren A, Bertolino P, Cogger VC, McLean AJ, Fraser R, Le Couteur DG. Hepatic pseudocapillarization in aged mice. Exp Gerontol. 2005;40:807–12.
39. Smedsrød B, Pertoft H, Gustafson S, Laurent TC. Scavenger functions of the liver endothelial cell. Biochem J. 1990;266:313–27.
40. Knook DL, Sleyster EC. Isolated parenchymal, Kupffer and endothelial rat liver cells characterized by their lysosomal enzyme content. Biochem Biophys Res Commun. 1980;96:250–7.
41. Malovic I, Sorensen KK, Elvevold KH, Nedredal GI, Paulsen S, Erofeev AV, et al. The mannose receptor on murine liver sinusoidal endothelial cells is the main denatured collagen clearance receptor. Hepatology. 2007;45:1454–61.
42. Martens JH, Kzhyshkowska J, Falkowski-Hansen M, Schledzewski K, Gratchev A, Mansmann U, et al. Differential expression of a gene signature for scavenger/lectin receptors by endothelial cells and macrophages in human lymph node sinuses, the primary sites of regional metastasis. J Pathol. 2006;208:574–89.
43. Blomhoff R, Drevon CA, Eskild W, Helgerud P, Norum KR, Berg T. Clearance of acetyl low density lipoprotein by rat liver endothelial cells. Implications for hepatic cholesterol metabolism. J Biol Chem. 1984;259:8898–903.
44. Nagelkerke JF, Barto KP, van Berkel TJ. In vivo and in vitro uptake and degradation of acetylated low density lipoprotein by rat liver endothelial, Kupffer, and parenchymal cells. J Biol Chem. 1983;258:12221–7.
45. Van Berkel TJ, De Rijke YB, Kruijt JK. Different fate in vivo of oxidatively modified low density lipoprotein and acetylated low density lipoprotein in rats. Recognition by various scavenger receptors on Kupffer and endothelial liver cells. J Biol Chem. 1991;266:2282–9.
46. Smedsrød B, Melkko J, Araki N, Sano H, Horiuchi S. Advanced glycation end products are eliminated by scavenger-receptor-mediated endocytosis in hepatic sinusoidal Kupffer and endothelial cells. Biochem J. 1997;322:567–73.
47. Mousavi SA, Sporstøl M, Fladeby C, Kjeken R, Barois N, Berg T. Receptor-mediated endocytosis of immune complexes in rat liver sinusoidal endothelial cells is mediated by Fc?RIIb2. Hepatology. 2007;46:871–84.
48. March S, Hui EE, Underhill GH, Khetani S, Bhatia SN. Microenvironmental regulation of the sinusoidal endothelial cell phenotype in vitro. Hepatology. 2009;50:920–8.
49. Ito Y, Sørensen KK, Bethea NW, Svistounov D, McCuskey MK, Smedsrød BH, et al. Age-related changes in the hepatic microcirculation in mice. Exp Gerontol. 2007;42:789–97.
50. Tamaki S, Ueno T, Torimura T, Sata M, Tanikawa K. Evaluation of hyaluronic acid binding ability of hepatic sinusoidal endothelial cells in rats with liver cirrhosis. Gastroenterology. 1996;111:1049–57.

51. DeLeve LD, Wang X, Guo Y. Sinusoidal endothelial cells prevent rat stellate cell activation and promote reversion to quiescence. Hepatology. 2008;48:920–30.
52. Xie G, Kanel GC, DeLeve LD. cGMP Signaling Regulates Liver Sinusoidal Endothelial Cell (SEC) Phenotype and Accelerates Reversal of Cirrhosis. Gastroenterology. 2010 (abstract);138.
53. Knolle PA, Schmitt E, Jin S, Germann T, Duchmann R, Hegenbarth S, et al. Induction of cytokine production in naive CD4+ T cells by antigen-presenting murine liver sinusoidal endothelial cells but failure to induce differentiation toward Th1 cells. Gastroenterology. 1999;116:1428–40.
54. Knolle PA, Gerken G. Local control of the immune response in the liver. Immunol Rev. 2000;174:21–34.
55. Limmer A, Ohl J, Kurts C, Ljunggren HG, Reiss Y, Groettrup M, et al. Efficient presentation of exogenous antigen by liver endothelial cells to CD8+ T cells results in antigen-specific T-cell tolerance. Nat Med. 2000;6:1348–54.
56. Klugewitz K, Blumenthal-Barby F, Schrage A, Knolle PA, Hamann A, Crispe IN. Immunomodulatory effects of the liver: deletion of activated CD4+ effector cells and suppression of IFN-gamma-producing cells after intravenous protein immunization. J Immunol. 2002;169:2407–13.
57. Uhrig A, Banafsche R, Kremer M, Hegenbarth S, Hamann A, Neurath M, et al. Development and functional consequences of LPS tolerance in sinusoidal endothelial cells of the liver.[Erratum appears in J Leukoc Biol. 2005 Jul;78(1):5A]. J Leukoc Biol. 2005;77:626–33.
58. Diehl L, Schurich A, Grochtmann R, Hegenbarth S, Chen L, Knolle PA. Tolerogenic maturation of liver sinusoidal endothelial cells promotes B7-homolog 1-dependent CD8+ T cell tolerance. Hepatology. 2008;47:296–305.
59. Schildberg FA, Hegenbarth SI, Schumak B, Limmer A, Knolle PA. Liver sinusoidal endothelial cells veto CD8 T cell activation by antigen-presenting dendritic cells. Eur J Immunol. 2008;38:957–67.
60. Onoe T, Ohdan H, Tokita D, Shishida M, Tanaka Y, Hara H, et al. Liver sinusoidal endothelial cells tolerize T cells across MHC barriers in mice. J Immunol. 2005;175:139–46.
61. Knolle PA, Limmer A. Neighborhood politics: the immunoregulatory function of organ-resident liver endothelial cells. Trends Immunol. 2001;22:432–7.
62. Steinberg P, Lafranconi WM, Wolf CR, Waxman DJ, Oesch F, Friedberg T. Xenobiotic metabolizing enzymes are not restricted to parenchymal cells in rat liver. Mol Pharmacol. 1987;32:463–70.
63. Steinberg P, Schramm H, Schladt L, Robertson LW, Thomas H, Oesch F. The distribution, induction and isoenzyme profile of glutathione S-transferase and glutathione peroxidase in isolated rat liver parenchymal, Kupffer and endothelial cells. Biochem J. 1989;264:737–44.
64. DeLeve LD. Dacarbazine toxicity in murine liver cells: a novel model of hepatic endothelial injury and glutathione defense. J Pharmacol Exp Ther. 1994;268:1261–70.
65. DeLeve LD, Wang X, Kaplowitz N, Shulman HM, Bart JA, van der Hoek A. Sinusoidal endothelial cells as a target for acetaminophen toxicity: direct action versus requirement for hepatocyte activation in different mouse strains. Biochem Pharmacol. 1997;53:1339–45.
66. DeLeve LD, Wang X, Kuhlenkamp JF, Kaplowitz N. Toxicity of azathioprine and monocrotaline in murine sinusoidal endothelial cells and hepatocytes: the role of glutathione and relevance to hepatic venoocclusive disease. Hepatology. 1996;23:589–99.
67. DeLeve LD. Glutathione defense in non-parenchymal cells. Semin Liver Dis. 1998;18:403–13.
68. Shulman HM, Fisher LB, Schoch HG, Henne KW, McDonald GB. Venoocclusive disease of the liver after marrow transplantation: histological correlates of clinical signs and symptoms. Hepatology. 1994;19:1171–80.
69. DeLeve LD, Shulman HM, McDonald GB. Toxic injury to hepatic sinusoids: sinusoidal obstruction syndrome (veno-occlusive disease). Semin Liver Dis. 2002;22:27–42.
70. Willmot FC, Robertson GW. Senecio disease, or cirrhosis of the liver due to senecio poisoning. Lancet. 1920;2:848–9.
71. McFarlane AL, Branday W. Hepatic enlargement with ascitic children. Br Med J. 1945;1:838–40.
72. Selzer G, Parker RGF. Senecio poisoning exhibiting as Chiari's syndrome: a report on twelve cases. Am J Pathol. 1950;27:885–907.
73. DeLeve LD. Cellular target of cyclophosphamide toxicity in the murine liver: role of glutathione and site of metabolic activation. Hepatology. 1996;24:830–7.
74. DeLeve LD, McCuskey RS, Wang X, Hu L, McCuskey MK, Epstein RB, et al. Characterization of a reproducible rat model of hepatic veno-occlusive disease. Hepatology. 1999;29:1779–91.
75. Lamé MW, Jones AD, Wilson DW, Dunston SK, Segall HJ. Protein targets of monocrotaline pyrrole in pulmonary artery endothelial cells. J Biol Chem. 2000;275:29091–9.
76. DeLeve LD, Wang X, Tsai J, Kanel GC, Strasberg SM, Tokes ZA. Prevention of sinusoidal obstruction syndrome (hepatic venoocclusive disease) in the rat by matrix metalloproteinase inhibitors. Gastroenterology. 2003;125:882–90.
77. DeLeve LD, Ito I, Bethea NW, McCuskey MK, Wang X, McCuskey RS. Embolization by sinusoidal lining cell obstructs the microcirculation in rat sinusoidal obstruction syndrome. Am J Physiol Gastrointest Liver Physiol. 2003;284:G1045–52.
78. DeLeve LD, Wang X, Kanel GC, Tokes ZA, Tsai J, Ito Y, et al. Decreased hepatic nitric oxide production contributes to the development of rat sinusoidal obstruction syndrome. Hepatology. 2003;38:900–8.
79. Eberhardt W, Beeg T, Beck KF, Walpen S, Gauer S, Bohles H, et al. Nitric oxide modulates expression of

matrix metalloproteinase-9 in rat mesangial cells. Kidney Int. 2000;57:59–69.
80. Gurjar MV, DeLeon J, Sharma RV, Bhalla RC. Mechanism of inhibition of matrix metalloproteinase-9 induction by NO in vascular smooth muscle cells. J Appl Physiol. 2001;91:1380–6.
81. Upchurch Jr GR, Ford JW, Weiss SJ, Knipp BS, Peterson DA, Thompson RW, et al. Nitric oxide inhibition increases matrix metalloproteinase-9 expression by rat aortic smooth muscle cells in vitro. J Vasc Surg. 2001;34:76–83.
82. Upadhya GA, Strasberg SM. Glutathione, lactobionate, and histidine: cryptic inhibitors of matrix metalloproteinases contained in University of Wisconsin and histidine/tryptophan/ketoglutarate liver preservation solutions. Hepatology. 2000;31:1115–22.
83. McDonald GB. Review article: management of hepatic disease following haematopoietic cell transplant. Aliment Pharmacol Ther. 2006;24:441–52.
84. McKoy JM, Angelotta C, Bennett CL, Tallman MS, Wadleigh M, Evens AM, et al. Gemtuzumab ozogamicin-associated sinusoidal obstructive syndrome (SOS): an overview from the research on adverse drug events and reports (RADAR) project. Leuk Res. 2007;31:599–604.
85. Rajvanshi P, Shulman HM, Sievers EL, McDonald GB. Hepatic sinusoidal obstruction following Gemtuzumab Ozogamicin (Mylotarg®). Blood. 2002;99:2310–4.
86. Wadleigh M, Richardson PG, Zahrieh D, Lee SJ, Cutler C, Ho V, et al. Prior gemtuzumab ozogamicin exposure significantly increases the risk of veno-occlusive disease in patients who undergo myeloablative allogeneic stem cell transplantation. Blood. 2003;102:1578–82.
87. Czauderna P, Katski K, Kowalczyk J, Kurylak A, Lopatka B, Skotnicka-Klonowicz G, et al. Venoocclusive liver disease (VOD) as a complication of Wilms' tumour management in the series of consecutive 206 patients. Eur J Pediatr Surg. 2000; 10:300–3.
88. Tornesello A, Piciacchia D, Mastrangelo S, Lasorella A, Mastrangelo R. Veno-occlusive disease of the liver in right-sided Wilms' tumours. Eur J Cancer. 1998;34:1220–3.
89. Jagt CT, Zuckermann M, Ten Kate F, Taminiau JAJM, Dijkgraaf MGW, Heij H, et al. Veno-occlusive disease as a complication of preoperative chemotherapy for Wilms tumor: a clinico-pathological analysis. Pediatr Blood Cancer. 2009;53:1211–5.
90. Bearman SI. The syndrome of hepatic veno-occlusive disease after marrow transplantation. Blood. 1995;85:3005–20.
91. Bornhauser M, Storer B, Slattery JT, Appelbaum FR, Deeg HJ, Hansen J, et al. Conditioning with fludarabine and targeted busulfan for transplantation of allogeneic hematopoietic stem cells. Blood. 2003; 102:820–6.
92. de Lima M, Couriel D, Thall PF, Wang X, Madden T, Jones R, et al. Once-daily intravenous busulfan and fludarabine: clinical and pharmacokinetic results of a myeloablative, reduced-toxicity conditioning regimen for allogeneic stem cell transplantation in AML and MDS. Blood. 2004;104:857–64.
93. Hogan WJ, Maris M, Storer B, Sandmaier BM, Maloney DG, Schoch HG, et al. Hepatic injury after nonmyeloablative conditioning followed by allogeneic hematopoietic cell transplantation: a study of 193 patients. Blood. 2004;103:78–84.
94. McCune JS, Batchelder A, Guthrie KA, Witherspoon R, Appelbaum FR, Phillips B, et al. Personalized dosing of cyclophosphamide in the total body irradiation-cyclophosphamide conditioning regimen: a phase II trial in patients with hematologic malignancy. Clin Pharmacol Ther. 2009;85:615–22.
95. McDonald GB, McCune JS, Batchelder A, Cole SL, Phillips B, Ren AG, et al. Metabolism-based cyclophosphamide dosing for hematopoietic cell transplant. Clin Pharmacol Ther. 2005;78:298–308.
96. Méresse V, Hartmann O, Vassal G, Benhamou E, Valteau-Couanet D, Brugieres L, et al. Risk factors for hepatic veno-occlusive disease after high-dose busulfan-containing regimens followed by autologous bone marrow transplantation: a study in 136 children. Bone Marrow Transplant. 1992;10:135–41.
97. Chevallier P, Prebet T, Turlure P, Hunault M, Vigouroux S, Harousseau JL, et al. Prior treatment with gemtuzumab ozogamicin and the risk of veno-occlusive disease after allogeneic haematopoietic stem cell transplantation. Bone Marrow Transplant. 2010;45:165–70.
98. Satti MB, Weinbren K, Gordon-Smith EC. 6-thioguanine as a cause of toxic veno-occlusive disease of the liver. J Clin Pathol. 1982;35:1086–91.
99. Kao NL, Rosenblate HJ. 6-Thioguanine therapy for psoriasis causing toxic hepatic venoocclusive disease. J Am Acad Dermatol. 1993;28:1017–8.
100. Dubinsky MC, Vasiliauskas EA, Singh H, Abreu MT, Papadakis KA, Tran T, et al. 6-thioguanine can cause serious liver injury in inflammatory bowel disease patients. Gastroenterology. 2003;125:298–303.
101. Ingold JA, Reed Jr GB, Kaplan HS, Bagshaw MA. Radiation hepatitis. Am J Roentgenol. 1965;93:200–8.
102. Fajardo LF, Colby TV. Pathogenesis of veno-occlusive liver disease after radiation. Arch Pathol Lab Med. 1980;104:584–8.
103. Lawrence TS, Robertson JM, Anscher MS, Jirtle RL, Ensminger WD, Fajardo LF. Hepatic toxicity resulting from cancer treatment. Int J Radiat Oncol Biol Phys. 1995;31:1237–48.
104. Hillaire S, Bonte E, Denninger MH, Casadevall N, Cadranel JF, Lebrec D, et al. Idiopathic non-cirrhotic intrahepatic portal hypertension in the West: a re-evaluation in 28 patients. Gut. 2002;51:275–80.
105. Ibarrola C, Colina F. Clinicopathological features of nine cases of non-cirrhotic portal hypertension: current definitions and criteria are inadequate. Histopathology. 2003;42:251–64.
106. Nakanuma Y, Hoso M, Sasaki M, Terada T, Katayanagi K, Nonomura A, et al. Histopathology of the liver in

non-cirrhotic portal hypertension of unknown aetiology. Histopathology. 1996;28:195–204.
107. Wanless IR. Micronodular transformation (nodular regenerative hyperplasia) of the liver: a report of 64 cases among 2, 500 autopsies and a new classification of benign hepatocellular nodules. Hepatology. 1990;11:787–97.
108. Shimamatsu K, Wanless IR. Role of ischemia in causing apoptosis, atrophy, and nodular hyperplasia in human liver. Hepatology. 1997;26:343–50.
109. Croquelois A, Blindenbacher A, Terracciano L, Wang X, Langer I, Radtke F, et al. Inducible inactivation of <I>Notch1</I> causes nodular regenerative hyperplasia in mice. Hepatology. 2005; 41:487–96.
110. Nakanuma Y, Ohta G, Sasaki K. Nodular regenerative hyperplasia of the liver associated with polyarteritis nodosa. Arch Pathol Lab Med. 1984;108:133–5.
111. Young ID, Segura J, Ford PM, Ford SE. The pathogenesis of nodular regenerative hyperplasia of the liver associated with rheumatoid vasculitis. J Clin Gastroenterol. 1992;14:127–31.
112. Scoazec JY, Marche C, Girard PM, Houtmann J, Durand-Schneider AM, Saimot AG, et al. Peliosis hepatis and sinusoidal dilation during infection by the human immunodeficiency virus (HIV). An ultrastructural study. Am J Pathol. 1988;131:38–47.
113. Goerdt S, Sorg C. Endothelial heterogeneity and the acquired immunodeficiency syndrome: a paradigm for the pathogenesis of vascular disorders. Clin Investig. 1992;70:89–98.
114. Leong SS, Cazen RA, Yu GS, LeFevre L, Carson JW. Abdominal visceral peliosis associated with bacillary angiomatosis. Ultrastructural evidence of endothelial destruction by bacilli. Arch Pathol Lab Med. 1992;116:866–71.

Pseudocapillarization and the Aging Liver

3

Dmitri Svistounov, Svetlana N. Zykova, Victoria C. Cogger, Alessandra Warren, Robin Fraser, Bård Smedsrød, Robert S. McCuskey, and David G. Le Couteur

Abstract

Old age is associated with changes in the cells of the hepatic sinusoid. The liver sinusoidal endothelial cell undergoes pseudocapillarization characterized by defenestration, thickening, and altered expression of endothelial and extracellular matrix antigens. Pseudocapillarization contributes to age-related dyslipidemia and reduction in hepatic perfusion and might also have a role in age-related changes in drug metabolism and susceptibility to autoimmune disease. Old age is also associated with impaired endocytosis activity by liver endothelial cells. With respect to the other cells of the hepatic sinusoid and aging, there are increased numbers of activated Kupffer cells but they respond less well to stimuli. Stellate cells become engorged with fat and do not appear to be activated. Such aging changes in the cells of the hepatic sinusoid are likely to impact on overall hepatic function.

Keywords

Aging • Endocytosis • Fenestrae • Kupffer cell • Liver sinusoidal endothelial cell • Pseudocapillarization • Stellate cell

The Structure of the Hepatic Sinusoid

The hepatic sinusoids are small blood vessels, comparable to capillaries that perfuse the hepatocytes. However, unlike the capillaries in other tissues, sinusoids are formed by discontinuous endothelium that lacks any significant underlying basement membrane. The liver sinusoidal endothelial cell (LSEC) is perforated by cytoplasmic holes called fenestrae, which do not have any intervening diaphragmatic membrane and thus are fully patent holes through the cell. This specialized lace-like morphology of the LSEC minimizes any barrier to the bidirectional transfer of solutes and particulate substrates between the sinusoidal blood and hepatocytes, while retaining the capacity and substantial surface area to undergo interactions with circulating blood cells including immune cells [1–3].

In mature animals, sinusoidal microcirculatory systems are found only in the liver, lymph nodes, bone marrow, and spleen. Of these, the liver has the most extensive sinusoidal network and only LSECs have the combination of nondiaphragmed fenestrae and the lack of an organized basement membrane. During initial

D.G. Le Couteur (✉)
Centre for Education and Research on Ageing,
The University of Sydney and Concord R.G. Hospital,
Sydney, NSW, Australia
e-mail: david.lecouteur@sydney.edu.au

L.D. DeLeve and G. Garcia-Tsao (eds.), *Vascular Liver Disease: Mechanisms and Management*,
DOI 10.1007/978-1-4419-8327-5_3,

hepatogenesis, the hepatic sinusoids are lined by a continuous endothelium. The LSEC only becomes fenestrated by approximately 15 days of gestation in mice, 17 days of gestation in rats, and after the 12th week of gestation in humans. Of note, basement membrane has not been identified in liver sinusoids at any developmental stage until old age [4–7].

Sinusoids are formed by LSECs that are separated from liver parenchyma by perisinusoidal extravascular space, called the space of Disse (Fig. 3.1). There are three other cell types that reside in the liver sinusoids apart from the LSEC: Kupffer cells, stellate cells, and pit cells. The space of Disse is the extravascular space that lies between the hepatocytes and LSECs. It contains some components of extracellular matrix and most components of blood plasma filtered through LSECs sieve plates. Extracellular matrix in the space of Disse includes fibronectin and collagen type I, III, V, and VI. Collagen type IV is also present, but unlike typical basement membranes, it appears in the form of discontinuous aggregates [7]. Membrane projections from the sinusoidal surface of the hepatocytes protrude into the space of Disse and increase the available surface area for the transport and diffusion of substrates [1–3].

LSECs represent about 2.8% of total liver volume and 15–20% of all liver cells [8–10]. LSECs differ substantially both structurally and functionally from the endothelial cells of capillaries in other tissues. Cytoplasmic extensions of LSECs are thin and perforated with fenestrae, which are circular and oval pores approximately 50–200 nm in diameter (see Fig. 3.1). Fenestrae occur frequently over the surface of LSEC (3–20 fenestrae per μm² and between 2 and 20% of the surface of the LSEC is covered by fenestrae, the so-called

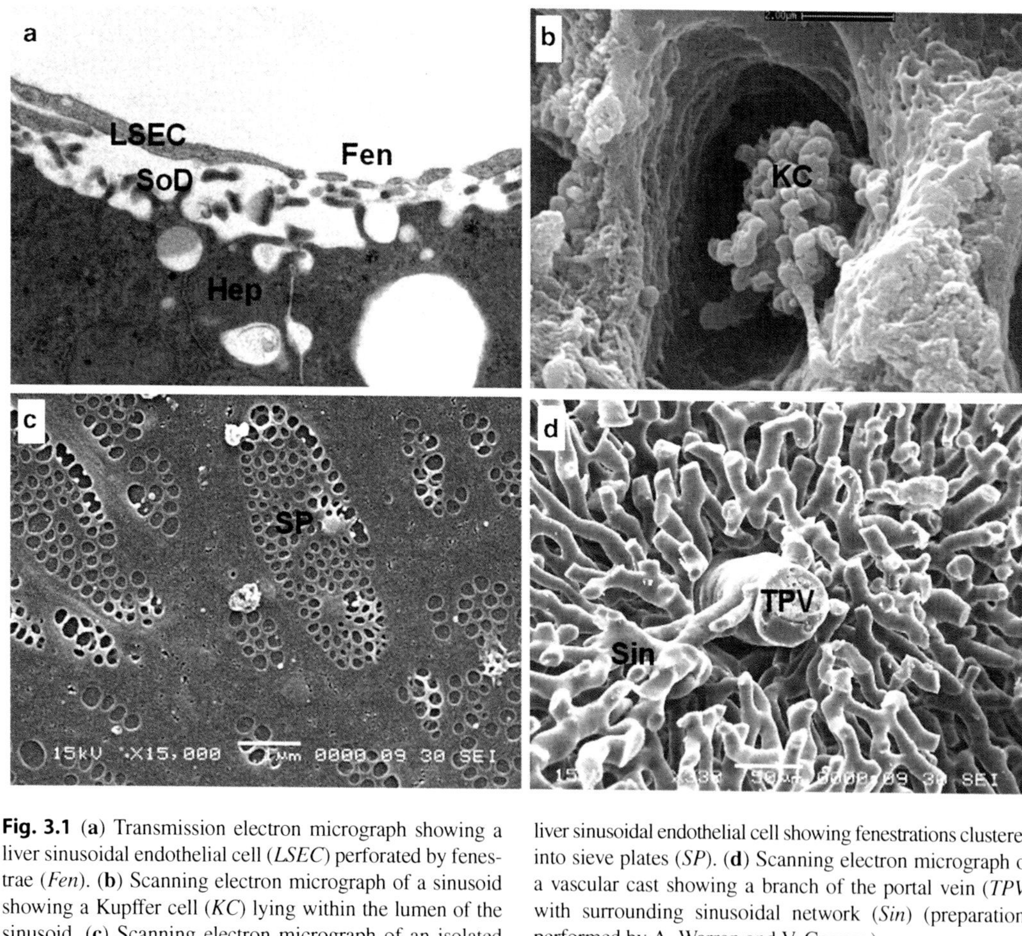

Fig. 3.1 (**a**) Transmission electron micrograph showing a liver sinusoidal endothelial cell (*LSEC*) perforated by fenestrae (*Fen*). (**b**) Scanning electron micrograph of a sinusoid showing a Kupffer cell (*KC*) lying within the lumen of the sinusoid. (**c**) Scanning electron micrograph of an isolated liver sinusoidal endothelial cell showing fenestrations clustered into sieve plates (*SP*). (**d**) Scanning electron micrograph of a vascular cast showing a branch of the portal vein (*TPV*) with surrounding sinusoidal network (*Sin*) (preparations performed by A. Warren and V. Cogger.)

"porosity") [2]. The diameter of fenestrae has a normal distribution but is skewed to the right by the presence of larger pores, sometimes called gaps [11, 12]. Dumbbell-shaped fenestra probably represents fusion of two adjacent fenestrae, while mesh-like structures similar to vesiculo-vacuolar organelles have also been reported [2, 13]. Fenestrae have been found in all species including such diverse species as man, rat, mouse, guinea pig, sheep, goat, rabbit, fowl, monkey, baboon, bat, kitten, dog, turtle, and gold fish [2]. They are sometimes found isolated on the LSEC surface, but more commonly fenestrae are clustered into groups of tens to hundreds called liver sieve plates. In fact, between 60 and 75% of fenestrae are found within sieve plates in rats [14]. In isolated LSECs, there are often many tens of sieve plates present in the cytoplasmic extension of a single cell, representing many hundreds or even thousands of fenestrae per cell [15, 16]. LSECs are rich in coated pits and vesicles and other organelles associated with endocytosis. Although the LSECs constitute only 2.8% of the total liver volume, they contain about 15% of the total lysosomal volume and about 45% of the pinocytic vesicle volume of the liver [10]. Moreover, specific activities of several lysosomal enzymes are higher in LSECs than in other liver cells [17]. LSECs express a set of high-affinity endocytic receptors for soluble macromolecular waste products, generated during normal tissue turnover, blood clotting, inflammatory processes, and pathological conditions [18–23]. Following receptor-mediated endocytosis in LSECs most of the ligands are rapidly degraded intralysosomally. Thus, LSECs represent a major site of scavenging and degradation of harmful waste macromolecules from the circulation.

Kupffer cells represent 20% of the population of liver sinusoidal cells and 80–90% of all fixed macrophages in the body (Fig. 3.1b) [24]. They generally reside within the lumen of the liver sinusoids and take up bacterial and other large particles such as cell debris from the circulation by phagocytosis. In response to bacterial infection, Kupffer cells produce cytokines and other soluble proinflammatory factors that promote influx and activation of neutrophils [4, 21]. Together, LSECs and Kupffer cells constitute the hepatic reticuloendothelial system (RES), the most powerful scavenger system of mammals and other terrestrial vertebrates. Stellate cells, or fat-storing cells, are located within the perisinusoidal space and represent the largest and most important storage of vitamin A in the body (Fig. 3.2). The cells

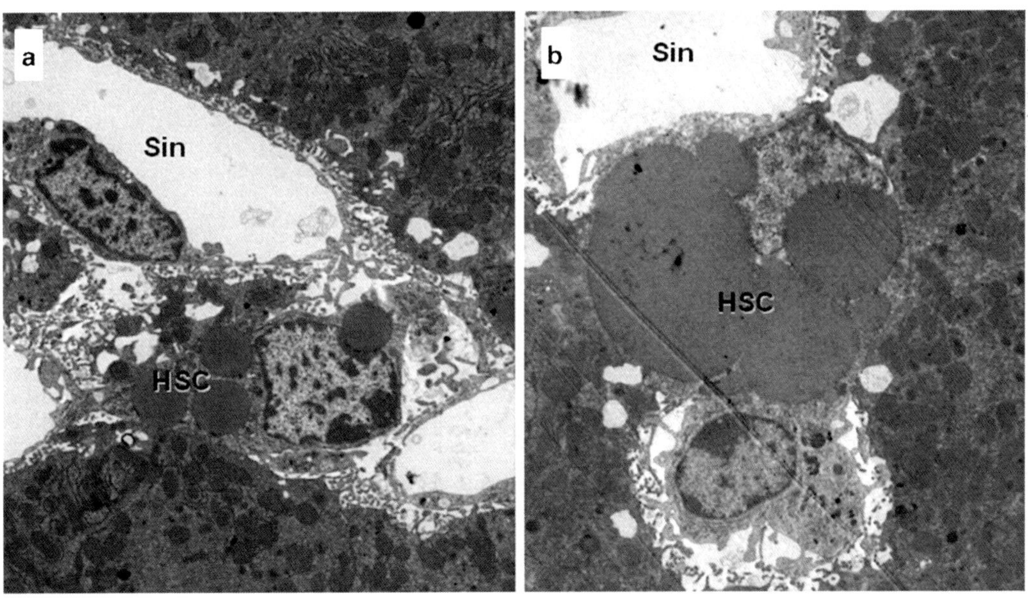

Fig. 3.2 Transmission electron micrographs of stellate cells from a young (**a**) and an old (**b**) mouse liver. The increased size and number of lipid droplets in the old stellate cells are apparent (*Sin*, sinusoid, *HSC* hepatic stellate cell) (preparations performed by A. Warren and V. Cogger.)

receive vitamin A from the neighboring hepatocytes. In response to liver injury or certain stimuli they acquire a myofibroblast-like phenotype, proliferate, and produce extracellular matrix components [25]. Pit cells represent less than 1% of the sinusoidal cells and are granular lymphocyte-like cells situated in the sinusoidal lumen that exhibit natural killer and neuroendocrine activities [26].

The Normal Function of the LSEC

The fenestrated endothelium is a filter and accordingly has been called "the liver sieve" [27, 28]. Fenestrae allow the transfer of a wide range of substrates including plasma and plasma molecules, plasma proteins including albumin, some lipoproteins, and colloidal particles [29]. Because the diameters of blood cells are greater than that of the sinusoids [12], it was hypothesized that fluid must be squeezed through the fenestrae as blood cells traverse the hepatic sinusoids. This process has been termed "endothelial massage." The fenestrated LSEC can be defined as an ultrafiltration system because it is a low-pressure system with pores approximately 100 nm in diameter. Specifically, the liver sieve can be described as a Loeb–Sourirajan ultrafiltration system, with the stellate cells providing the supporting layer and the LSECs providing the thin porous layer [30]. The transfer of fluid across an ultrafiltration system can be calculated using the Hagen Poiseuille equation for ultrafiltration where the flux of fluid is proportional to the number of pores and the radius of the pores to the power of four [30–32]. Therefore, small changes in the size of fenestrae can have profound effects on the size and number of substrates and macromolecules that can gain passage into the space of Disse. Indeed, manipulation of fenestration diameter might have a role in regulating the transfer of substrates in response to physiological changes such as feeding and fasting.

LSECs also have an extraordinary endocytic activity. Because of this activity, LSECs are often termed "scavenger endothelial cells" [33]. LSECs remove many of the macromolecular waste products from the systemic circulation and are the most active endocytic cells in the body [18, 22]. Connective tissue macromolecules including hyaluronan, chondroitin sulphate, collagen α-chain, PICP, PINP, and PIIINP are exclusively cleared from the blood circulation by mannose receptor-mediated or scavenger receptor-mediated endocytosis in LSECs [18, 22, 34]. Other substrates include oxidized and acetylated low-density lipoproteins (LDLs), advanced glycation end products, immune complexes, and microbial CpG motifs [20, 23, 35].

LSECs interact with circulating leukocytes and lymphocytes [36, 37]. LSECs have a possible role in antigen presentation [38] and are involved in the development of immunotolerance by inducing apoptosis in lymphocytes [39]. Fenestrae mediate interactions between circulating immune cells and hepatocytes in that naïve T cells make contact with hepatocytes through fenestrae in the LSEC (transendothelial hepatocyte lymphocyte interactions) [40].

Aging and the Liver

Although the liver is not typically considered to be a major target of senescence-related degeneration and morbidity like the brain or cardiovascular system, subtle ultrastructural changes in the liver vasculature that occur in midlife probably initiate a sequence of detrimental events leading to development of atherosclerosis and other age-related phenotypes [41].

Previously it has generally been considered that the liver does not undergo significant aging changes because of its large functional reserve, regenerative capacity, and dual blood supply [42]. Conversely, age-related changes in hepatic function are significant and influence systemic exposure to xenobiotics, endogenous substrates associated with disease and medications [43]. Thus such changes in the liver have implications for many diseases of aging and the aging process itself. One of the earliest descriptions of the aging liver was "brown atrophy," which is the reduction in liver mass associated with deposition of the aging pigment, lipofuscin [42]. The reduction in liver size as a fraction of body weight is usually in the order of 25–35% [44] and this is associated with fewer hepatocytes, probably secondary to an age-related increase in apoptosis. In addition, most studies show that total hepatic blood flow is reduced by about 30–50% [44]. Liver perfusion, which is the flow per mass of liver, is also reduced in old age but to a lesser extent than total blood flow. Recently it has been found that the reduction in hepatic perfusion is secondary to blocking of the hepatic sinusoids by increased numbers of leukocytes attached to the endothelium as a result of age-related up-regulation of ICAM1 [45]. The clearance of highly extracted substrates, including most medications, is dependent on blood flow, therefore the age-related reduction in hepatic blood flow has a dramatic effect on its overall function [44]. In addition, hepatocytes increase in size with aging and there are increased polyploid and binucleate cells [46].

In terms of gene expression, there is much less age-related change in gene expression in the liver compared with other tissues [47]. However, there does appear to be decreased expression of genes involved with xenobiotic metabolism, mitochondria, apoptosis, and cell cycle/nucleic acid metabolism, whereas there is increased expression of genes involved with inflammation. These are increased markers of oxidative stress and oxidative injury, while endogenous antioxidant systems such as superoxide dismutase, catalase, glutathione peroxidase, ascorbic acid, reduced glutathione tend to decrease with age. Old age is associated with reduced expression of many hepatic antioxidant enzymes and increased evidence of oxidative stress in most studies, but such results are variable and probably influenced by species, strain, and gender [41].

Aging and the Hepatic Sinusoid

Although most studies have shown that changes in the structure of the hepatocytes with old age are subtle, recent studies have focused on changes in the sinusoidal cells and these have generally revealed quite marked changes in their morphology and activity [48]. One of the first studies of aging and hepatic sinusoid was that of Hinton and Williams in 1968. They noted some perisinusoidal fibrosis detected with reticulin staining in the livers of aged mice [49]. A later study in 1990 found no major structural changes in isolated LSECs with old age [50].

It has now been reported that old age is associated with substantial ultrastructural changes in the LSEC and space of Disse from intact livers of the rat [51, 52], human [53], mouse [31, 45], and the nonhuman primate, *Papio hamadryas* (Fig. 3.3) [54]. The findings have now been replicated in three centers around the world [45, 51, 55]. These changes have been termed "pseudocapillarization" because the aging LSEC is similar to capillaries seen in other nonfenestrated vascular beds [51]. Unlike "capillarization" seen in the

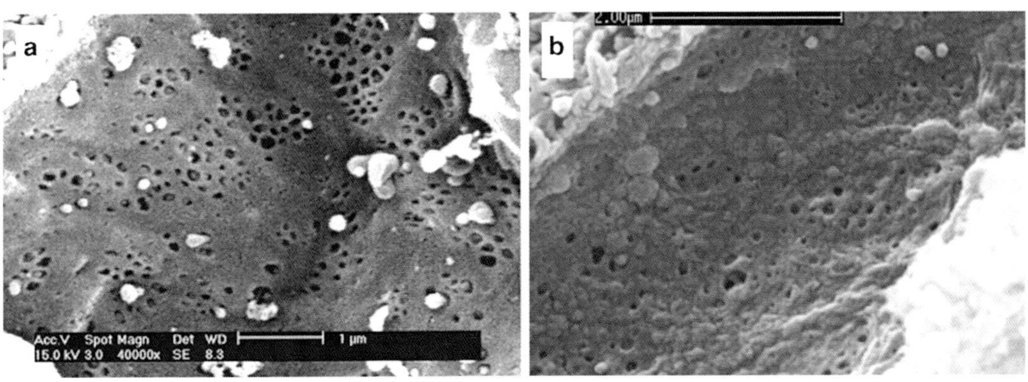

Fig. 3.3 Scanning electron micrographs of the liver sinusoid of a young (**a**) and an old (**b**) rat. The loss of fenestrae perforating the endothelial cell surface in the old liver is apparent (preparations performed by A. Warren and V. Cogger.)

hepatic sinusoid in cirrhosis, aging is not associated with cirrhosis-related changes on light microscopy such as bridging fibrosis and nodular regeneration [48, 51]. With old age, LSEC thickness is increased by approximately 50% and there is a similar reduction of about 50% in the porosity and number of fenestrae. These changes are associated with perisinusoidal basal lamina deposition in many old livers and some scattered collagen in the space of Disse. The effect of aging on the diameter of fenestrae has been inconsistent between species; however, there is a trend towards a reduction in the diameter of around 5–10% [48]. Isolated LSECs retain some of these ultrastructural changes. Fenestration diameter was reduced in old age from 194 ± 1 to 185 ± 1 nm in isolated rat LSECs and there was an age-related increase in the number of fused fenestrae and large gaps [13]. This suggests that this age-related change may be intrinsic to the LSEC and/or irreversible.

The electron microscopic changes are associated with altered expression of various markers used to study blood vessels. For example, the endothelial marker, von Willebrand's factor (vWf), is not normally expressed in healthy young liver sinusoids; yet most studies report that the perisinusoidal expression of vWf is increased in old age [48]. There is also reduced caveolin-1 expression [52] and increased ICAM-1 expression [45]. There is variable up-regulation of markers of extracellular matrix, mostly collagen IV and Sirius red (a general stain for collagen). These findings, together with the occasional observation of collagen in the space of Disse on electron microscopy, are consistent with the presence of at least some perisinusoidal fibrosis in old age. Although old age was associated with some deposition of lipofuscin and multinucleate cells in the hepatic parenchyma in these studies, there was no other indication of liver disease [31, 45, 51, 53, 54].

Although the dimensions of the sinusoids do not change significantly with old age in mice, there are some subtle changes in the architecture of the microcirculation. There was a slight reduction in the fractal dimension for the branching structure of the sinusoids and also a reduction in the degree of anisotropy. However, this was not sufficient to generate any change in the vascular dispersion number (a measure of substrate mixing within sinusoids) as determined by the multiple indicator dilution technique [56].

A reduction of caloric intake by about 40% increases maximum life expectancy by a similar amount associated with a delay in the onset of most age-associated disorders and pathology [57]. It has been found that caloric restriction also delays the onset of pseudocapillarization in rats. In old caloric-restricted rats, endothelial thickness was significantly less and fenestration porosity was significantly greater than in old *ad libitum* fed rats. Caloric restriction prevented the age-related decrease in caveolin-1 expression and increase in perisinusoidal collagen IV staining [52]. The finding that caloric restriction influences pseudocapillarization suggests that this is secondary to the aging process and is potentially reversible.

Fenestrae have a role in the transfer of lipoproteins from blood to the hepatocyte, therefore it is likely that pseudocapillarization will impair lipoprotein clearance by the liver and contribute to dyslipidemia in older people [58]. Atherosclerosis increases dramatically with old age and its complications affect mostly older people [59]. The clearance of chylomicron remnants is significantly impaired in older people [60, 61] and in people aged 65 years and older, remnant-like lipoprotein cholesterol is associated with the development of coronary artery disease [62]. To determine whether age-related defenestration impairs the transfer of lipoproteins across the LSEC, multiple indicator dilution method was used to study lipoprotein disposition in perfused rat livers [63]. In young livers, lipoproteins (approximately 50 nm diameter) entered the entire extracellular space whereas in old livers, the lipoproteins were confined to the vascular space. This confirmed that age-related pseudocapillarization impairs the hepatic disposition of lipoproteins and thus plays a role in age-related dyslipidemia. As a consequence, modulation of LSEC fenestrae might be a therapeutic target for the treatment of age-related dyslipidemia and prevention of vascular disease.

In addition, pseudocapillarization might influence the hepatic clearance of medications and uptake of oxygen by hepatocytes, thus contributing to the age-related impairment of xenobiotic metabolism and associated adverse drug reactions [29]. It is also possible that the loss of fenestrae might contribute to autoimmune disease in older people by impeding the interactions between naïve T lymphocytes and hepatocytes that are thought to induce immunotolerance [40].

Pseudocapillarization also contributes to age-related reduction in hepatic blood flow. Most studies show that total hepatic blood flow is reduced in the order of 30–50% and parallels the age-related reduction in liver mass [44, 46]. Mechanisms for this change remain unclear; however, a recent study using high-resolution in vivo microscopy has shown how pseudocapillarization might contribute to this phenomena. There was a 14% reduction in the numbers of perfused sinusoids with old age and a 35% reduction in sinusoidal blood flow [45]. This was associated with a marked increase in the perisinusoidal expression of ICAM-1 and an increase in leukocyte adhesion. Narrower sinusoids with thickened LSECs and swollen stellate cells with abundant lipid droplets were also observed. It was concluded that these changes caused age-related reduction in hepatic perfusion and hepatic blood flow by blocking the sinusoids [45]. Vollmar et al. [64] used in vivo microscopy to study sinusoidal perfusion in the rat. They reported a minor reduction of sinusoidal density to 87% over life but concluded that there were no aging changes in sinusoidal perfusion, leukocyte adhesion or sinusoidal diameter. However, there was a reduction in sinusoidal flow between 3 and 24 months of age.

The morphological changes in the LSEC in old age might also affect its role in endocytosis. Recently, in vivo microscopy was used to examine LSEC uptake of two scavenger receptors ligands: advanced glycation end product (AGE)-modified albumin and formaldehyde-treated albumin [45]. Endocytosis was diminished in old mice, particularly in the pericentral zone. This change might increase the risk of extrahepatic deposition and adverse effects of circulating waste macromolecules. Advanced glycation end products are linked with aging and many age-related diseases [65].

In addition to changes in the LSEC and space of Disse, there have been some reports of the effects of aging on Kupffer cells and stellate cells [48]. Two early studies of Kupffer cells in humans noted an increase in their numbers and activity in old age [66, 67], while another reported a reduction in their volume density [68]. Kupffer cells from old rat livers have fewer pseudopodia, reduced actin and myosin cytoskeleton [69], and an increased number of lysosomes [70]. The effects of age on Kupffer cell phagocytic activity are inconsistent. For example, the uptake of large microspheres by Kupffer cells is either largely unchanged [64, 71], decreased [69] or increased [72]. Overall, the responsiveness of Kupffer cells to stimuli is diminished in old age while there appears to be an increase in basal activity consistent with the proinflammatory nature of the aging process.

Finally, old age is associated with the development of fat engorged stellate cells (see Fig. 3.2) [31, 45, 54, 64, 68, 73, 74]. These cells can even be identified on light microscopy by their signet ring appearance [31, 54]. It has also been reported that vitamin A autofluorescence is increased in old age which is further evidence that stellate cells increase in number and vitamin A content in old age [64]. Some of the stellate cells are so swollen that they protrude into the sinusoidal lumen and potentially could reduce sinusoidal blood flow [48].

Conclusions

In conclusion, old age is associated with morphological changes in the hepatic sinusoidal endothelium and the extracellular space of Disse. These changes have been called "pseudocapillarization." There is an increase in endothelial thickness and a reduction in the porosity and number of fenestrae. The age-related reduction in fenestration and porosity is substantial (around 50%) and has several implications. In particular, the effect of the loss of fenestrae on the hepatic disposition of lipoproteins such as chylomicron remnants and consequent risk of systemic vascular disease has been reported. The loss of fenestrae and altered diffusional properties of the aged sinusoidal endothelium and space of Disse also influence the hepatic clearance of medications, thus contributing to adverse drug reactions. These structural changes are associated with impaired endocytosis, further contributing to the risk of disease in old age. The liver sinusoid also contains Kupffer cells and stellate cells. In old age, there are increased numbers of Kupffer cells and increased basal activity of these cells, but their responses to antigenic challenge are reduced and stellate cells become swollen and engorged with fat. The liver sinusoid has proven to be a fruitful site for aging research and may generate novel therapeutic targets for the prevention of age-related disease.

References

1. Wisse E, Braet F, Luo D, et al. Structure and function of sinusoidal lining cells in the liver. Toxicol Pathol. 1996;24:100–11.
2. Cogger VC, Le Couteur DG. Fenestrations in the liver sinusoidal endothelial cell. In: Arias I, Wolkoff A, Boyer J, et al., editors. The liver: biology and pathobiology. 5th ed. Hokoben, NJ: Wiley; 2009. p. 387–404.
3. Fraser R, Dobbs BR, Rogers GW. Lipoproteins and the liver sieve: the role of fenestrated sinusoidal endothelium in lipoprotein metabolism, atherosclerosis, and cirrhosis. Hepatology. 1995;21:863–74.
4. Smedsrod B, Le Couteur D, Ikejima K, et al. Hepatic sinusoidal cells in health and disease. Liver Int. 2009;29:490–501.
5. Nonaka H, Tanaka M, Suzuki K, Miyajima A. Development of murine hepatic sinusoidal endothelial cells characterized by the expression of hyaluronan receptors. Dev Dyn. 2007;236:2258–67.
6. Enzan H, Himeno H, Hiroi M, Kiyoku H, Saibara T, Onishi S. Development of hepatic sinusoidal structure with special reference to the Ito cells. Microsc Res Tech. 1997;39:336–49.
7. Martinez-Hernandez A, Amenta PS. The hepatic extracellular matrix. I. Components and distribution in normal liver. Virchows Arch A Pathol Anat Histopathol. 1993;423:1–11.
8. Arias IM. The biology of hepatic endothelial cell fenestrae. Prog Liver Dis. 1990;9:11–26.
9. Arii S, Imamura M. Physiological role of sinusoidal endothelial cells and Kupffer cells and their implication in the pathogenesis of liver injury. J Hepatobiliary Pancreat Surg. 2000;7:40–8.
10. Blouin A, Bolender RP, Weibel ER. Distribution of organelles and membranes between hepatocytes and nonhepatocytes in the rat liver parenchyma. A stereological study. J Cell Biol. 1977;72:441–55.
11. Wisse E, De Zanger RB, Jacobs R, McCuskey RS. Scanning electron microscope observations on the structure of portal veins, sinusoids and central veins in rat liver. Scan Electron Microsc. 1983;3:1441–52.
12. Wisse W, De Zanger RB, Charels K, Van Der Smissen P, McCuskey RS. The liver sieve: considerations concerning the structure and function of endothelial fenestrae, the sinusoidal wall and the space of Disse. Hepatology. 1985;5:683–92.
13. O'Reilly JN, Cogger VC, Le Couteur DG. Old age is associated with ultrastructural changes in isolated rat liver sinusoidal endothelial cells. J Electron Microsc (Tokyo). 2009;59(1):65–9.
14. Vidal-Vanaclocha F, Barbera-Guillem E. Fenestration patterns in endothelial cells of rat liver sinusoids. J Ultrastruct Res. 1985;90:115–23.
15. Funyu J, Mochida S, Inao M, Matsui A, Fujiwara K. VEGF can act as vascular permeability factor in the hepatic sinusoids through upregulation of porosity of endothelial cells. Biochem Biophys Res Commun. 2001;280:481–5.
16. DeLeve LD, Wang X, McCuskey MK, McCuskey RS. Rat liver endothelial cells isolated by anti-CD31 immunomagnetic separation lack fenestrae and sieve plates. Am J Physiol. 2006;291:G1187–9.
17. Knook DL, Sleyster EC. Isolated parenchymal, Kupffer and endothelial rat liver cells characterized by their lysosomal enzyme content. Biochem Biophys Res Commun. 1980;96:250–7.
18. Smedsrod B. Clearance function of scavenger endothelial cells. Comp Hepatol. 2004;3 Suppl 1:S22.
19. Smedsrod B, Elvevold K, Martinez I. The liver sinusoidal endothelial cell: a cell type of controversial and confusing identity. 13th International symposium on cells of the hepatic sinusoid. 2006. p. 61–2.
20. Smedsrod B, Melkko J, Araki N, Sano H, Horiuchi S. Advanced glycation end products are eliminated by scavenger-receptor-mediated endocytosis in hepatic sinusoidal Kupffer and endothelial cells. Biochem J. 1997;322(Pt 2):567–73.
21. Smedsrod B, De Bleser PJ, Braet F, et al. Cell biology of liver endothelial and Kupffer cells. Gut. 1994;35:1509–16.
22. Smedsrod B, Pertoft H, Gustafson S, Laurent TC. Scavenger functions of the liver endothelial cell. Biochem J. 1990;266:313–27.
23. Skogh T, Blomhoff R, Eskild W, Berg T. Hepatic uptake of circulating IgG immune complexes. Immunology. 1985;55:585–94.
24. Knook DL, Sleyster EC. Separation of Kupffer and endothelial cells of the rat liver by centrifugal elutriation. Exp Cell Res. 1976;99:444–9.

25. Atzori L, Poli G, Perra A. Hepatic stellate cell: a star cell in the liver. Int J Biochem Cell Biol. 2009;41: 1639–42.
26. Wisse E, Luo D, Vermijlen D, Kanellopoulou C, De Zanger R, Braet F. On the function of pit cells, the liver-specific natural killer cells. Semin Liver Dis. 1997;17:265–86.
27. Fraser R, Bosanquet AG, Day WA. Filtration of chylomicrons by the liver may influence cholesterol metabolism and atherosclerosis. Atherosclerosis. 1978;29:113–23.
28. Wisse E. An electron microscopic study of the fenestrated endothelial lining of rat liver sinusoids. J Ultrastruct Res. 1970;31:125–50.
29. Le Couteur DG, Fraser R, Hilmer S, Rivory LP, McLean AJ. The hepatic sinusoid in aging and cirrhosis – effects on hepatic substrate disposition and drug clearance. Clin Pharmacokinet. 2005;44:187–200.
30. Baker RW. Membrane technology and applications. 2nd ed. Hokoben, NJ: Wiley; 2004.
31. Warren A, Bertolino P, Cogger VC, McLean AJ, Fraser R, Le Couteur DG. Hepatic pseudocapillarization in aged mice. Exp Gerontol. 2005;40:807–12.
32. Le Couteur DG, Cogger VC, Hilmer SN, et al. Aging, atherosclerosis and the liver sieve. In: Clark LV, editor. New research on atherosclerosis. New York: Nova Science; 2006. p. 19–44.
33. Seternes T, Sorensen K, Smedsrod B. Scavenger endothelial cells of vertebrates: a nonperipheral leukocyte system for high-capacity elimination of waste macromolecules. Proc Natl Acad Sci USA. 2002;99: 7594–7.
34. Malovic I, Sorensen KK, Elvevold KH, et al. The mannose receptor on murine liver sinusoidal endothelial cells is the main denatured collagen clearance receptor. Hepatology. 2007;45:1454–61.
35. Martin-Armas M, Simon-Santamaria J, Pettersen I, Moens U, Smedsrod B, Sveinbjornsson B. Toll-like receptor 9 (TLR9) is present in murine liver sinusoidal endothelial cells (LSECs) and mediates the effect of CpG-oligonucleotides. J Hepatol. 2006;44:939–46.
36. Enomoto K, Nishikawa Y, Omori Y, et al. Cell biology and pathology of liver sinusoidal endothelial cells. Med Electron Microsc. 2004;37:208–15.
37. Lalor PF, Lai WK, Curbishley SM, Shetty S, Adams DH. Human hepatic sinusoidal endothelial cells can be distinguished by expression of phenotypic markers related to their specialised functions in vivo. World J Gastroenterol. 2006;12:5429–39.
38. Limmer A, Ohl J, Kurts C, et al. Efficient presentation of exogenous antigen by liver endothelial cells to CD8+ T cells results in antigen-specific T-cell tolerance. Nat Med. 2000;6:1348–54.
39. Karrar A, Broome U, Uzunel M, Qureshi AR, Sumitran-Holgersson S. Human liver sinusoidal endothelial cells induce apoptosis in activated T cells: a role in tolerance induction. Gut. 2007;56:243–52.
40. Warren A, Le Couteur DG, Fraser R, Bowen DG, McCaughan GW, Bertolino P. T lymphocytes interact with hepatocytes through fenestrations in murine liver sinusoidal endothelial cells. Hepatology. 2006;44: 1182–90.
41. Le Couteur DG, Everitt A, Lebel M. The aging liver. Geriatr Aging. 2009;12:319–22.
42. Popper H. Aging and the liver. Prog Liver Dis. 1986;8:659–83.
43. McLean AJ, Le Couteur DG. Aging biology and geriatric clinical pharmacology. Pharmacol Rev. 2004;56: 163–84.
44. Le Couteur DG, McLean AJ. The aging liver – drug clearance and an oxygen diffusion barrier hypothesis. Clin Pharmacokinet. 1998;34:359–73.
45. Ito Y, Sorensen KK, Bethea NW, et al. Age-related changes in the hepatic microcirculation of mice. Exp Gerontol. 2007;48:789–97.
46. Schmucker DL. Aging and the liver: an update. J Gerontol. 1998;53A:B315–20.
47. Zahn JM, Poosala S, Owen AB, et al. AGEMAP: a gene expression database for aging in mice. PLoS Genet. 2007;3:e201.
48. Le Couteur DG, Warren A, Cogger VC, et al. Old age and the hepatic sinusoid. Anat Rec (Hoboken). 2008; 291:672–83.
49. Hinton DE, Williams WL. Hepatic fibrosis associated with aging in four stocks of mice. J Gerontol. 1968; 23:205–11.
50. De Leeuw AM, Brouwer A, Knook DL. Sinusoidal endothelial cells of the liver: fine structure and function in relation to age. J Electron Microsc Tech. 1990;14:218–36.
51. Le Couteur DG, Cogger VC, Markus AMA, et al. Pseudocapillarization and associated energy limitation in the aged rat liver. Hepatology. 2001;33:537–43.
52. Jamieson H, Hilmer SN, Cogger VC, et al. Caloric restriction reduces age-related pseudocapillarization of the hepatic sinusoid. Exp Gerontol. 2007;42:374–8.
53. McLean AJ, Cogger VC, Chong GC, et al. Age-related pseudocapillarization of the human liver. J Pathol. 2003;200:112–7.
54. Cogger VC, Warren A, Fraser R, Ngu M, McLean AJ, Le Couteur DG. Hepatic sinusoidal pseudocapillarization with aging in the non-human primate. Exp Gerontol. 2003;38:1101–7.
55. Stacchiotti A, Lavazza A, Ferroni M, et al. Effects of aluminium sulphate in the mouse liver: similarities to the aging process. Exp Gerontol. 2008;43:330–8.
56. Warren A, Chaberek S, Ostrowski K, et al. Effects of old age on vascular complexity and dispersion of the hepatic sinusoidal network. Microcirculation. 2008;15: 191–202.
57. Everitt A, Roth GS, Le Couteur DG, Hilmer SN. Calorie restriction versus drug therapy to delay the onset of aging diseases and extend life. Age. 2005;27:1–10.
58. Le Couteur DG, Fraser R, Cogger VC, McLean AJ. Hepatic pseudocapillarisation and atherosclerosis in ageing. Lancet. 2002;359:1612–5.
59. Lakatta EG, Levy D. Arterial and cardiac aging: major shareholders in cardiovascular disease enterprises: part I: aging arteries: a 'set up' for vascular disease. Circulation. 2003;107:139–46.

60. Krasinski SD, Cohn JS, Schaefer EJ, Russell RM. Postprandial plasma retinyl ester response is greater in older subjects compared with younger subjects. Evidence for delayed plasma clearance of intestinal lipoproteins. J Clin Invest. 1990;85:883–92.
61. Borel P, Mekki N, Boirie Y, et al. Comparison of postprandial plasma vitamin A response in young and older adults. J Gerontol. 1998;53:B133–40.
62. Simons LA, Simons J, Friedlander Y, McCallum J. Cholesterol and other lipids predict coronary heart disease and ischemic stroke in the elderly, but only in those below 70 years. Atherosclerosis. 2001;159:201–8.
63. Hilmer SN, Cogger VC, Fraser R, McLean AJ, Sullivan D, Le Couteur DG. Age-related changes in the hepatic sinusoidal endothelium impede lipoprotein transfer in the rat. Hepatology. 2005;42:1349–54.
64. Vollmar B, Pradarutti S, Richter S, Menger MD. In vivo quantification of ageing changes in the rat liver from early juvenile to senescent life. Liver. 2002;22:330–41.
65. Singh R, Barden A, Mori T, Beilin L. Advanced glycation end-products: a review. Diabetologia. 2001;44:129–46.
66. Findor J, Perez V, Bruch Igartua E, Giovanetti M, Fioravanti N. Structure and ultrastructure of the liver in aged persons. Acta Hepatogastroenterol (Stuttg). 1973;20:200–4.
67. Schaffner F, Popper H. Nonspecific reactive hepatitis in aged and infirm people. Am J Dig Dis. 1959;4:389–99.
68. Martin G, Sewell B, Yeomans ND, Smallwood RA. Ageing has no effect on the volume density of hepatocytes, reticulo-endothelial cells or the extracellular space in livers of female Sprague–Dawley rats. Clin Exp Pharmacol Physiol. 1992;19:537–9.
69. Sun WB, Han BL, Peng ZM, et al. Effect of aging on cytoskeleton system of Kupffer cell and its phagocytic capacity. World J Gastroenterol. 1998;4:77–9.
70. Knook DL, Sleyster EC. Lysosomal enzyme activities in parenchymal and nonparenchymal liver cells isolated from young, adult and old rats. Mech Ageing Dev. 1976;5:389–98.
71. De Leeuw AM, Brouwer A, Barelds RJ, Knook DL. Maintenance cultures of Kupffer cells isolated from rats of various ages: ultrastructure, enzyme cytochemistry, and endocytosis. Hepatology. 1983;3:497–506.
72. Hilmer SN, Cogger VC, Le Couteur DG. Basal activity of Kupffer cells increases with old age. J Gerontol A Biol Sci Med Sci. 2007;62:973–8.
73. Grizzi F, Franceschini B, Gagliano N, et al. Mast cell density, hepatic stellate cell activation and TGF-beta1 transcripts in the aging Sprague–Dawley rat during early acute liver injury. Toxicol Pathol. 2003;31:173–8.
74. Durham SK, Brouwer A, Barelds RJ, Horan MA, Knook DL. Comparative endotoxin-induced hepatic injury in young and aged rats. J Pathol. 1990;162:341–9.

Stellate Cells and the Microcirculation

4

Massimo Pinzani

Abstract

Activation of hepatic stellate cells (HSCs) within hepatic sinusoids during chronic liver diseases is a key feature of the capillarization of sinusoids. This latter feature likely represents an initial cause of portal hypertension during the early development of hepatic fibrosis. Contraction of activated HSC occurs in vitro in response to different vasoconstrictors, and this feature may have important implications in the pathogenesis of portal hypertension and in the contraction of mature scar tissue. In cirrhotic liver, portal blood flow is largely diverted toward the systemic circulation through portal-central anastomoses. These neoformed vascular structures, although representing direct connections between the portal and the systemic circulation, follow irregular patterns, are site of thrombotic events, and are embedded in developing scar tissue. This tissue is characterized by the presence of different types of ECM-producing cells, all potentially able to contract in response to vasocostrictors (e.g., ET-1) released within cirrhotic liver tissues. It is implicit that cell contraction in response to these agents could be antagonized by autologous vasodilators (e.g., NO) or by drugs provided with vasodilator properties.

Keywords

Hepatic stellate cells • Myofibroblasts • Pericytes • Cell contraction • Liver fibrosis • Cirrhosis • Portal hypertension

Research performed in the last two decades suggests that hepatic stellate cells (HSCs) are involved in the regulation of the liver microcirculation and portal hypertension. Activated HSCs have the necessary machinery to contract or relax in response to a number of vasoactive substances. Because stellate cells play a role in both fibrosis and portal hypertension, they are currently regarded as therapeutic targets to prevent and treat the complications of chronic liver disease.

M. Pinzani (✉)
Dipartimento di Medicina Interna, Center for Research, High Education and Transfer DENOThe, Università degli Studi di Firenze, Viale G.B. Morgagni, 85, 50134 Firenze, Italy
e-mail: m.pinzani@dmi.unifi.it

Anatomy and Ultrastructure

HSCs are located in the space of Disse in close contact with hepatocytes and sinusoidal endothelial cells. In human liver, HSCs are distributed along the sinusoids with a nucleus-to-nucleus

L.D. DeLeve and G. Garcia-Tsao (eds.), *Vascular Liver Disease: Mechanisms and Management*, DOI 10.1007/978-1-4419-8327-5_4, © Springer Science+Business Media, LLC 2011

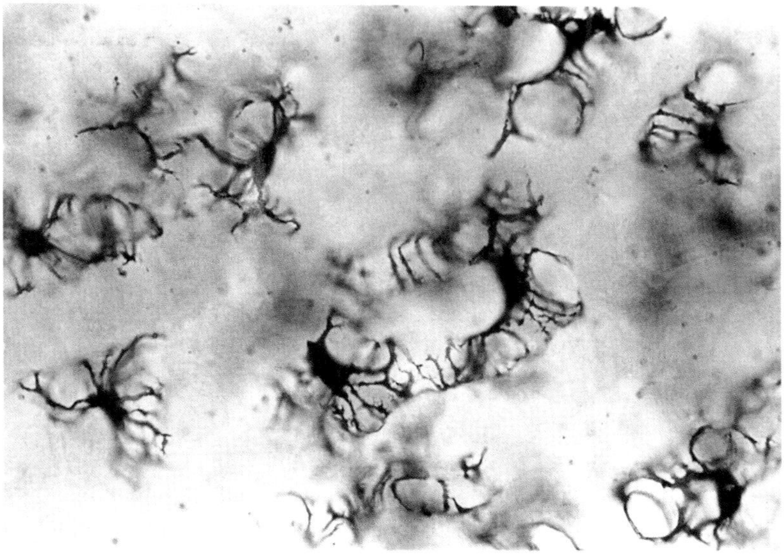

Fig. 4.1 Stellate cells in the porcine liver. The long cytoplasmic processes encompass sinusoids at regular intervals. Golgi's silver method. ×840 [80] (Courtesy of Prof. Kenjiro Wake)

distance of 40 μm, indicating that the sinusoids contain HSCs at certain fixed distances [1]. Therefore, although the total number of HSCs constitutes a small percentage of the total number of liver cells (approximately 5–8%), their spatial disposition and spatial extension may be sufficient to cover the entire hepatic sinusoidal microcirculatory network. The three-dimensional structure of HSC consists of the cell body and several long and branching cytoplasmic processes (Fig. 4.1). Two main types of cytoplasmic processes are recognized according to their spatial disposition: the *intersinusoidal* or *interhepatocellular* processes and the *perisinusoidal* or *subendothelial* processes. The interhepatocellular processes penetrate the hepatic cell plates and extend to nearby sinusoids [1]. A single HSC may provide interhepatocellular processes to two or more neighboring sinusoids (Fig. 4.2). The perisinusoidal processes encircle the sinusoid located on the same cell plate by means of a series of adjacent periodic side-branches extending subendothelially. In general, the subendothelial processes appear to adhere to the sinusoidal wall by narrow strands of material resembling a basement membrane. These latter structures, although not continuously distributed, seem to ensure a strong connection between HSC and the sinusoidal endothelium [2]. The minute thorn-like microprojections or spines, termed *hepatocyte-contacting* processes [3], are an important and distinctive element of this cell type. These spines face the microvillous facet of hepatocytes and establish close intercellular contacts between HSC and parenchymal cells [4]. Although the functions of these microprojections are presently unknown, several lines of evidence suggest that they may play a role in epithelial–mesenchymal interactions that promote cell differentiation [4, 5].

Considering the classic division of the liver lobule in three zones (zone 1: periportal; zone 2: intermediate; zone 3: pericentral), several characteristics of HSC vary according to their location within the liver lobule [6–8] (Fig. 4.3). HSCs located in zone 1 appear small and contain minute vitamin A lipid droplets. Perisinusoidal branching processes are short and smoothly contoured with few hepatocyte-contacting processes, whereas desmin immunoreactivity is present but not particularly intense. HSCs located in lobular zone 2 store abundant vitamin A lipid droplets and extend encompassing processes that show intense desmin immunoreaction (in the rat). These processes display conspicuous branching and abundant hepatocyte-contacting spines. Proceeding toward the centrilobular vein, HSCs become more elongated assuming a dendritic appearance, whereas their desmin immunoreactivity and vitamin A storage are progressively reduced becoming virtually absent around the center of the lobule. Therefore, the

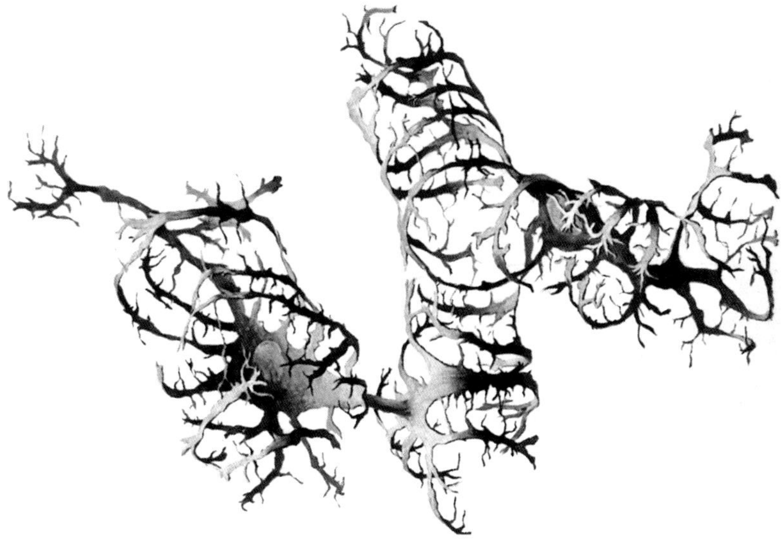

Fig. 4.2 Drawing of the 3-D structure of two hepatic stellate cells of porcine liver. The drawing was made according to the findings obtained by the Golgi's silver method [81] (Courtesy of Prof. Kenjiro Wake)

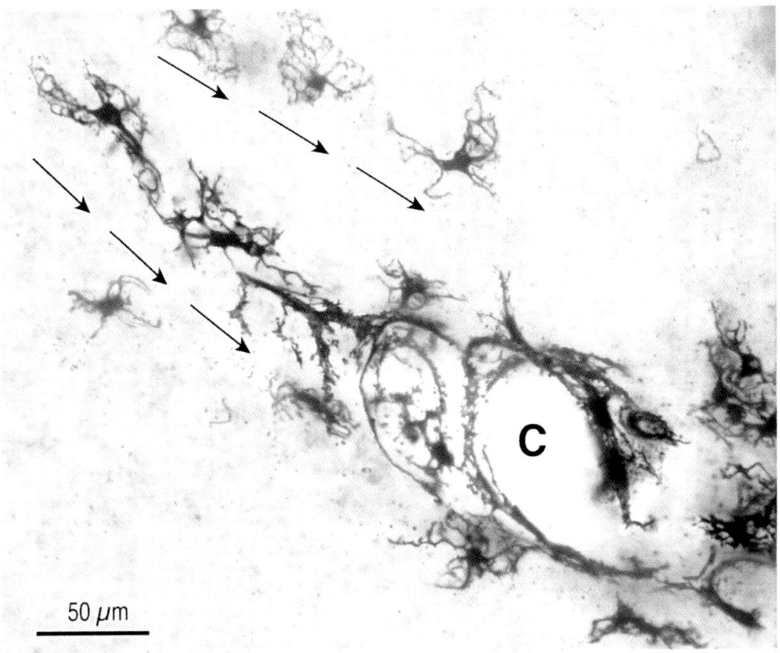

Fig. 4.3 Panzonal polymorphism of hepatic stellate cell population. HSCs located in zone 1 appear small and contain minute vitamin A lipid droplets. Perisinusoidal branching processes are short and smoothly contoured with few hepatocyte-contacting processes. HSCs located in lobular zone 2 extend encompassing processes that show intense desmin immunoreaction (in the rat). These processes display conspicuous branching and abundant hepatocyte-contacting spines. Proceeding toward the centrilobular vein, HSCs become more elongated assuming a dendritic appearance. *C* centrolobular vein (Courtesy of Prof. Wichai Ekataksin)

intralobular heterogeneity of HSC may reflect, at least, differences in the metabolic handling of vitamin A and in the regulation of sinusoidal blood pressure in different areas of the liver lobule.

The most relevant ultrastructural feature of HSC in adult normal liver is the presence of cytoplasmic lipid droplets ranging in diameter from 1 to 2 μm. This feature is related to one of the main known physiological functions of HSC, i.e., the hepatic storage of retinyl esters. Numerous microtubular structures are present in the cytoplasm together with bundles of microfilaments (5 nm thick), particularly along the subsurface cytoplasmic matrix apposed to the neighboring sinusoidal endothelial cell. Other 10-nm-thick filaments are widely distributed in the cytoplasm, especially around the nucleus and among the rough endoplasmic reticulum area. These microtubules and microfilaments may function as the cytoskeleton of dendritic processes and play a role in lipid synthesis and/or transport. Finally, ultrastructural analysis of the subendothelial processes revealed that these peculiar structures are equipped with massive 5-nm actin-like filaments, thus leading to the hypothesis that they may contribute to reinforce the endothelial lining and/or enhance the efficiency of contraction of sinusoidal capillaries [9].

HSC as Liver-Specific Pericytes

The role of HSC as liver-specific pericytes is suggested by their anatomical location and ultrastructural features. In addition, HSCs are characterized by a close relationship with the autonomous nervous system. Branches of the autonomic nerve fibers coursing through the space of Disse are in contact with HSC [10], and nerve endings containing substance P and vasoactive intestinal peptide have been demonstrated in the vicinity of HSC [11]. In both normal and fibrotic liver, the expression of N-CAM, a typical central nervous system adhesion molecule detected in hepatic nerves, and the expression of glial fibrillary acidic protein (GFAP) are restricted among liver cell types to HSC [12]. These observations raise a still unresolved issue concerning the origin of this cell type previously considered to be of myogenic origin because of the expression of desmin and smooth muscle α-actin (α-SMA). Along these lines, activated HSCs express nestin, a class VI intermediate filament protein originally identified as a marker for neural stem cells [13]. Remarkably, the expression of this cell marker appears to be restricted to HSC and pericytes of brain parenchyma vessels, among all organ-specific pericytes. Another neuroendocrine marker suggesting a combination of mesenchymal and neural/neuroendocrine features in HSC is synaptophysin, a protein involved in neurotransmitter exocytosis. Synaptophysin reactivity is present in perisinusoidal stellate cells in normal human and rat liver, and the number of synaptophysin-reactive perisinusoidal cells is increased in pathological conditions [14]. Additional experimental evidence indicates that rat and human HSC express neurotrophins (including nerve growth factor-NGF, brain-derived neurotrophin, neurotrophin 3, and neurotrophin 4/5) and neurotrophin receptors [15]. In aggregate, these observations suggest a complex interaction between the pathophysiological role of HSC and the function of the peripheral nervous system.

The recognition that HSCs have contractile properties was a key milestone in our understanding of the biology of this cell type. Several studies have shown that HSCs isolated from rat or human liver and maintained in culture contract in response to several vasoconstricting stimuli [16]. Contraction of HSC in response to these stimuli has been demonstrated independently from the cell attachment substrata (glass, plastic, silicone membranes, or collagen lattices). Importantly, following stimulation with thrombin, endothelin-1, and angiotensin II, cell contraction is coupled with an increase in intracellular calcium concentration [17]. These observations greatly contribute to categorizing HSC as pericytes. It should be noted, however, that cultured HSCs are characterized by an activated phenotype resembling transitional or myofibroblast-like cells rather than quiescent HSCs. Therefore, the contractile properties demonstrated in these experiments are likely to be more representative of HSC contractile status in fibrotic liver. Whether or not HSCs contract in normal liver tissue is still open to discussion. From the morphological standpoint, some observations argue against the role of HSC in the regulation of sinusoidal blood flow [18]. First, in their *in vivo* tridimensional orientation HSCs do not have a stellate form (typical of their aspect in bidimensional culture on plastic) but rather a "spider-like" appearance ("arachnocytes") with a small cell body and a series of radiating and parallel slender processes. According to the authors of these observations, cells with this tridimensional appearance are not likely to be "contraction ready." Additional limitations to effective cell contraction are offered by the spatial limitation of the space of Disse, by the intracytoplasmic presence of lipid droplets that prevent microfilaments from assembly in a long span, and by ultrastructural evidence of limited development of contractile filaments in quiescent HSC. Regardless of this, the studies evaluating the hepatic microcirculation by intravital microscopy techniques have suggested that HSC could be involved in the regulation of sinusoidal tone in normal liver [19, 20]. An additional matter of debate is provided by studies aimed at quantifying HSC contraction with techniques able to detect the development of contractile forces in response to vasoconstrictors [21]. The results of these studies indicate that the magnitude and kinetics of contraction and relaxation are consistent with the hypothesis that HSC may affect sinusoidal resistance. However, for understandable technical reasons, these data were obtained in rat HSC in primary culture 7 days after isolation, when a certain degree of activation in culture has already occurred. In conclusion, although HSCs could be proposed as liver-specific pericytes based on their location, spatial distribution, relationship with the peripheral nervous system, and ultrastructural features, no conclusive evidence establishes a role in regulating normal sinusoidal blood flow. Overall, it is likely that in normal liver HSCs contribute to the regulation of sinusoidal blood flow in conjunction with other relevant sites of circulatory modulation equipped with inlet and outlet sphincters such as: (i) portal venules, (ii) hepatic arterioles, (iii) central venules, and with sinusoidal endothelial cells, which are able to influence sinusoidal pressure through the regulation of the size of fenestrae.

Contractility of Activated HSCs

Following two pioneering studies [17, 22] demonstrating the contraction of HSC in response to different vasoconstrictors (Fig. 4.4), the potential involvement of this cell type in the genesis and progression of portal hypertension was postulated. Available experimental evidence suggests that

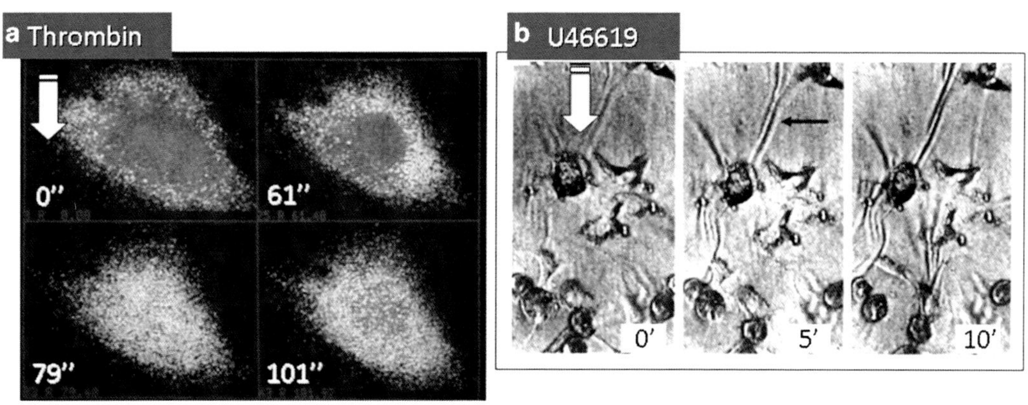

Fig. 4.4 Contraction of activated hepatic stellate cells. (**a**) Time-sequence changes in intracellular calcium concentration in a single Fura-2-loaded human hepatic stellate cell responding to 0.3 NIH units/ml of thrombin. Note the reduction of cell area associated with intracellular calcium increase [17]. From Pinzani et al. [17]. (**b**) Effect of the thromboxane A_2 agonist U46619 on rat stellate cell contraction. Stellate cells were cultured for 7 days on silicone membranes and then stimulated with 2 μm M-U46619 for 5 and 10 min. Note that wrinkle appearance on the silicone membrane was associated with diminution of cell size (×200) [22]. From Kawada N, Klein H, and Decker K. Eicosanoid-mediated contractility of hepatic stellate cells. Biochem J 1992; 285: 367-371. Reprinted with permission from the Biochemical Society (http://www.biochemi.org)

although HSC may constitute resident contractile structures in hepatic sinusoids in normal liver, a remarkable increase in their contractile properties is likely a key feature of their activated state [17, 22–24]. HSCs in their "myofibroblast-like" phenotype have been shown to express a large number of voltage-operated calcium channels, the activation of which is associated with increased intracellular calcium concentration followed by marked cell contraction [25]. These changes may be dependent on intra- and extracellular factors. First, complete transition to the "myofibroblast-like" phenotype is ultrastructurally characterized by the appearance of massive contractile structures including dense bodies and patches of myofilaments present diffusely throughout the cytoplasm (Fig. 4.5). Second, HSC activation is accompanied by increased expression of α-SMA, and it is likely that this change in the cytoskeletal structure is linked to increased cell contractility. Interestingly, both profibrogenic agents and vasoconstrictors represent potential regulators of the α-SMA gene, and, in this context, the transcription factor c-myb has been shown to form complexes with a regulatory element of the α-SMA gene, suggesting that induction of this gene may be transcriptionally regulated [26]. Among "external" factors that could affect HSC contractility, the modified ECM pattern typical of fibrotic liver is likely to play an important role. Indeed, the presence of an abnormal amount of fibrillar ECM, typical of "capillarized" sinusoids, may condition the expression and function of integrin receptors supporting a cytoskeletal organization more suitable for cell contraction, at least when compared with the situation present in normal liver. Engagement of integrin receptors with ECM results in the assembly of focal adhesion plaques with the phosphorylation of key proteins such as focal adhesion kinase (FAK). This interaction is necessary for the polymerization of actin filaments. Stimulation with a variety of stimuli, particularly with vasoconstrictors, causes the phosphorylation of myosin light chain, which in turn interacts with actin filaments thus leading to the formation of stress fibers. In this context, recent data suggest that activation of integrin-related intracellular signaling pathways including Rho, a small GTP-binding protein belonging to the Ras superfamily, directs activation-associated changes in rat HSC morphology via regulation of the actin cytoskeleton [27]. Interestingly, inhibition of integrin signaling with Arg-Gly-Asp motifs in activated rat HSC results in a disturbance of actin stress fiber organization and focal adhesion assembly and in a reduction of cell activation markers, including α-SMA expression [28]. Finally, it is logical to hypothesize that HSC contractile status could be conditioned by the presence of vasoactive substances present in the microenvironment of hepatic tissue undergoing active fibrogenesis.

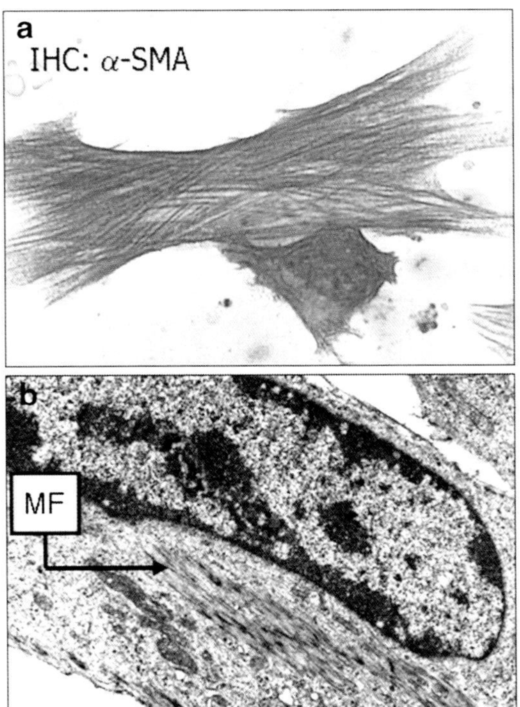

Fig. 4.5 Contractile machinery of activated human hepatic stellate cells. (**a**) Immunohistochemistry staining for alpha-smooth muscle actin. (**b**) Electronmicrophotograph showing massive contractile structures including dense bodies and patches of myofilaments diffuse throughout the cytoplasm

It is clear that both Ca^{2+}-dependent and independent mechanisms are involved in HSC contraction. It has been speculated that, as HSCs are activated and exhibit "smooth muscle-like features," Ca^{2+} signaling could become more important [29]. However, this has been challenged more recently as it was demonstrated that both pathways are necessary for maximal contraction of HSC, but that Ca^{2+}-independent pathways predominate in activated HSC and in cirrhotic liver [30]. At least two different types of Ca^{2+} channels have been described in activated HSC: voltage-operated calcium channels and store-operated channels. It has been demonstrated that the activation of HSC is associated with both an up-regulation of L-type voltage-operated Ca^{2+}channels that mediate Ca^{2+} influx and KCl-induced contraction [31]. However, as HSCs have not been shown to be excitable, it will be important to establish the physiological relevance of these channels. Some of the changes in $[Ca^{2+}]i$ are mediated by means of store-operated calcium channels [32]. Depletion of Ca^{2+} in the $[Ca^{2+}]i$ stores will lead to activation of these calcium channels. Furthermore, some G protein-coupled receptors such as endothelin can directly activate receptor-gated Ca^{2+} channels, but this mechanism has not been proven to be present in HSC. Whatever the mechanism of increased $[Ca^{2+}]i$, it will result in cell contraction. Indeed, it has been demonstrated that reductions in HSC area, a marker of contractile force generation, correlate with the height of the increased $[Ca^{2+}]i$ peak [17, 33].

Rho is a member of the Ras superfamily, and a number of rho effectors have been identified. The two serine/threonine kinases (rho kinase/ROKa/ROCK-II and p160ROCK/ROCKb), commonly referred to as rho kinase, are the best characterized [34]. Rho regulates cell morphology through organizing the actin cytoskeleton and control of actomyosin-dependent cellular processes [35]. Rho kinase has been shown to participate in the induction of stress fiber and focal adhesion formation and cell contraction [36]. Furthermore, rho kinase phosphorylates intermediate filaments, such as GFAP and vimentin [37]. In HSC, rho and rho kinase have been shown to enhance myosin activation suggesting a role in the generation of contractile force [38]. This possibility has been supported by the demonstration that rho-signaling pathways regulate agonist-induced (for example, ET-1, lysophosphatidic acid (LPA)) shrinkage of collagen gels [38, 39]. Moreover, HSC activation is associated with rho-induced formation of actin stress fibers and focal adhesions [27].

Vasoactive Substances Affecting HSC Contractility

The effects of vasoactive substances have been extensively studied in activated HSC (Table 4.1). One of the most potent and certainly the most studied vasoconstrictors is endothelin (ET)-1.

Table 4.1 Vasoactive agents acting on hepatic stellate cells

AGENT	Contraction	Relaxation	$[Ca^{2\pm}]i$ Increase
Endothelin-1	++++		Coupled
Thrombin	++++		Coupled
Angiotensin II	+++		Coupled
Substance P	+++		
Adenosine	+++		Coupled
Thromboxane	+++		
Vasopressin	++++		Coupled
Platelet-activating factor	+		Coupled
Cysteinyl leukotrienes	+++		Coupled
Adrenomedullin		++	[a]
Nitric oxide		++	[a]
Carbon monoxide		++	(Indirect evidence)
Hydrogen sulfide		++	(Indirect evidence)
cAMP increasing agents		+++	[a]
Lipo PGE_1		++	
Atrial natriuretic peptide		+++	[a]
C-type natriuretic peptide		+++	[a]

[a] Relaxation associated with an inhibition of vasoconstrictor-induced $[Ca^{2+}]i$ increase

Endothelins are a family of three homologous oligopeptides of 21 amino acid polypeptides (ET-1, ET-2, and ET-3) which are cleavage products of larger precursor proteins, cleaved by endothelin-converting enzyme [40, 41]. The peptides act through at least two G protein-coupled receptors, termed type A (ETA) and type B (ETB), with ETB receptor having two isoforms: ETB1 and ETB2. The affinity of ET-1 for the ETA receptor is 100-fold higher than that of ET-3, whereas the ETB receptor has similar affinity for ET-1, ET-2, and ET-3. The ETA receptor is mainly localized on smooth muscle cells and mediates principally vasoconstriction while ETB receptors are present on a variety of cells and have several biological effects. The ETB1 receptor induces endothelial cell nitric oxide synthetase (eNOS) resulting in NO release and relaxation, whereas ETB2 receptors cause vasoconstriction [42–44]. Both ETA and ETB receptors were present on HSC and hepatocytes while only ETB receptors were present on sinusoidal endothelial cells and Kupffer cells [45–47]. It is overall evident that the process of HSC activation and phenotypical modulation is characterized by a close and complex relationship with the ET system. The ability to synthesize and release ET-1 is associated with a progressive shift in the relative predominance of ETA and ETB receptors observed during serial subculture: ETA receptors are predominant in the early phases of activation, whereas ETA receptors become increasingly more abundant in "myofibroblast-like" cells [48–50]. The shift in the relative ET receptor densities may be directed at differentiating the possible paracrine and autocrine effects of ET-1 on HSC during the activation process. Indeed, when HSCs are provided with a majority of ETA receptors (early phases of activation), stimulation with ET-1 causes a dose-dependent increase in cell growth, ERK activity, and expression of *c-fos*. These effects, likely related to the activation of the Ras–ERK pathway, are completely blocked by pretreatment with BQ-123, a specific ETA receptor antagonist [48]. Conversely, in later stages of activation, when the number of ETB receptors increases, ET-1 appears to induce a predominantly antiproliferative effect linked to the activation of this receptor subtype [51]. In this setting the activation of the ETB receptor stimulates the production of prostaglandins, leading to an increase in intracellular cAMP, which in turn reduces the activation of both ERK and JNK [52]. In addition, both cAMP and prostaglandins upregulate ETB-binding sites, thus suggesting the possibility of a positive feedback regulatory loop. In aggregate these observations suggest that ET-1 may act as a potent vasoconstrictor agonist regulating intrahepatic blood flow in cirrhotic liver with a potential role in the pathogenesis of portal hypertension. Along these lines, morphological studies have clearly indicated that ET-1 (both at mRNA and protein levels) is markedly overexpressed in different cellular elements present within cirrhotic liver tissue, and particularly in sinusoidal endothelial and HSC in their activated phenotype located in the sinusoids of the regenerating nodules, at the edges of fibrous septa, and in the ECM embedding neoformed vessels within fibrous bands [48]. Recently, fibronectin has been demonstrated to stimulate activated HSC to produce endothelin-1 and contract, via an ERK-dependent signaling pathway. The resulting autocrine functional effects of endothelin-1 are likely to be important in the wound-healing process in chronically injured liver [53]. In addition, clinical studies indicate that a direct relationship exists between ET receptor mRNA abundance and the degree of portal hypertension in cirrhotic patients [54].

It is well established that the renin-angiotensin system is implicated in portal hypertension and its complications. Studies performed in the past decade have shown the presence of AT1 receptors in activated rat and human HSC [54, 55]. Activation of AT1 receptors by angiotensin II elicited a marked contraction of activated human HSCs by an increase in intracellular $[Ca^{2+}]_i$ [17, 56]. The same group of investigators demonstrated that activated HSC express renin, angiotensinogen, and angiotensin-converting enzyme and synthesize angiotensin II [57]. These observations suggested that the local renin-angiotensin system could be implicated in portal hypertension. Angiotensin II, in addition to its vasoconstrictor action, has been shown to act as a pleiotropic cytokine with important profibrogenic effects in different organs including the liver [58]. Accordingly, drugs blocking the renin-angiotensin system have been proposed as antifibrotic agents. Indeed, inhibition of the renin-angiotensin system at different levels attenuates fibrosis progression in animal models of liver fibrosis [59].

Nitric oxide is a small, relatively stable, free-radical gas that readily diffuses into cells and membranes wherein it reacts with molecular targets. Importantly, the precise biochemical reactions, which are realized in any biological setting, depend on the concentration of NO achieved and often on subtle variations in the composition of the intra- and extracellular milieu. Accordingly, the biological actions of NO are often defined as a "double-edged sword." NO may act as a key signaling molecule in physiological processes as diverse as host-defense, neuronal communication, and regulation of vascular tone. It is a potent vasodilator, acting in a paracrine manner by directly stimulating soluble guanylate cyclase, resulting in increased levels of cGMP and consequently decreased $[Ca^{2+}]i$ and vasorelaxation [60]. In cirrhosis, systemic and splanchnic vascular NO production is increased, but intrahepatic NO production is deficient. Nitric oxide was shown to modulate the contractile effect of endothelin-1 on cultured HSC [61]. Moreover, an intrahepatic NO-donor decreased HSC contractility in vitro and reduced portal hypertension in cirrhotic rats [61]. These observations suggest a role of HSC in NO-induced regulation of intrahepatic vascular resistance [62]. Interestingly, the effects of NO on activated human HSC do not seem related to the activation of the classic soluble guanylate cyclase (sGC)/cGMP pathway, whose expression progressively decreases with the process of activation, but rather to an increased synthesis of prostaglandin E_2 associated with an increase in intracellular cAMP levels [63], thus indicating a predominant activation of the adenylate cyclase/cAMP pathway (Fig. 4.6).

Studies, demonstrating the correction of the hyperresponsiveness to vasoconstrictors by Rho kinase inhibitors, imply a causal role of the RhoA/Rho kinase pathway for the increased vasoconstrictor sensitivity and the elevated intrahepatic resistance of cirrhotic livers [64]. Most recently, adenosine has been shown to be a physiological inhibitor of the Rho pathway in HSC. Thus the loss of adenosine-induced contraction of HSC seen with more advanced liver disease might contribute to the substantial functional benefit seen in patients with cirrhosis in the presence of adenosine-induced hepatic arterial dilatation [65]. Treatment with nitroflurbiprofen, an NO-releasing cyclooxygenase inhibitor, seems to be a particularly interesting approach to counteract the imbalance in vasoreactivity, because nitroflurbiprofen improves portal hypertension in cirrhotic rats by inhibition of the hyperresponsiveness to vasoconstrictors through the inhibition of COX and by the supply of NO to the intrahepatic circulation [66]. Recent work has shown that adenosine inhibits endothelin-1- and LPA-mediated HSC contraction, and it has been postulated that adenosine is a physiological inhibitor of the Rho pathway in HSCs with functional consequences, including loss of HSC contraction [67].

Carbon monoxide is a gaseous molecule produced by degradation of heme, mediated by activity of heme oxygenase (HO). Carbon monoxide activates soluble guanylate cyclase to produce cGMP, thereby causing smooth muscle relaxation. Two isoforms (HO-1 and HO-2) are expressed in normal liver (HO-1 in Kupffer cells and HO-2 in hepatocytes), but both isoforms were undetectable in normal rat HSC [68]. Heme oxygenase-1 gene expression was upregulated in hepatocytes and Kupffer cells of rats and patients with cirrhosis and portal hypertension [69–71]. In rats, increased HO-1 expression resulted in increased CO production and a reduction of hepatic vascular resistance [72]. In vivo microscopy demonstrated that HO-1 directly acts by means of HSC in rat livers [73]. HO-1 seems to play a role in counteracting the vasoconstrictor effect of ET-1 in the stressed liver. Up to now, it remains unknown whether this mediator system is relevant in patients with portal hypertension.

In contrast to CO and NO, much less is reported about the role of H_2S in the regulation of hepatic microvascular blood flow. H_2S is a gaseous neuromodulator that exerts potent vasodilatory effects in both the systemic and the

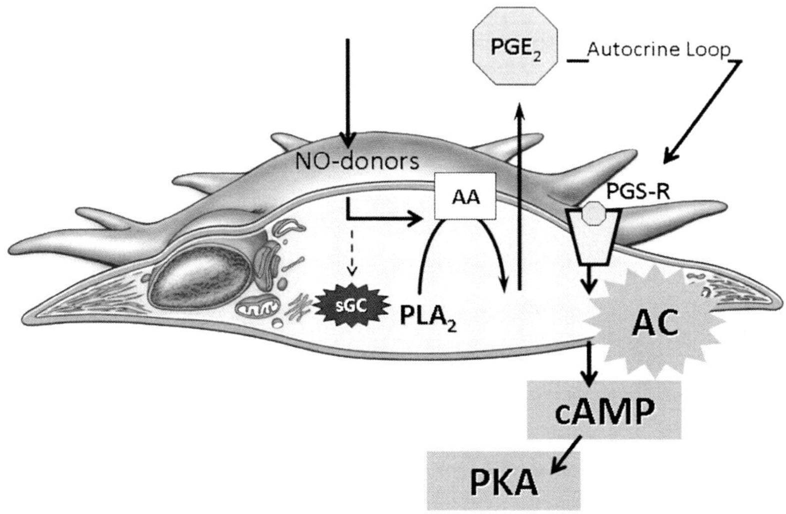

Fig. 4.6 Defective soluble guanylate cyclase (sGC)/cGMP pathway in activated human stellate cells (Failli et al. [64]). The effects of NO on activated human HSC do not seem to be related to the activation of the classic soluble guanylate cyclase (sGC)/cGMP pathway, whose expression progressively decreases with the process of activation but rather to an increased synthesis of prostaglandin E_2 associated with an increase in intracellular cAMP levels, thus indicating a predominant activation of the adenylate cyclase/cAMP pathway (modified from original cartoon courtesy of Prof. V.J. Shah)

splanchnic circulation [74, 75]. In normal livers, H_2S treatment, from either exogenous (NaHS supplementation) or endogenous (l-cysteine supplementation) sources, reverses the norepinephrine-induced increase of portal pressure [74]. Unlike NO, H_2S is not produced by sinusoidal endothelial cells (SEC), as they express none of the two H_2S-generating enzymes (cystathionine-lyase (CSE) and cystathionine-synthetase (CBS)), but is released from the CSE-expressing stellate cells [74]. The fact that H_2S released by normal rat livers is not modified by increased shear stress underscores that sites different from that of SEC are involved in the synthesis of H_2S [74]. This is in agreement with the observation that modulation of intrahepatic resistance by H_2S is not dependent on NO [74]. Although endothelial dysfunction caused by hyperhomocysteinemia leads to defective NO bioavailability, homocysteine-induced impairment of NO release can be reversed by H_2S in an NO-independent manner, indicating that NO and H_2S exert additive effects in the liver microcirculation [76].

Somatostatin is able to reduce portal pressure by several mechanisms [77]. In addition to direct effects on portal blood flow, activation of the somatostatin receptor subtype 1 induces partial inhibition of endothelin-1-induced contraction of rat HSC [78]. More recently, intravital fluorescence microscopy experiments have shown that somatostatin, but not octreotide, induces dilatation of hepatic sinusoids at the site of HSC, thereby reducing intrahepatic vascular resistance [79].

References

1. Wake K. Liver perivascular cells revealed by gold and silver impregnation methods and electron microscopy. In: Motta P, editor. Biopathology of the liver, an ultrastructural approach. Dordrecht: Kluwer; 1988. p. 23–6.
2. Wake K. Hepatic stellate cells. In: Tanikawa K, Ueno T, editors. Liver diseases and hepatic sinusoidal cells. Tokyo: Springer; 1999. p. 56–65.
3. Wake K. Structure of the sinusoidal wall in the liver. In: Wisse E, Knook DL, Wake K, editors. Cells of the hepatic sinusoid. Leiden: The Kupffer Cell Foundation; 1995. p. 241–6.

4. Wake K, Motomatsu K, Ekataksin W. Postnatal development of the perisinusoidal stellate cells in the rat liver. In: Wisse E, Knook DL, McCuskey RS, editors. Cells of the hepatic sinusoid. Leiden: The Kupffer Cell Foundation; 1991. p. 269–75.
5. Gressner AM, Lofti S, Gressner G, Lahme B. Identification and partial characterization of a hepatocyte-derived factor promoting proliferation of cultured fat-storing cells (parasinusoidal lipocytes). Hepatology. 1992;16:1250–66.
6. Ballardini G, Groff P, Badiali de Giorgi L, Schuppan D, Bianchi FB. Ito cell heterogeneity: desmin-negative Ito cells in normal rat liver. Hepatology. 1994; 19:440–6.
7. Zou Z, Ekataksin W, Wake K. Zonal and regional differences identified from precision mapping of vitamin A-storing lipid droplets of the hepatic stellate cells in pig liver: a novel concept of addressing the intralobular area of heterogeneity. Hepatology. 1998;27:1098–108.
8. Higashi N, Senoo H. Distribution of vitamin A-storing lipid droplets in hepatic stellate cells in liver lobules-a comparative study. Anat Rec A Discov Mol Cell Evol Biol. 2003;271:240–8.
9. Wake K. Perisinusoidal stellate cells (fat-storing cells, interstitial cells, lipocytes), their related structure in and around the liver sinusoids, and vitamin A-storing cells in extrahepatic organs. Int Rev Cytol. 1980; 66:303–53.
10. Lafon ME, Bioulac-Sage P, LeBail N. Nerves and perisinusoidal cells in human liver. In: Wisse E, Knook DL, Decker K, editors. Cells of hepatic sinusoid. Riswijk: Kupffer Cell Foundation; 1989. p. 230–4.
11. Ueno T, Inuzuka S, Torimura T, Sakata R, Sakamoto M, Gondo K, et al. Distribution of substance P and vasoactive intestinal peptide in the human liver. Light and electron immunoperoxidase methods of observation. Am J Gastroenterol. 1991;138:1233–42.
12. Knittel T, Aurisch S, Neubauer K, Eichhorst S, Ramadori G. Cell-type-specific expression of neural cell adhesion molecule (N-CAM) in Ito cells of rat liver. Am J Pathol. 1996;149:449–62.
13. Niki T, Pekny M, Hellemans K, De Bleser P, Van Den Berg K, Vaeyens F, et al. Class VI intermediate filament protein nestin is induced during activation of rat hepatic stellate cells. Hepatology. 1999;29:520–7.
14. Cassiman D, Denef C, Desmet V, Roskams T. Human and rat hepatic stellate cells express neurotrophins and neurotrophin receptors. Hepatology. 2001;33:148–58.
15. Geerts A. On the origin of stellate cells: mesodermal, endodermal or neuro-ectodermal? J Hepatol. 2004; 40:331–4.
16. Pinzani M, Gentilini P. Biology of hepatic stellate cells and their possible relevance in the pathogenesis of portal hypertension in cirrhosis. Semin Liver Dis. 1999;19:397–410.
17. Pinzani M, Failli P, Ruocco C, Casini A, Milani S, Baldi E, et al. Fat-storing cells as liver-specific pericytes. Spatial dynamics of agonist-stimulated intracellular calcium transients. J Clin Invest. 1992;90:642–6.
18. Ekataksin W, Kaneda K. Liver microvascular architecture: an insight into the pathophysiology of portal hypertension. Sem Liv Dis. 1999;19:359–82.
19. Zhang JX, Pegoli Jr W, Clemens MG. Endothelin-1 induces direct constriction of hepatic sinusoids. Am J Physiol. 1994;266:G624–32.
20. Zhang JX, Bauer M, Clemens MG. Vessel- and target cell-specific actions of endothelin-1 and endothelin-3 in rat liver. Am J Physiol. 1995;269:G269–77.
21. Thimgan MS, Yee Jr HF. Quantitation of rat hepatic stellate cell contraction: stellate cells' contribution to sinusoidal tone. Am J Physiol. 1999;277:G137–43.
22. Kawada N, Klein H, Decker K. Eicoesanoid-mediated contractility of hepatic stellate cells. Biochem J. 1992;285:367–71.
23. Rockey DC, Housset CN, Friedman SL. Activation-dependent contractility of rat hepatic lipocytes in culture and in vivo. J Clin Invest. 1993;92:1795–804.
24. Rockey DC, Weisiger RA. Endothelin induced contractility of stellate cells from normal and cirrhotic rat liver: implications for regulation of portal pressure and resistance. Hepatology. 1996;24:233–40.
25. Bataller R, Nicolas JM, Gines P, Gorbig N, Garcia-Ramallo E, Lario S, et al. Contraction of human hepatic stellate cells activated in culture: a role for voltage-operated calcium channels. J Hepatol. 1998;29:398–408.
26. Lee KS, Buck M, Houglum K, Chojkier M. Activation of hepatic stellate cells by TGF alpha and collagen type I is mediated by oxidative stress through c-myb expression. J Clin Invest. 1995;96:2461–8.
27. Yee Jr HF. Rho directs activation-associated changes in rat hepatic stellate cell morphology via regulation of the actin cytoskeleton. Hepatology. 1998;28:843–50.
28. Iwamoto H, Sakai H, Nawata H. Inhibition of integrin signaling with Arg-Gly-Asp motifs in rat hepatic stellate cells. J Hepatol. 1998;29:752–9.
29. Yee Jr HF. Ca^{2+} and rho signaling pathways: two paths to hepatic stellate cell contraction. Hepatology. 2001;33:1007–8.
30. Laleman W, Van Landeghem L, Severi T, Vander Elst I, Zeegers M, Bisschops R, et al. Both Ca^{2+} -dependent and -independent pathways are involved in rat hepatic stellate cell contraction and intrahepatic hyperresponsiveness to methoxamine. Am J Physiol Gastrointest Liver Physiol. 2007;292:G556–64.
31. Bataller R, Gasull X, Gines P, Hellemans K, Gorbig MN, Nicolas JM, et al. In vitro and in vivo activation of rat hepatic stellate cells results in de novo expression of L-type voltage-operated calcium channels. Hepatology. 2001;33:956–62.
32. Tao J, Mallat A, Gallois C, Belmadani S, Mery PF, Tran-Van Nhieu J, et al. Biological effects of C-type natriuretic peptide in human myofibroblastic stellate cells. J Biol Chem. 1999;274:23761–9.
33. Bataller R, Nicolas JM, Ginees P, Gorbig MN, Garcia-Ramallo E, Lario S, et al. Contraction of human hepatic stellate cells activated in culture: a role for voltage-operated calcium channels. J Hepatol. 1998; 29:398–408.

34. Sah VP, Seasholtz TM, Sagi SA, Brown JH. The role of Rho in G protein-coupled receptor signal transduction. Annu Rev Pharmacol Toxicol. 2000;40:459–89.
35. Ridley AJ, Hall A. The small GTP-binding protein rho regulates the assembly of focal adhesions and actin stress fibers in response to growth factors. Cell. 1992;70:389–99.
36. Amano M, Chihara K, Kimura K, et al. Formation of actin stress fibers and focal adhesions enhanced by Rho-kinase. Science. 1997;275:1308–11.
37. Amano M, Fukata Y, Kaibuchi K. Regulation and functions of Rho-associated kinase. Exp Cell Res. 2000;261:44–51.
38. Yanase M, Ikeda H, Matsui A, et al. Lysophosphatidic acid enhancescollagen gel contraction by hepatic stellate cells: association with rho-kinase. Biochem Biophys Res Commun. 2000;277:72–8.
39. Kawada N, Seki S, Kuroki T, et al. ROCK inhibitor Y-27632 attenuates stellate cell contraction and portal pressure increase induced by endothelin-1. Biochem Biophys Res Commun. 1999;266:296–300.
40. Barton M, Yanagisawa M. Endothelin: 20 years from discovery to therapy. Can J Physiol Pharmacol. 2008;86:485–98.
41. Kedzierski RM, Yanagisawa M. Endothelin system: the double-edged sword in health and disease. Annu Rev Pharmacol Toxicol. 2001;41:851–76.
42. Bauer M, Bauer I, Sonin NV, Kresge N, Baveja R, Yokoyama Y, et al. Clemens MG.Functional significance of endothelin B receptors in mediating sinusoidal and extrasinusoidal effects of endothelins in the intact rat liver. Hepatology. 2000;31:937–47.
43. Clozel M, Gray GA, Breu V, Breu V, Löffler BM, Osterwalder R. The endothelin ETB receptor mediates both vasodilation and vasoconstriction in vivo. Biochem Biophys Res Commun. 1992;186:867–73.
44. Higuchi H, Satoh T. Endothelin-1 induces vasoconstriction and nitric oxide release via endothelin ET(B) receptors in isolated perfused rat liver. Eur J Pharmacol. 1997;328:175–82.
45. Housset C, Rockey DC, Bissell DM. Endothelin receptors in rat liver: lipocytes as a contractile target for endothelin 1. Proc Natl Acad Sci USA. 1993;90: 9266–70.
46. Serradeil-Le Gal C, Jouneaux C, Sanchez-Bueno A, Raufaste D, Roche B, Préaux AM, et al. Endothelin action in rat liver. Receptors, free Ca2+ oscillations, and activation of glycogenolysis. J Clin Invest. 1991;87:133–8.
47. Kuddus RH, Nalesnik MA, Subbotin VM, Rao AS, Gandhi CR. Enhanced synthesis and reduced metabolism of endothelin-1 (ET-1) by hepatocytes – an important mechanism of increased endogenous levels of ET-1 in liver cirrhosis. J Hepatol. 2000;33: 725–32.
48. Pinzani M, Milani S, DeFranco R, Grappone C, Caligiuri A, Gentilini A, et al. Endothelin 1 is overexpressed in human cirrhotic liver and exerts multiple effects on activated hepatic stellate cells. Gastroenterology. 1996;110: 534–48.
49. Rockey DC, Fouassier L, Chung JJ, Carayon A, Vallee P, Rey C, et al. Cellular localization of endothelin-1 and increased production in liver injury in the rat: potential for autocrine and paracrine effects on stellate cells. Hepatology. 1998;27:472–80.
50. Reinehr RM, Kubitz R, Peters-Regehr T, Bode JG, Haussinger D. Activation of rat hepatic stellate cells in culture is associated with increased sensitivity to endothelin 1. Hepatology. 1998;28:1566–77.
51. Mallat A, Fouassier F, Preaux AM, Serradeil-Le Gal C, Raufaste D, Rosembaum J, et al. Growth inhibitory properties of endothelin-1 in human hepatic myofibroblastic Ito cells: an endothelin B receptor-mediated pathway. J Clin Invest. 1995;96:42–9.
52. Mallat A, Preaux A-M, Serradeil-Le Gal C, Raufaste D, Gallois C, Brenner DA, et al. Growth inhibitory properties of endothelin-1 in activated human hepatic stellate cells: a cyclic adenosine monophosphate-mediated pathway. J Clin Invest. 1996;98:2771–8.
53. Zhan S, Chan CC, Serdar B, Rockey DC. Fibronectin stimulates endothelin-1 synthesis in rat hepatic myofibroblasts via a Src/ERK-regulated signaling pathway. Gastroenterology. 2009;136:2345–55.
54. Leivas A, Jimenez W, Bruix J, Boix L, Bosch J, Arroyo V, et al. Gene expression of endothelin-1 and ET(A) and ET(B) receptors in human cirrhosis: relationship with hepatic hemodynamics. J Vasc Res. 1998;35:186–93.
55. Bataller R, Gines P, Nicolas JM, Gorbig MN, Garcia-Ramallo E, Gasull X, et al. Angiotensin II induces contraction and proliferation of human hepatic stellate cells. Gastroenterology. 2000;118:1149–56.
56. Zhang Y, Yang X, Wu P, Xu L, Liao G, Yang G. Expression of angiotensin II type 1 receptor in rat hepatic stellate cells and its effects on cell growth and collagen production. Horm Res. 2003;60:105–10.
57. Bataller R, Sancho-Bru P, Gines P, Lora JM, Al Garawi A, Sole M, et al. Activated human hepatic stellate cells express the renin-angiotensin system and synthesize angiotensin II. Gastroenterology. 2003;125:117–25.
58. Moreno M, Bataller R. Cytokines and renin-angiotensin system signaling in hepatic fibrosis. Clin Liver Dis. 2008;12:825–52.
59. Bataller R, Sancho-Bru P, Gines P, et al. Liver fibrogenesis: a new role for the renin-angiotensin system. Antioxid Redox Signal. 2007;7:1346–55.
60. Wiest R, Groszmann RJ. Nitric oxide and portal hypertension: its role in the regulation of intrahepatic and splanchnic vascularresistance. Semin Liver Dis. 1999;19:411–26.
61. Kawada N, Tran-Thi TA, Klein H, Decker K. The contraction of hepatic stellate (Ito) cells stimulated with vasoactive substances. Possible involvement of endothelin 1 and nitric oxide in the regulation of the sinusoidal tonus. Eur J Biochem. 1993;213:815–23.
62. Rockey DC, Chung JJ. Inducible nitric oxide synthase in rat hepatic lipocytes and the effect of nitric oxide on lipocyte contractility. J Clin Invest. 1995;95: 1199–206.

63. Failli P, De Franco RM, Caligiuri A, Gentilini A, Romanelli RG, Marra F, et al. Nitrovasodilators inhibit platelet-derived growth factor-induced proliferation and migration of activated human hepatic stellate cells. Gastroenterology. 2000;119:479–92.
64. Zhou Q, Hennenberg M, Trebicka J, Jochem K, Leifeld L, Biecker E, et al. Intrahepatic upregulation of RhoA and Rho-kinase signalling contributes to increased hepatic vascular resistance in rats with secondary biliary cirrhosis. Gut. 2006;55:1296–305.
65. Zipprich A, Steudel N, Behrmann C, Meiss F, Sziegoleit U, Fleig WE, et al. Functional significance of hepatic arterial flow reserve in patients with cirrhosis. Hepatology. 2003;37:385–92.
66. Laleman W, Van Landeghem L, Van der Elst I, Zeegers M, Fevery J, Nevens F. Nitroflurbiprofen, a nitric oxide-releasing cyclooxygenase inhibitor, improves cirrhotic portal hypertension in rats. Gastroenterology. 2007;132:709–19.
67. Sohail MA, Hashmi AZ, Hakim W, Watanabe A, Zipprich A, Groszmann RJ, et al. Adenosine induces loss of actin stress fibers and inhibits contraction in hepatic stellate cells via Rho inhibition. Hepatology. 2009;49:185–94.
68. Goda N, Suzuki K, Naito M, Takeoka S, Tsuchida E, Ishimura Y, et al. Distribution of heme oxygenase isoforms in rat liver. Topographic basis for carbon monoxide-mediated microvascular relaxation. J Clin Invest. 1998;101:604–12.
69. Fernandez M, Bonkovsky HL. Increased heme oxygenase-1 gene expression in liver cells and splanchnic organs from portal hypertensive rats. Hepatology. 1999;29:1672–9.
70. Makino N, Suematsu M, Sugiura Y, Morikawa H, Shiomi S, Goda N, et al. Altered expression of heme oxygenase-1 in the livers of patients with portal hypertensive diseases. Hepatology. 2001;33:32–42.
71. Matsumi M, Takahashi T, Fujii H, Ohashi I, Kaku R, Nakatsuka H, et al. Increased heme oxygenase-1 gene expression in the livers of patients with portal hypertension due to severe hepatic cirrhosis. J Int Med Res. 2002;30:282–8.
72. Wakabayashi Y, Takamiya R, Mizuki A, Kyokane T, Goda N, Yamaguchi T, et al. Carbon monoxide overproduced by heme oxygenase-1 causes a reduction of vascular resistance in perfused rat liver. Am J Physiol. 1999;277:G1088–96.
73. Rensing H, Bauer I, Zhang JX, Paxian M, Pannen BH, Yokoyama Y, et al. Endothelin-1 and heme oxygenase-1 as modulators of sinusoidal tone in the stress-exposed rat liver. Hepatology. 2002;36:1453–65.
74. Rizzo G, Distrutti E, Shah V, Morelli A. The third gas: H2S regulates perfusion pressure in both the isolated and perfused normal rat liver and in cirrhosis. Hepatology. 2005;42:539–48.
75. Fiorucci S, Distrutti E, Cirino G, Wallace JL. The emerging roles of hydrogen sulfide in the gastrointestinal tract and liver. Gastroenterology. 2006;131:259–71.
76. Distrutti E, Mencarelli A, Santucci L, Renga B, Orlandi S, Donini A, et al. The methionine connection: homocysteine and hydrogen sulfide exert opposite effects on hepatic microcirculation in rats. Hepatology. 2008;47:659–67.
77. Reynaert H, Geerts A. Pharmacological rationale for the use of somatostatin and analogues in portal hypertension. Aliment Pharmacol Ther. 2003;18:375–86.
78. Reynaert H, Vaeyens F, Qin H, Hellemans K, Chatterjee N, Winand D, et al. Somatostatin suppresses endothelin-1-induced rat hepatic stellate cell contraction via somatostatin receptor subtype 1. Gastroenterology. 2001;121:915–30.
79. Vanheule E, Geerts AM, Reynaert H, Van Vlierberghe H, Geerts A, De Vos M, et al. Influence of somatostatin and octreotide on liver microcirculation in an experimental mouse model of cirrhosis studied by intravital fluorescence microscopy. Liver Int. 2008;28:107–16.
80. Wake K, Sato T. Intralobular heterogeneity of perisinusoidal stellate cells in porcine liver. Cell Tissue Res. 1993;273:227–37.
81. Wake K. In: Vidal-Vanaclocha F, editor. Functional heterogeneity of liver tissue. Austin: RG Landes Co; 1977.

Circulatory Injury in Liver Transplantation

5

Ashraf Mohammad El-Badry, Philipp Dutkowski, and Pierre-Alain Clavien

Abstract

Optimum graft function after liver transplantation is dependent on adequate sinusoidal perfusion. Hepatic microcirculation may be compromised by several factors such as cold ischemia, quality of the liver graft, handling of the organ during surgery, surgical procedure, and reperfusion injury. This chapter will focus on the pathological consequences of cold preservation and reperfusion injury on hepatic microcirculation. Microcirculatory dysfunction in grafts donated after cardiac death as well as steatotic grafts will be underlined. We will summarize the effects of graft manipulation and denervation during surgery. Furthermore, we will discuss the contribution of microcirculatory failure to graft rejection. Finally, recent advances in visualization and assessment of human hepatic microcirculation will be highlighted.

Keywords

Liver transplantation • Microcirculation • Ischemia/reperfusion • Liver steatosis • Graft rejection

Abbreviations

DCD	Donation after cardiac death
I/R	Ischemia/reperfusion
OLT	Orthotopic liver transplantation
PG	Prostaglandin
TNF	Tumor necrosis factor
ROS	Reactive oxygen species
TX	Thromboxane

P.-A. Clavien (✉)
Department of Surgery, University Hospital of Zurich, Ramistrase 100, CH-8091 Zurich, Switzerland
e-mail: clavien@access.uzh.ch

Introduction

Among several features that render the liver a "unique" organ are the dual blood supply and the distinctive microcirculation. Therefore, adequate hepatic circulation is mandatory for appropriate graft function after transplantation. Ischemia/reperfusion (I/R)-induced impairment of hepatic microcirculation during cold preservation and subsequent implantation of the liver graft is associated with high morbidity and occasional mortality. In addition, a number of other factors are substantially implicated in jeopardizing sinusoidal perfusion such as donation after cardiac death, the quality of the liver graft parenchyma, graft handling and denervation, and rejection.

L.D. DeLeve and G. Garcia-Tsao (eds.), *Vascular Liver Disease: Mechanisms and Management*,
DOI 10.1007/978-1-4419-8327-5_5,

Numerous techniques for assessment of the hepatic microcirculation were examined in experimental animal models and enabled a more thorough understanding of the physiology and pathophysiology of hepatic microvascular perfusion. The introduction of new techniques such as orthogonal polarization spectral (OPS) imaging and its successor sidestream dark field (SDF) imaging may extend the potential of early diagnosis and treatment of microcirculatory derangements in the experimental and clinical settings.

Impact of Ischemia/Reperfusion on Microcirculation of the Liver Graft

Reperfusion of the liver after ischemic insults triggers a cascade of pathological events including disintegration of the sinusoidal endothelial cells, sinusoidal constriction, an inflammatory reaction, stagnation of leukocytes and platelet aggregation with microthrombi formation. Eventually, these alterations result in microcirculatory and hepatocellular damage and consequently liver failure [1].

Liver transplantation encompasses two forms of liver ischemia, namely cold and rewarming ischemia; both induce hepatocellular injury even though the mechanisms are different. Cold ischemia occurs during organ retrieval; when the liver is cooled, perfused and then stored in a cold preservation solution. Several morphologic alterations in the sinusoidal endothelial cells, including cell swelling and loss of cytoplasmic processes, have been described during cold preservation [2]. These structural changes result from pathological processes involving the cytoskeleton and extracellular matrix [3]. While most of the sinusoidal endothelial cells survive during the period of cold ischemia, they rapidly slough into the sinusoidal lumen on reperfusion [4]. The extent of this endothelial cell detachment is directly related to the duration of cold ischemia [5].

On the other hand, rewarming ischemia is encountered during back table graft preparation and also at the stage of implantation while performing the vascular anastomoses. Rapid decrease in cellular energy stores and accumulation of electron donors occur during this stage.

Afterwards, exposure of ischemic liver tissue to oxygen at normothermic temperature (37°C) leads to severe aggravation of injury, termed reperfusion injury. All hepatic cells, including Kupffer cells, hepatocytes, endothelial cells and stellate cells appear to be activated at this stage by different mechanisms. Importantly, a synergistic action of blood elements (platelets), Kupffer cells, and hepatocytes is mandatory [6], but the exact sequence of reactions remains unknown. However, current evidence points to the release of reactive oxygen species (ROS) as a decisive initiating factor [7]. All hepatic cells can generate ROS, but they use different mechanisms and different cellular compartments. Kupffer cells and endothelial cells produce vascular ROS by activation of membrane bound NADPH oxidase [8]. Hepatocytes release intracellular ROS through mitochondria or xanthine oxidase [8]. Activated Kupffer cells release soluble inflammatory mediators such as tumor necrosis factor (TNF)-α and interleukin-6 and also vasoactive molecules such as nitric oxide and endothelin-1 [9]. Importantly, hepatocytes may activate Kupffer cells through activation of NF-κB by mitochondrial ROS [10]. Several consequences have been described following these initial events. The high amount of ROS results in an imbalance of endothelin and nitric oxide, leading to a relative excess of endothelin. These endothelins are most likely released by Kupffer cells and stellate cells in response to hypoxia, ROS, proinflammatory cytokines, and bacterial lipopolysaccharides. The imbalance between endothelins and vascular nitric oxide levels narrows sinusoids and reduces microcirculatory perfusion [11]. Consequently, hepatic cellular oxygen supply is decreased resulting in intracellular edema, decreased erythrocyte velocity, and extravasation of red blood cells due to loss of endothelial integrity. Blood stasis causes further progressive ischemia and activation of leukocytes. Simultaneously, alterations of the sinusoidal endothelial cell surface also activates first platelets [12] and later leukocytes [5], resulting in clogging of the sinusoidal lumen and impairment of microvascular perfusion [13]. Mitochondrial damage, either by electron transfer interruption due to electron leakage and opening of the mitochondrial permeable transition pore or by receptor activation of t-bid, induces further reduction of cellular ATP levels and initiation of the complex apoptotic machinery [14].

I/R injury provokes two distinctive manifestations of microvascular damage known as capillary "no-reflow" and the "reflow-paradox." The "no-reflow" phenomenon is characterized by lack of blood flow upon onset of reperfusion, most likely due to swelling of the microvascular endothelium, hemoconcentration, and imbalance between vasoactive mediators [15]. The "reflow-paradox" refers to leukocyte stasis and adherence to the lining endothelium in postcapillary and collecting venules and occurs after the reestablishment of microvascular perfusion and reoxygenation following reperfusion [15]. Among other contributors to the "reflow-paradox" are complement, thromboxane A_2, platelet-activating factor, TNF-α(alpha), interleukin-1, endothelin-1, and fatty acid components of hepatic lipids [2, 16].

Microcirculatory Dysfunction in Grafts Donated after Cardiac Death

During procurement, sufficient microvascular perfusion of the donor liver with preservation solution is essential to achieve appropriate graft function after implantation. The use of liver allografts donated after cardiac death (DCD) can be lifesaving for patients with end-stage liver disease. However, experience in human DCD liver transplantation is limited because of the high risk of primary graft failure or later biliary complications, which are reported in up to 55% of cases [17]. While the use of such donors may have the potential to substantially increase donor pools, these grafts obviously require an improved preservation and implantation strategy due to severe impairment of hepatic microcirculation. A number of strategies, mostly experimental in nature, have been proposed for amelioration of hepatic microcirculation. So far three different approaches can be distinguished: first, improvement of liver microcirculation during initial flush by thrombolysis and vasodilatation; second, oxygenation of the graft before organ procurement or during preservation; and third, cytoprotective strategies in the donor and/or recipient.

Refinement of Microcirculation During Organ Procurement

The administration of streptokinase during the cold flush of the ischemic liver has been shown to improve microvascular perfusion and to reduce hepatocellular enzyme release in rat ex vivo reperfusion after warm ischemia [18, 19]. The vasodilatory effect of a warm preflush in DCD liver grafts is reported by several groups. These effects can even be enhanced by adding prostaglandins in the flush perfusate. Also, the use of low viscosity cold flush solutions (polysol, celsior) has led to lower vascular resistance and improved survival of DCD livers if applied directly after harvest with minimal cold storage time [20–22].

Oxygenation of the Graft

Either in situ warm or ex situ warm or cold machine perfusion has successfully rescued warm or cold ischemia-damaged livers. Several interesting approaches have been recently published. The group from Barcelona described an approach where potential human donors are put on cardiopulmonary oxygenated support before organ procurement for several hours to maintain organ function. The results show, however, that many grafts treated by this technique had to be turned down after procurement because of heterogeneous flush. Ten out of 40 grafts were transplanted, five recipients survived [23]. Alternatively, the group of P. Friend in Oxford recently demonstrated that an extracorporeal normothermic machine perfusion through the hepatic artery and the portal vein with diluted donor blood was able to protect DCD pig livers against 40 min of warm in situ ischemia. In this model, the ischemic liver was subjected to 20 h of normothermic machine perfusion resulting in 5-day survival of five out of six animals after OLT [24].

One general disadvantage of the normothermic approach is that perfusion needs to be initiated immediately after organ procurement, i.e., before organ transport. Our group has therefore put a major emphasis on the practicability of machine perfusion. With this aim, we developed a hypothermic concept favoring end-ischemic hypothermic oxygenated perfusion (HOPE) through the portal vein only, which can easily be applied after organ transport and back table preparation. Recent results showed protection of pig liver grafts after 60 min of warm in situ ischemia combined with 6 h of cold storage [25]. In spite of all this experimental success, long-term data on human graft function are urgently needed. For example, it is unclear whether the high incidence of bile duct injury associated with DCD donors can be prevented with any kind of perfusion approach.

Cytoprotective Strategies

Pharmacological treatment of donors has been reported to be effective in various animal models [26–29], but donor conditioning in humans is limited due to ethical reasons. A few studies describe improvement of DCD livers without pretreatment of the donor. These studies target recipient Kupffer cell activation (glycine, p38 mitogen-acivated protein kinase (MAPK) inhibitor, and pentoxifylline), release of ROS (glutathione, tocopherol, apotransferrin) or vasodilatation (endothelin antagonist, nitric oxide donor). In this context, Gu et al. [30] reported porcine liver graft protection after 45 min of warm in situ ischemia and 8 h of cold storage by applying an endothelin antagonist (TAK-044) and a platelet-activating factor antagonist (E5880) to the preservation solution and the recipient [30]. While most studies focus on one specific cell type or molecule, current approaches favor a multifactorial approach combining the advantages of many studies. A very recent example of this promising approach of multifactorial biological modulation is the use of a cocktail including streptokinase, epoprostenol, glycine, glutathione, apotransferrin, α(alpha)1-acid glycoprotein, α(alpha)-tocopherol, and MAPK inhibitor. Applying these substances during flush, before, and during implantation led to improved survival in a clinical relevant pig liver DCD model [31]. Combinations of substances, such as sevoflurane, steroids, caspase inhibitors, and pentoxifylline, are conceivable [32]. However, translating all these strategies to the clinic still requires more understanding of the mechanisms of ischemia–reperfusion injury in normal and especially in marginal organs.

Liver Steatosis and Graft Microcirculatory Failure

Impairment of hepatic microcirculation in fatty liver grafts increases their susceptibility to I/R injury. The reduction of sinusoidal perfusion has long been thought to arise from enlargement of hepatic parenchymal cells due to accumulated lipid, widening of the parenchymal cell plates, and narrowing and distortion of the sinusoidal lumen which eventually reduces the intrasinusoidal volume [33]. However, studies demonstrating that the sinusoidal diameter in the fatty liver of Zucker rats is not significantly narrowed compared with their lean littermates [34] and similar data from steatotic ob/ob mice [35] do not support this theory. Alternatively, there is emerging evidence on the impact of the composition of hepatic lipids on the liver microcirculation and reperfusion injury [36].

The effect of steatosis on the liver microcirculation and hepatocellular injury remains a matter of debate since the assessment of the grade and stage of nonalcoholic fatty liver disease traditionally relies on microscopic evaluation by pathologists [16]. Consequently, several studies have demonstrated that hepatic steatosis represents a substantial risk factor for poor outcome after major liver resection [37–40] and OLT [41–45], while other reports did not document a negative effect [46–50]. The microscopic diagnosis of hepatic steatosis has several pitfalls, which may considerably hamper the pathologist's interpretation. The number of biopsy samples has been shown to significantly influence the histological assessment of steatosis [51]. Certain variants of hepatic steatosis, such as focal steatosis, hypersteatosis and hepatic fatty sparing [52], may confound the pathologist's evaluation when a single biopsy is used for the histological assessment. Moreover, different fixatives can modify the diagnosis of hepatic steatosis by induction of artifactual fusions or collapse of lipid droplets. Cold methanol enhances fusion of lipid droplets while acetone fixation leads to their disintegration [53]. Furthermore, visualization of lipid droplets is obviously prejudiced by the staining method. Lipid droplets stained with Nile red have a different appearance than those stained by Sudan III, and oil red O [54]. In an interesting study on liver transplant donors, marked hepatic steatosis (>30%) was identified in 49% of patients when sections were stained with Sudan III compared with 38% and 21% of patients, respectively, using frozen or deparaffinated hematoxylin and eosin (H & E)-stained sections [55].

Lack of agreement was recently reported among different pathologists performing histological evaluation of liver steatosis. High interobserver disagreement was documented among expert pathologists regarding both the quantitative and qualitative estimation of steatosis and steatohepatitis [56]. The assessment of liver sections by four prominent pathologists from well-known centers in Europe and North America showed poor concordance regarding the degree of total macro- and microsteatosis. Lack of agreement also was noted for the semiquantitative assessment; for instance, the diagnosis of marked steatosis (≥30%) varied from 22% to 46%. Disagreement among pathologists was also apparent with regard to the assessment of the parameters of steatohepatitis (lobular and portal inflammation, hepatocyte ballooning, and Mallory's hyaline) as well as its overall diagnosis [56]. These astonishing results probably clarify the discrepancy among numerous published studies on the relevance of liver steatosis to liver surgery and transplantation. Given the failure of histological evaluation of hepatic steatosis to predict clinical outcome, this directs attention to the potential role of the chemical composition of hepatic lipids, particularly fatty acids [16, 36, 56].

Mouse models of hepatic steatosis have broadened our knowledge of the hepatic microcirculation. Significant baseline microcirculatory impairment was demonstrated in a mouse model of macrosteatosis (ob/ob mice). Impaired hepatic microcirculation was evidenced by reduced functional sinusoidal density in comparison with lean and microsteatotic liver models (wild-type mice on control or choline-deficient diet, respectively). Defective sinusoidal perfusion in livers with predominance of macrosteatosis was associated with more pronounced hepatic damage after warm I/R. Amelioration of sinusoidal perfusion by means of prolonged dietary supplementation of ob/ob mice with Ω(omega)-3 fatty acids resulted in significant improvement of hepatic microvascular perfusion before ischemia, which markedly protected the liver against microcirculatory and hepatocellular damage after reperfusion [36]. In another study, hepatic arterial and microcirculatory flow were significantly lower in steatotic compared with lean rat liver. Both parameters could be significantly improved by intravenous bolus administrations of L-arginine [57], through its action as precursor of nitric oxide [58]. Similarly, prolonged supplementation of Ω(omega)-3 fatty acids in patients with hepatic steatosis improved biochemical and ultrasonographic features of liver steatosis and decreased serum transaminases and triglycerides. Concomitantly, Doppler perfusion index was increased compared with control patients [59]. In the setting of human OLT, a multichannel laser Doppler flowmeter was used to assess microcirculatory alterations due to hepatic fatty infiltration. Sinusoidal perfusion was documented to be significantly reduced in fatty compared to lean liver grafts [60].

The impact of fat composition, particularly, content of Ω(omega)-3 and Ω-6 fatty acids, on sinusoidal perfusion and I/R injury was recently demonstrated [16]. Metabolism of dihomo-γ(gamma)-linolenic, arachidonic (Ω-6), and eicosapentaenoic (Ω-3) acids results in the synthesis of vasoactive mediators with a significant effect on the liver microcirculation. These long-chain fatty acids are released from cell membranes by phospholipase A_2 and serve as substrates for cyclooxygenase and lipoxygenase enzymes.

Each enzymatic pathway results in synthesis of specific Ω-6 and Ω-3 prostanoids. Products of the cyclooxygenase pathway include prostaglandins and thromboxanes while leukotrienes are synthesized through lipooxygenase-mediated reactions. With an elevated Ω-6:Ω-3 FA ratio, the metabolite profile is altered [16]. Studies on rodents showed that prostaglandin E_1 (PGE_1) suppresses leukocyte adhesion to the sinusoidal endothelium and protects against I/R injury. Moreover, PGE_1 has an antiapoptotic effect on cultured human liver sinusoidal endothelial cells. Another mechanism of hepatocellular protection by PGE_1 has been shown in cultured rat hepatocytes treated with tert-butyl hydroperoxide, where PGE_1 reduced the oxidative stress-induced hepatocyte injury [16]. PGE_2 is another arachidonic acid-derived hepato-protective prostaglandin that is mainly released by Kupffer cells. Inhibition of PGE_2 synthesis contributes to hepatocyte damage [16]. TXA_2 is a strong vasoactive metabolite of arachidonic acid with powerful proaggregatory and proinflammatory properties. In a rat model of I/R, selective inhibition of TXA_2 synthase and specific blockage of TXA_2 receptors conferred protection of the sinusoidal lining cells, ameliorated liver necrosis, blunted serum transaminase levels, restored hepatic tissue blood flow and improved survival [61]. In humans, levels of circulating TXB_2, a downstream metabolite of TXA_2, were remarkably increased during hepatic resection. Intravenous administration of TXA_2 synthase inhibitor intraoperatively reduced plasma TXB_2 and concomitantly reduced serum transaminase levels [62]. Working in balance with TXA_2, prostacyclin (PGI_2) triggers several biological effects which oppose those of TXA_2. PGI_2 decreases platelet aggregation and leukocyte adhesion to the endothelial surface. In rats, a PGI_2 analog significantly reduced the microcirculatory impairment after reperfusion, reduced leukocyte adhesion, and improved flow velocity [16]. Very recently, a few live liver donors with moderate steatosis were treated with oral administration of Ω-3 fatty acids prior to right hemi-hepatectomy. This approach resulted in a remarkable reduction of steatosis grade and extent of macrosteatosis, and an uncomplicated postoperative course that could be attributed to improvement of the hepatic microcirculation [63]. This strategy may pave the way for safe expansion of the live liver donor pool from one of the most common marginal donors.

The Impact of Liver Denervation and Manipulation on Graft Microcirculation

Explantation of liver mandates transsection of the entire hepatic nerve supply of the graft. However, there is no evidence that denervation of the liver allograft significantly influences the outcome of OLT. To date, several studies on the effect of hepatic denervation on hepatic microcirculation have reported conflicting results [64]. Denervation of the rat liver was demonstrated to induce reduction of sinusoidal perfusion for 20 min with partial recovery afterwards [65]. Other studies demonstrated increased hepatic artery blood flow, a steady venous hepatic blood flow, or increased total hepatic blood flow [64]. In the situation of OLT, liver denervation before organ explanation was shown to prevent circulatory failure and primary nonfunction [66]. Thus, the impact of hepatic innervation on the hepatic microcirculation and the clinical outcome after OLT remains debatable.

Rat models of OLT have shown that retraction, touching and manipulation of the liver induces evident injury of the microcirculation, which contributes to increased tissue hypoxia, parenchymal cell injury and decrease of recipient survival [67]. Liver manipulation seems to activate Kupffer cells, increase the release of reactive oxygen, and subsequently induce microcirculatory impairment. Depletion of Kupffer cells by gadolinium chloride significantly rescues sinusoidal perfusion, protects against tissue hypoxia, and therefore improves recipient survival [68]. In the steatotic rat liver graft, organ manipulation before OLT resulted in pronounced reduction of graft survival [69]. Therefore, it appears that the extent of posttransplant microcirculatory derangements is triggered by a combination of cold and rewarming ischemia, the degree and type of intrahepatic lipids, and the surgical manipulation of the graft.

Thus, cautious handling of the liver graft appears to be imperative for graft function and, more importantly, to support the pharmacological strategies that could be applied to improve the graft function, particularly in the presence of steatosis.

Liver Circulation and Graft Rejection

The adequacy of sinusoidal perfusion seems to be intimately related to liver graft rejection. Microcirculatory derangements may represent the initial manifestation of rejection. Therefore, the hepatic microcirculation is considered a key target of immune-response-mediated graft destruction [15].

The relation between the hepatic microcirculation and acute graft rejection was studied in 43 patients who underwent OLT in Heidelberg. Using a thermodiffusion probe, the hepatic microcirculation was assessed during the first postoperative week after OLT. Graft rejection was diagnosed on the basis of increased serum aminotransferase levels and liver biopsy. Among the study group, acute rejection was confirmed in 15 patients. A significant reduction of sinusoidal perfusion was noted 36 h before the rise of serum aminotransferases. Interestingly, the impairment of sinusoidal perfusion correlated closely with the histological grade of graft rejection [70].

This phenomenon could be explained by the dual impact of intracellular adhesion molecule-I (ICAM-I) on the hepatic microcirculation and acute rejection. Up-regulation of ICAM-I occurs after reperfusion in conjunction with injury of the endothelial lining, particularly that of the postsinusoidal venules, and promotes adhesion of leukocytes and induction of hepatic microperfusion failure [2]. Likewise, it is known that T-cell activation, the cornerstone of liver graft rejection, partly results from increased expression of ICAM-I on hepatocytes [71]. Therefore, it is plausible to explain the cascade of impaired microcirculation-graft rejection by assuming that ICAM-I induces microvascular perfusion impairment and subsequent promotion of T-cell activation. Of note, in addition to I/R injury as the main determinant of impaired hepatic microcirculation, the rejection process is obviously involved in sinusoidal perfusion failure. In a rat model of OLT, graft rejection was associated with microcirculatory failure, leukocyte stagnation and adhesion. In addition, significant enhancement of the hepatic cord width, most probably due to swelling of parenchymal and sinusoidal lining cells, was noted [72]. In a model of isolated perfused rat liver, studies using intravital microscopy demonstrated that perfusion of rat liver with human blood induces microcirculatory derangements. Complement depletion by cobra venom factor and immunoabsorption and administration of acetylsalicylate and platelet-activating factor antagonists effectively ameliorate rejection-induced sinusoidal perfusion failure. Fucoidin, which inhibits selectin-dependent interactions white blood cells and platelets with the vascular endothelium, effectively improved sinusoidal perfusion failure and reduced platelet and leukocyte accumulation [15].

Alternatively, acute vascular rejection may be accentuated by impairment of the hepatic microcirculation. Based on experiments that show persistent impairment of the hepatic microcirculation in nonrearterialized liver grafts [73], the influence of defective graft microperfusion was studied in a model of rearterialized versus nonrearterialized hamster-to-rat OLT. With a short course of immunosuppression, recipients of rearterialized grafts exhibited significantly prolonged survival. Acute rejection was evident in nonrearterialized liver xenografts even under immunosuppressive therapy. The authors concluded that graft rejection may be accelerated by impaired hepatic microcirculation secondary to the lack of a hepatic arterial supply [74]. Furthermore, pharmacological prevention of I/R-induced microvascular reperfusion failure seems to reduce primary nonfunction and reduce the incidence of late graft rejection [15].

Assessment of Human Hepatic Microcirculation

Intravital fluorescence microscopy is successfully used for microcirculatory analysis of rodent liver. However, the use of the intravital microscope in human liver is limited by the large size, complex setup, and the need to inject toxic fluorescent dyes for contrast enhancement [15].

In 1999, Groner et al. published their report on OPS imaging, which allowed noninvasive visualization of the microcirculation. In OPS imaging, the liver is illuminated with linearly polarized light and imaged via a polarizer, which is placed orthogonal to the plane of the illuminating light. Only depolarized photons that are scattered in the liver contribute to the image [75].

In a validation study, the microcirculation of the rat liver was studied using OPS imaging and intravital fluorescence microscopy. Identical microvascular regions were examined before and after warm lobar ischemia. OPS imaging showed accurate quantification of the sinusoidal perfusion rate, vessel diameter, and venular red blood cell velocity with significant agreement with the data obtained by intravital microscopy at the same time points [76].

Two years later, a report on the first attempt to study the hepatic microcirculation in humans using OPS imaging was published. Hepatic microperfusion parameters were assessed in 11 healthy individuals undergoing partial liver resection for living-donor liver transplantation. The study demonstrated that OPS imaging enables direct in vivo visualization and quantification of the human hepatic microcirculation and provides significant insight into the physiology of the human liver microcirculation [77].

Furthermore, the relevance of the human liver microcirculation for early graft function was investigated using OPS imaging. Sinusoidal perfusion was assessed 27 recipients undergoing full-size OLT and compared with 32 healthy live liver donors. The hepatic microcirculation was dramatically impaired after implantation compared with the control subjects. The increase of volumetric blood flow within the initial 30 min after reperfusion correlated significantly with postoperative transaminase levels and bilirubin elimination. These data indicate that sinusoidal hyperperfusion may confer protection against postischemic liver injury in the setting of OLT [78].

SDF imaging was recently introduced as the successor of OPS imaging. The device consists of a light guide surrounded by diodes, emitting 530 nm light, which is absorbed by the hemoglobin of red blood cells, allowing their observation as dark cells in the microcirculation. The diodes at the tip of the light guide are optically isolated from the inner image-conducting core, and pump light deep into the tissue, thereby illuminating the microcirculation from within. The application of dark-field illumination from the side eliminates tissue surface reflections. Consequently, SDF imaging generates high-quality images of the microcirculation with visualization of red blood cells and possibly leukocytes [11]. Currently, only one study on the use of SDF imaging for the study of rat liver microcirculation is available [79].

References

1. Selzner M, Rudiger HA, Sindram D, Madden J, Clavien PA. Mechanisms of ischemic injury are different in the steatotic and normal rat liver. Hepatology. 2000;32:1280–8.
2. Selzner N, Rudiger H, Graf R, Clavien P-A. Protective strategies against ischemic injury of the liver. Gastroenterology. 2003;125:917–36.
3. Upadhya GA, Strasberg SM. Evidence that actin disassembly is a requirement for matrix metalloproteinase secretion by sinusoidal endothelial cells during cold preservation in the rat. Hepatology. 1999;30: 169–76.
4. Miyagawa Y, Imamura H, Soeda J, Matsunaga K, Mochida S, Fujiwara K, et al. Fate of hepatocyte and sinusoidal lining cell function and kinetics after extended cold preservation and transplantation of the rat liver. Liver Transpl. 2002;8:370–81.
5. Clavien PA, Morgan GR, Sanabria JR, Petrunka C, Levy GA, Robert P, et al. Effect of cold preservation on lymphocyte adherence in the perfused rat liver. Transplantation. 1991;52:412–7.
6. Sindram D, Porte RJ, Hoffman MR, Bentley RC, Clavien PA. Synergism between platelets and leukocytes in inducing endothelial cell apoptosis in the cold ischemic rat liver: a Kupffer cell-mediated injury. FASEB J. 2001;15:1230–2.
7. Abe Y, Hines I, Zibari G, Grisham MB. Hepatocellular protection by nitric oxide or nitrite in ischemia and reperfusion injury. Arch Biochem Biophys. 2009;484: 232–7.
8. Novo E, Parola M. Redox mechanisms in hepatic chronic wound healing and fibrogenesis. Fibrogenesis Tissue Repair. 2008;1:5.
9. Jaeschke H. Molecular mechanisms of hepatic ischemia-reperfusion injury and preconditioning. Am J Physiol Gastrointest Liver Physiol. 2003;284:G15–26.

10. Younis HS, Parrish AR. Glenn Sipes I. The role of hepatocellular oxidative stress in Kupffer cell activation during 1, 2-dichlorobenzene-induced hepatotoxicity. Toxicol Sci. 2003;76:201–11.
11. Vollmar B, Menger MD. The hepatic microcirculation: mechanistic contributions and therapeutic targets in liver injury and repair. Physiol Rev. 2009;89:1269–339.
12. Sindram D, Porte RJ, Hoffman MR, Bentley RC, Clavien PA. Platelets induce sinusoidal endothelial cell apoptosis upon reperfusion of the cold ischemic rat liver. Gastroenterology. 2000;118:183–91.
13. Marzi I, Knee J, Menger MD, Harbauer G, Buhren V. Hepatic microcirculatory disturbances due to portal vein clamping in the orthotopic rat liver transplantation model. Transplantation. 1991;52:432–6.
14. Rudiger HA, Kang KJ, Sindram D, Riehle HM, Clavien PA. Comparison of ischemic preconditioning and intermittent and continuous inflow occlusion in the murine liver. Ann Surg. 2002;235:400–7.
15. Menger MD, Vollmar B. Role of microcirculation in transplantation. Microcirculation. 2000;7:291–306.
16. El-Badry AM, Graf R, Clavien PA. Omega 3 – omega 6: what is right for the liver? J Hepatol. 2007;47:718–25.
17. Dutkowski P, De Rougemont O, Mullhaupt B, Clavien PA. Current and future trends in liver transplantation in Europe. Gastroenterology. 2010;138: 802–9; e801–4.
18. Yamauchi J, Richter S, Vollmar B, Menger MD, Minor T. Microcirculatory perfusion pattern during harvest of livers from non-heart-beating donors: beneficial effect of warm preflush with streptokinase. Transplant Proc. 2000;32:21–2.
19. Minor T, Hachenberg A, Tolba R, Pauleit D, Akbar S. Fibrinolytic preflush upon liver retrieval from non-heart beating donors to enhance postpreservation viability and energetic recovery upon reperfusion. Transplantation. 2001;71:1792–6.
20. Tojimbara T, Wicomb WN, Garcia-Kennedy R, Burns W, Hayashi M, Collins G, et al. Liver transplantation from non-heart beating donors in rats: influence of viscosity and temperature of initial flushing solutions on graft function. Liver Transpl Surg. 1997;3:39–45.
21. Ohwada S, Sunose Y, Aiba M, Tsutsumi H, Iwazaki S, Totsuka O, et al. Advantages of Celsior solution in graft preservation from non-heart-beating donors in a canine liver transplantation model. J Surg Res. 2002;102:71–6.
22. Bessems M, Doorschodt BM, Albers PS, van Vliet AK, van Gulik TM. Wash-out of the non-heart-beating donor liver: a comparison between ringer lactate, HTK, and polysol. Transplant Proc. 2005;37:395–8.
23. Fondevila C, Hessheimer AJ, Ruiz A, Calatayud D, Ferrer J, Charco R, et al. Liver transplant using donors after unexpected cardiac death: novel preservation protocol and acceptance criteria. Am J Transplant. 2007;7:1849–55.
24. Brockmann J, Reddy S, Coussios C, Pigott D, Guirriero D, Hughes D, et al. Normothermic perfusion: a new paradigm for organ preservation. Ann Surg. 2009;250:1–6.
25. de Rougemont O, Breitenstein S, Leskosek B, Weber A, Graf R, Clavien PA, et al. One hour hypothermic oxygenated perfusion (HOPE) protects nonviable liver allografts donated after cardiac death. Ann Surg. 2009;250:674–83.
26. Xu HS, Stevenson WC, Pruett TL, Jones RS. Donor lazaroid pretreatment improves viability of livers harvested from non-heart-beating rats. Am J Surg. 1996;171:113–6; discussion 116–7.
27. Richter S, Yamauchi J, Minor T, Menger MD, Vollmar B. Heparin and phentolamine combined, rather than heparin alone, improves hepatic microvascular procurement in a non-heart-beating donor rat-model. Transpl Int. 2000;13:225–9.
28. Astarcioglu H, Karademir S, Unek T, Ozer E, Menekay S, Coker A, et al. Beneficial effects of pentoxifylline pretreatment in non-heart-beating donors in rats. Transplantation. 2000;69:93–8.
29. Ikegami T, Nishizaki T, Hiroshige S, Ohta R, Yanaga K, Sugimachi K. Experimental study of a type 3 phosphodiesterase inhibitor on liver graft function. Br J Surg. 2001;88:59–64.
30. Gu M, Takada Y, Fukunaga K, Ishiguro S, Taniguchi H, Seino K, et al. Pharmacologic graft protection without donor pretreatment in liver transplantation from non-heart-beating donors. Transplantation. 2000;70: 1021–5.
31. Monbaliu D, Vekemans K, Hoekstra H, Vaahtera L, Libbrecht L, Derveaux K, et al. Multifactorial biological modulation of warm ischemia reperfusion injury in liver transplantation from non-heart-beating donors eliminates primary nonfunction and reduces bile salt toxicity. Ann Surg. 2009;250:808–17.
32. de Rougemont O, Dutkowski P, Clavien PA. Biological modulation of liver ischemia-reperfusion injury. Curr Opin Organ Transplant. 2010;15(2):183–9.
33. Farrell GC, Teoh NC, McCuskey RS. Hepatic microcirculation in fatty liver disease. Anat Rec (Hoboken). 2008;291:684–92.
34. Sun CK, Zhang XY, Zimmermann A, Davis G, Wheatley AM. Effect of ischemia-reperfusion injury on the microcirculation of the steatotic liver of the Zucker rat. Transplantation. 2001;72:1625–31.
35. Hasegawa T, Ito Y, Wijeweera J, Liu J, Malle E, Farhood A, et al. Reduced inflammatory response and increased microcirculatory disturbances during hepatic ischemia-reperfusion injury in steatotic livers of ob/ob mice. Am J Physiol Gastrointest Liver Physiol. 2007;292:G1385–95.
36. El-Badry AM, Moritz W, Contaldo C, Tian Y, Graf R, Clavien PA. Prevention of reperfusion injury and microcirculatory failure in macrosteatotic mouse liver by omega-3 fatty acids. Hepatology. 2007;45: 855–63.
37. Behrns KE, Tsiotos GG, DeSouza NF, Krishna MK, Ludwig J, Nagorney DM. Hepatic steatosis as a potential risk factor for major hepatic resection. J Gastrointest Surg. 1998;2:292–8.
38. Belghiti J, Hiramatsu K, Benoist S, Massault P, Sauvanet A, Farges O. Seven hundred forty-seven

hepatectomies in the 1990s: an update to evaluate the actual risk of liver resection. J Am Coll Surg. 2000;191:38–46.
39. Kooby DA, Fong Y, Suriawinata A, Gonen M, Allen PJ, Klimstra DS, et al. Impact of steatosis on perioperative outcome following hepatic resection. J Gastrointest Surg. 2003;7:1034–44.
40. McCormack L, Petrowsky H, Jochum W, Furrer K, Clavien PA. Hepatic steatosis is a risk factor for postoperative complications after major hepatectomy: a matched case-control study. Ann Surg. 2007;245: 923–30.
41. Marsman WA, Wiesner RH, Rodriguez L, Batts KP, Porayko MK, Hay JE, et al. Use of fatty donor liver is associated with diminished early patient and graft survival. Transplantation. 1996;62:1246–51.
42. Urena MA, Ruiz-Delgado FC, Gonzalez EM, Segurola CL, Romero CJ, Garcia IG, et al. Assessing risk of the use of livers with macro and microsteatosis in a liver transplant program. Transplant Proc. 1998;30:3288–91.
43. Hayashi M, Fujii K, Kiuchi T, Uryuhara K, Kasahara M, Takatsuki M, et al. Effects of fatty infiltration of the graft on the outcome of living-related liver transplantation. Transplant Proc. 1999;31:403.
44. Verran D, Kusyk T, Painter D, Fisher J, Koorey D, Strasser S, et al. Clinical experience gained from the use of 120 steatotic donor livers for orthotopic liver transplantation. Liver Transpl. 2003;9:500–5.
45. Briceno J, Ciria R, Pleguezuelo M, de la Mata M, Muntane J, Naranjo A, et al. Impact of donor graft steatosis on overall outcome and viral recurrence after liver transplantation for hepatitis C virus cirrhosis. Liver Transpl. 2009;15:37–48.
46. Fishbein TM, Fiel MI, Emre S, Cubukcu O, Guy SR, Schwartz ME, et al. Use of livers with microvesicular fat safely expands the donor pool. Transplantation. 1997;64:248–51.
47. Jarnagin WR, Gonen M, Fong Y, DeMatteo RP, Ben-Porat L, Little S, et al. Improvement in perioperative outcome after hepatic resection: analysis of 1,803 consecutive cases over the past decade. Ann Surg. 2002;236:397–406; discussion 406–7.
48. Soejima Y, Shimada M, Suehiro T, Kishikawa K, Yoshizumi T, Hashimoto K, et al. Use of steatotic graft in living-donor liver transplantation. Transplantation. 2003;76:344–8.
49. Cho JY, Suh KS, Kwon CH, Yi NJ, Lee KU. Mild hepatic steatosis is not a major risk factor for hepatectomy and regenerative power is not impaired. Surgery. 2006;139:508–15.
50. Angele MK, Rentsch M, Hartl WH, Wittmann B, Graeb C, Jauch KW, et al. Effect of graft steatosis on liver function and organ survival after liver transplantation. Am J Surg. 2008;195:214–20.
51. Vuppalanchi R, Unalp A, Van Natta ML, Cummings OW, Sandrasegaran KE, Hameed T, et al. Effects of liver biopsy sample length and number of readings on sampling variability in nonalcoholic fatty liver disease. Clin Gastroenterol Hepatol. 2009;7:481–6.
52. Karcaaltincaba M, Akhan O. Imaging of hepatic steatosis and fatty sparing. Eur J Radiol. 2007; 61:33–43.
53. DiDonato D, Brasaemle DL. Fixation methods for the study of lipid droplets by immunofluorescence microscopy. J Histochem Cytochem. 2003;51:773–80.
54. Fukumoto S, Fujimoto T. Deformation of lipid droplets in fixed samples. Histochem Cell Biol. 2002;118:423–8.
55. Garcia Urena MA, Colina Ruiz-Delgado F, Moreno Gonzalez E, Jimenez Romero C, Garcia Garcia I, Loinzaz Segurola C, et al. Hepatic steatosis in liver transplant donors: common feature of donor population? World J Surg. 1998;22:837–44.
56. El-Badry AM, Breitenstein S, Jochum W, Washington K, Paradis V, Rubbia-Brandt L, et al. Assessment of hepatic steatosis by expert pathologists: the end of a gold standard. Ann Surg. 2009;250(5):691–7.
57. Ijaz S, Winslet MC, Seifalian AM. The effect of consecutively larger doses of L-arginine on hepatic microcirculation and tissue oxygenation in hepatic steatosis. Microvasc Res. 2009;78:206–11.
58. Cottart CH, Do L, Blanc MC, Vaubourdolle M, Descamps G, Durand D, et al. Hepatoprotective effect of endogenous nitric oxide during ischemia-reperfusion in the rat. Hepatology. 1999;29:809–13.
59. Capanni M, Calella F, Biagini MR, Genise S, Raimondi L, Bedogni G, et al. Prolonged n-3 polyunsaturated fatty acid supplementation ameliorates hepatic steatosis in patients with non-alcoholic fatty liver disease: a pilot study. Aliment Pharmacol Ther. 2006;23:1143–51.
60. Seifalian AM, Chidambaram V, Rolles K, Davidson BR. In vivo demonstration of impaired microcirculation in steatotic human liver grafts. Liver Transpl Surg. 1998;4:71–7.
61. Shirabe K, Kin S, Shinagawa Y, Chen S, Payne WD, Sugimachi K. Inhibition of thromboxane A2 activity during warm ischemia of the liver. J Surg Res. 1996;61:103–7.
62. Shirabe K, Takenaka K, Yamamoto K, Kitamura M, Itasaka H, Matsumata T, et al. The role of prostanoid in hepatic damage during hepatectomy. Hepatogastroenterology. 1996;43:596–601.
63. Clavien PA, Oberkofler C, Raptis DA, Lehmann K, Rickenbacher A, El-Badry AM. What is critical for liver surgery and partial liver transplantation:size or quality? Hepatology. 2010;52(2):715–29.
64. Colle I, Van Vlierberghe H, Troisi R, De Hemptinne B. Transplanted liver: consequences of denervation for liver functions. Anat Rec A Discov Mol Cell Evol Biol. 2004;280:924–31.
65. Pedrosa ME, Montero EF, Nigro AJ. Liver microcirculation after selective denervation. Microsurgery. 2001;21:163–5.
66. Schemmer P, Bunzendahl H, Raleigh JA, Thurman RG. Graft survival is improved by hepatic denervation before organ harvesting. Transplantation. 1999;67:1301–7.

67. Schemmer P, Schoonhoven R, Swenberg JA, Bunzendahl H, Thurman RG. Gentle in situ liver manipulation during organ harvest decreases survival after rat liver transplantation: role of Kupffer cells. Transplantation. 1998;65:1015–20.
68. Schemmer P, Connor HD, Arteel GE, Raleigh JA, Bunzendahl H, Mason RP, et al. Reperfusion injury in livers due to gentle in situ organ manipulation during harvest involves hypoxia and free radicals. J Pharmacol Exp Ther. 1999;290:235–40.
69. Schemmer P, Schoonhoven R, Swenberg JA, Bunzendahl H, Raleigh JA, Lemasters JJ, et al. Gentle organ manipulation during harvest as a key determinant of survival of fatty livers after transplantation in the rat. Transpl Int. 1999;12:351–9.
70. Klar E, Angelescu M, Zapletal C, Kraus T, Herfarth C. Impairment of hepatic microcirculation as an early manifestation of acute rejection after clinical liver transplantation. Transplant Proc. 1999;31:385–7.
71. Adams DH, Hubscher SG, Shaw J, Rothlein R, Neuberger JM. Intercellular adhesion molecule 1 on liver allografts during rejection. Lancet. 1989;2: 1122–5.
72. Kawano K, Bowers JL, Kruskal JB, Clouse ME. In vivo microscopic assessment of hepatic microcirculation during liver allograft rejection in the rat. Transplantation. 1995;59:1241–8.
73. Tawadrous MN, Zimmermann A, Zhang XY, Wheatley AM. Persistence of impaired hepatic microcirculation after nonarterialized liver transplantation in the rat. Microcirculation. 2002;9:363–75.
74. Fudaba Y, Ohdan H, Tashiro H, Miyata Y, Shibata S, Shintaku S, et al. Rearterialization of hepatic xenografts in the combination of hamster-to-rat. Transplant Proc. 2000;32:1127–8.
75. Groner W, Winkelman JW, Harris AG, Ince C, Bouma GJ, Messmer K, et al. Orthogonal polarization spectral imaging: a new method for study of the microcirculation. Nat Med. 1999;5:1209–12.
76. Langer S, Harris AG, Biberthaler P, von Dobschuetz E, Messmer K. Orthogonal polarization spectral imaging as a tool for the assessment of hepatic microcirculation: a validation study. Transplantation. 2001;71: 1249–56.
77. Puhl G, Schaser KD, Vollmar B, Menger MD, Settmacher U. Noninvasive in vivo analysis of the human hepatic microcirculation using orthogonal polorization spectral imaging. Transplantation. 2003;75:756–61.
78. Puhl G, Schaser KD, Pust D, Kohler K, Vollmar B, Menger MD, et al. Initial hepatic microcirculation correlates with early graft function in human orthotopic liver transplantation. Liver Transpl. 2005;11: 555–63.
79. Cerny V, Turek Z, Parizkova R. In situ assessment of the liver microcirculation in mechanically ventilated rats using sidestream dark-field imaging. Physiol Res. 2009;58:49–55.

Portal Hypertension: Intrahepatic Mechanisms

6

Alexander Zipprich and Roberto J. Groszmann

Abstract

Portal hypertension is one of the most life-threatening complications of cirrhosis, leading to the development of ascites and esophageal varices. Increased intrahepatic resistance is the initial event in the development of portal hypertension. Anatomical lesions contribute approximately to 70% of the increased intrahepatic vascular resistance. These include regenerative nodules, capillarization of sinusoids, sinusoidal collapse, and hepatocyte enlargement. The remaining 30% represents the dynamic component of the increased intrahepatic vascular resistance. Hepatic stellate cells play a central role in the regulation of sinusoidal resistance. These cells are transformed to a myofibroblast-like cell type with increased constrictive properties. Increased levels of vasoconstrictors and decreased levels of vasodilators lead to HSC constriction and subsequently to an increase in intrahepatic vascular resistance. On the other hand, higher concentrations of vasodilators induce hepatic arterial vasodilatation and a lower vascular resistance of the hepatic artery in cirrhosis. Additionally, vascular architectural changes are present in cirrhosis and recent investigations have focused on the presence of neoangiogenesis and vascular remodeling in the intrahepatic circulation.

Keywords

Intrahepatic circulation • Portal pressure • Intrahepatic vascular resistance • Portal hypertension • Cirrhosis • Hepatic stellate cells • Nitric oxide

Introduction

The complications associated with portal hypertension are among the main causes of morbidity and mortality in patients with cirrhosis [1]. The initial event leading to portal hypertension in liver cirrhosis is the increase in intrahepatic vascular resistance [2]. Thus, understanding the pathophysiology and the abnormalities of the intrahepatic circulation are necessary to develop successful therapies. This chapter gives an overview of the intrahepatic mechanisms involved in the development of portal hypertension.

R.J. Groszmann (✉)
Department of Medicine-Digestive Diseases,
Yale University School of Medicine, PO Box 208019,
New Haven, CT 06520-8019, USA
e-mail: roberto.groszmann@yale.edu

L.D. DeLeve and G. Garcia-Tsao (eds.), *Vascular Liver Disease: Mechanisms and Management*,
DOI 10.1007/978-1-4419-8327-5_6, © Springer Science+Business Media, LLC 2011

Etiology of Portal Hypertension

Portal venous pressure is determined by portal venous *flow* and the *resistance* to this flow [3]. According to Ohm's law, the relation of these three factors is described in the following equation:

$$P = Q \times R$$

(P = portal pressure, Q = portal venous flow, and R = portal venous resistance).

The portal venous circulation can be separated into prehepatic, intrahepatic (which in turn can be divided into presinusoidal, sinusoidal and postsinusoidal) and posthepatic territories [4]. Any abnormalities in each of these territories can lead to an increase in vascular resistance and therefore portal hypertension. Most hepatic diseases lead to an increase of intrahepatic portal venous resistance. Although there is a wide range of causes of liver diseases, they all lead to a final common stage, cirrhosis. Cirrhosis is defined by the presence of fibrous tissue and development of nodules and is the main cause of increased intrahepatic portal venous resistance.

Intrahepatic Circulation in the Normal Liver

Liver Cells Involved in the Intrahepatic Circulation

The liver has different cell types, such as hepatocytes, hepatic stellate cells, Kupffer cells, and sinusoidal endothelial cells with different functional properties. Hepatocytes are the main functional cells in the liver. However, hepatocytes play only a minor role in the regulation of intrahepatic blood flow.

The most important cell types involved in the changes in the intrahepatic circulation are the hepatic stellate cells (HSC) [5]. HSC are mainly located around the sinusoids. Their contractile properties have been demonstrated in normal livers, underscoring the role they play in regulating sinusoidal blood flow [5, 6].

Kupffer cells are the macrophages of the liver and have first contact with bacteria, bacterial endotoxins, and microbiological debris derived from the gut. Activated Kupffer cells produce a large amount of nitric oxide but these cells are not involved in the regulation of the intrahepatic circulation of normal livers [7].

Sinusoidal endothelial cells have no basement membrane and the walls are characterized by fenestrae that allow passage of smaller, noncorpuscular blood components into the space of Disse [8]. These fenestrae allow further supply of oxygen and substrates to the hepatocytes [9–12]. Sinusoidal endothelial cells are the inner layer of the sinusoid. They have direct contact with the different elements of the blood and produce vasoactive mediators. Interestingly, sinusoidal endothelial cells from normal livers seem to be important in the regulation of the functional status of HSC.

Mediators that Regulate the Intrahepatic Circulation

Regulation of intrahepatic blood flow in the normal liver is mediated by the interaction between vasoconstrictors and, more importantly, vasodilators. One of the most important vasoconstrictors in the intrahepatic circulation is endothelin. Three different endothelins (endothelin-1, endothelin-2, and endothelin-3) are known, each with 21 amino acids [13]. The endothelin that mediates vasoconstriction in the intrahepatic circulation is endothelin-1 via the endothelin-A receptor [13].

In the early 1990s, it was demonstrated that nitric oxide (NO) regulates intrahepatic resistance in normal livers [14]. Sinusoidal endothelial cells respond to increases in shear stress with an increase in NO production [14]. Furthermore, vascular endothelial growth factor (VEGF) stimulates NO production by the sinusoidal endothelial cells. NO promotes HSC quiescence and reversal of activated stellate cells to a quiescent phenotype and is therefore crucial in maintaining a normal intrahepatic circulation [15].

Site of Resistance in the Intrahepatic Circulation and Hepatic Arterial Buffer Response

Blood entering the portal system is not regulated by liver metabolic requirements but by changes in vascular resistance at the level of the splanchnic arterioles. This is particularly important since blood flow changes in the splanchnic circulation are needed so that the liver can maintain a stable nutrient and oxygen supply [16]. The liver is unique in that it has a dual blood supply through the portal vein and hepatic artery (see Fig. 6.1). Both vessels supply blood to the sinusoids, which are the "capillary" network of the liver. The intrahepatic circulation can be divided into a presinusoidal, sinusoidal, and postsinusoidal circulatory region [17]. The site of resistance of the portal venous territory is located in the sinusoidal area while the site of resistance for the hepatic artery is located in the presinusoidal area [18]. To maintain a stable supply of oxygen and nutrients to the liver, changes in portal venous blood flow are balanced by opposite changes in hepatic arterial blood flow [19]. This mechanism is known as the hepatic arterial buffer response and seems to be mediated by local production of adenosine [20]. Adenosine is produced by tissue in the site of resistance of the hepatic artery, i.e., the presinusoidal area. This locally produced adenosine can either diffuse into the portal vein and be washed away, or it can remain locally and act on adenosine receptors on the hepatic artery and cause vasodilatation [21]. For example, with decreasing portal venous blood flow, adenosine accumulates and leads to hepatic arterial vasodilatation and therefore higher blood supply via the hepatic artery that counteracts the decreased portal venous blood supply. However, the hepatic arterial buffer response seems to be more important in stabilizing oxygen and nutrient delivery to the liver rather than total liver blood flow [16].

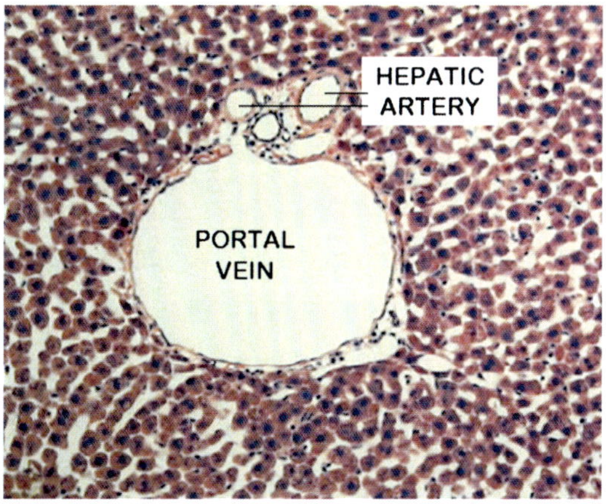

Fig. 6.1 Histological picture of a normal liver. Both, portal vein and hepatic artery drain into the sinusoids, the "capillary" network of the liver. The liver has therefore a unique dual blood supply. To maintain a stable supply of oxygen and nutrients to the liver, changes in portal venous blood flow are balanced by opposite changes in hepatic arterial blood flow. Also note the normal architecture of the liver parenchyma

Intrahepatic Changes in Cirrhosis

In cirrhosis, changes of the anatomy as well as functional properties of the vessels and sinusoids lead to major disturbances of the intrahepatic circulation. Anatomical changes contribute to around 70% of the increased portal venous pressure and therefore represent the main cause of increased intrahepatic vascular resistance. Indeed, in patients with cirrhosis portal pressure (measured by hepatic venous pressure gradient [HVPG]) correlates well with hepatic anatomical changes [22]. However, the initial study by Bhathal and Grossman demonstrated that vasodilators could decrease the hepatic vascular resistance in cirrhosis. They suggested that up to 30% of the increase in intrahepatic resistance in cirrhosis is due to an increased vascular tone. Although the magnitude of this functional component in patients with cirrhosis has not been yet quantified, this finding set the rationale for the treatment of portal hypertension using vasodilators.

Anatomical Lesions in Cirrhosis

Different anatomical lesions have been implicated in the development of an increased vascular resistance in cirrhosis. The main lesions are the accumulation of fibrous tissue and the

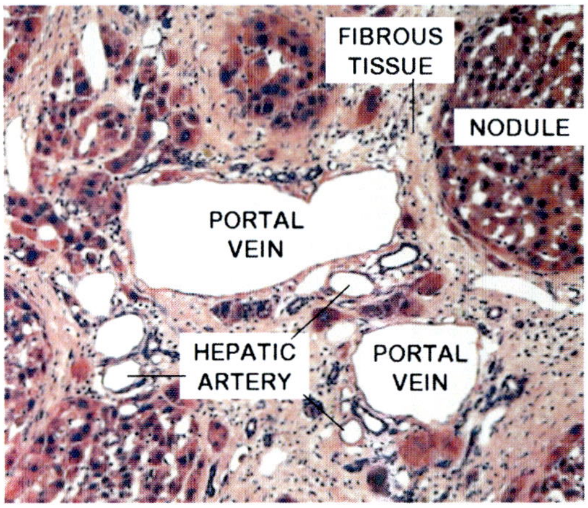

Fig. 6.2 Histological picture of a cirrhotic liver. The architecture of the liver is altered due to accumulation of fibrous tissue with formation of septa and nodules. Anatomical changes contribute to approximately 70% of the increased intrahepatic vascular resistance

development of regenerative nodules resulting in vascular obliteration and subsequently increased vascular resistance (see Fig. 6.2). HSC are the most important cells involved in the regulation of the intrahepatic circulation and production of fibrous tissue [5]. Activation of the HSC is the essential event that leads to the production of extracellular matrix and development of fibrous tissue around the sinusoids [15]. In the early stages of liver fibrosis this sinusoidal fibrous tissue leads to sinusoidal capillarization. Capillarized sinusoids are characterized by accumulation of extracellular matrix in the space of Disse, and sinusoidal endothelial cells that lose their fenestrae and their typical phenotype [15]. The matrix production of the activated HSC seems to be the initial event of capillarization of the sinusoids. Furthermore, sinusoidal endothelial cells also have an influence in the activation of HSC capillarization, leading to lower NO production by sinusoidal endothelial cells and thereby activation of HSC [15].

Later, the development of fibrous septa and regenerative nodules markedly alters the hepatic architecture and hepatic vascularization [23]. Moreover, it was suggested that thrombosis of the small portal and hepatic venules could contribute to increased hepatic vascular resistance and could be an important factor in the progression of the architectural disturbances of cirrhosis. Additionally, sinusoidal collapse and hepatocyte enlargement are anatomical changes that are detected during the development of fibrosis and cirrhosis. All these anatomical changes lead to a narrowing of the sinusoids, an increase in intrahepatic vascular resistance and therefore an increase in portal pressure.

Dynamic Components of the Increased Intrahepatic Vascular Resistance in Cirrhosis

Activation of Hepatic Stellate Cells in Cirrhotic Livers

The dynamic component of the increased hepatic vascular resistance reflects the existence of contractile structures in the liver that modulate hepatic resistance in response to endogenous or pharmacological vasoactive substances. After liver injury, the contractile capacity of HSC is particularly important. HSC transition occurs from a quiescent phenotype to a myofibroblast-like phenotype during the development of cirrhosis [23]. Activated HSC have a higher amount of alpha-smooth muscle actin, myosin, and cytosolic proteins essential for contractility which are absent in quiescent HSC [23].

In addition to the greater constrictive capacity, activated HSC also express different receptors that mediate constriction. For example, it has been shown that L-type operated Ca^{2+} channels (VOCC) are not present in HSC isolated from normal rats, whereas they are present in those isolated from cirrhotic animals [24]. Furthermore, high-conductance Ca^{2+}-activated K^{+} channels (BKCa), also involved in the regulation of intrahepatic Ca^{2+}-concentration, are also expressed in activated HSC [25]. These data suggest that in HSC these channels participate in the regulation of Ca^{2+} mobilization and cell contraction by modulating the effects of vasoactive substances such as endothelin-1 and NO [25]. However, HSC contraction is a multifactorial process that also involves the participation of calcium-independent mechanisms [26].

In summary, HSC are located around the hepatic sinusoids. These cells are activated in cirrhosis leading to sinusoidal vasoconstriction and therefore to an increase in intrahepatic vascular resistance. Different vasoconstrictive and vasodilatory mediators are involved in the activation as well as constriction of the HSC.

Increased Concentration of Vasoconstrictive Mediators

Increased vascular resistance in the portal venous vascular bed is a multifactorial process. The vasoconstrictors involved are endothelin, eicosanoids, angiotensin II, arginine vasopressin, and RhoA.

Endothelin

Endothelins are involved in the regulation of the intrahepatic circulation in normal livers (see above) and are particularly important in cirrhotic livers. The plasma concentrations of endothelin-1 and 3 are increased in patients with cirrhosis [27]. However, the effect of endothelin depends on the specific receptor that is activated. There are two different receptors, the endothelin-A receptor and the endothelin-B receptor [13]. The endothelin-A receptor is a G protein-dependent receptor that mediates vasoconstriction while the endothelin-B receptor mediates vasodilatation through an NO-dependent pathway [27]. The former receptor is in general located on the vascular smooth muscle cells. It seems to be the responsible receptor for endothelin-1 mediated vasoconstriction of HSC in cirrhosis as its expression is increased in cirrhosis, particularly on these cells [13]. The endothelins are produced by the injured liver itself, mainly by HSC and endothelial cells. In addition, in cirrhosis there is an increase in mediators, such as epinephrine, angiotensin II, vasopressin, and interleukin 1 and in shear stress, which may further stimulate the production of endothelins [27].

Eicosanoids

Eicosanoids are a group of vasoactive mediators that can lead to both vasoconstriction and vasodilatation. In cirrhosis, sinusoidal endothelial cells synthesize vasoconstrictive prostanoids via the COX-1 pathway [28]. Activation of cytosolic phospholipase A2 (PLA2) by a G protein-coupled receptor-dependent mechanism promotes the release of arachidonic acid from membrane phospholipids. Arachidonic acid is further metabolized to prostaglandin H2 (PGH2) by COX. PGH2 is the common precursor for prostaglandin and thromboxane [28]. Thromboxane A2 is a vasoconstrictive mediator involved in the intrahepatic vasoconstriction of cirrhosis [29]. Interestingly, thromboxane A2 is not only produced by sinusoidal endothelial cells but also by activated Kupffer cells. Thromboxane production by activated Kupffer cells has been observed in livers after induction of inflammation as well as in cirrhotic animals [30].

Angiotensin II

Patients with advanced cirrhosis show a marked activation of the renin-angiotensin system that correlates with the severity of portal hypertension and results in increased plasma concentrations of angiotensin II. In experimental studies using the isolated perfused liver model, angiotensin II infusion increases intrahepatic resistance. The vasoconstrictive effects of angiotensin II are mediated by the angiotensin II type I receptors on activated HSC. The stimulation of the angiotensin II type I receptor by angiotensin II leads to an increase in Ca^{2+}-concentration through L-type Ca channels and subsequently to contraction [31, 32]. Further evidence supporting the relevance of this pathway is shown by the effect of losartan on HSC [31]. This angiotensin II type I receptor blocker abolishes the effect of angiotensin II on these cells. Moreover, activated HSC express all the components of the renin-angiotensin system, i.e., angiotensinogen, renin, and angiotensin converting enzyme [33]. Activated HSC demonstrate renin and angiotensin converting enzyme activities and produce angiotensin II especially in the presence of the precursor angiotensinogen [33]. This suggests that not only circulating angiotensin but also locally produced angiotensin II has a role in the increased resistance in cirrhosis. Furthermore, other mediators are involved in angiotensin II synthesis by HSC. Endothelin-1 induces its synthesis, while NO reduces it [33] and, as mentioned previously, both endothelin-1 and NO are involved in the regulation of the intrahepatic circulation in cirrhotic livers. Endothelin-1 levels are increased and NO levels are decreased in the intrahepatic circulation leading to a higher production of angiotensin II by HSC. Nevertheless, administration of angiotensin II type I receptor blockers has not led to a reduction in portal pressure in patients with cirrhosis [34, 35].

RhoA

Another vasoconstrictive pathway that is activated in cirrhosis is the RhoA/Rho kinase pathway. Rho is a small, monomeric guanosine triphosphate-binding protein from the Ras super family. A number of studies have established Rho activity as a key regulator of actin organization, cell morphology, chemotaxis, and contraction in a wide range of cells including HSC [36]. Rho stimulates the Rho-associated coiled-coil forming protein kinase (ROCK) triggering the assembly of cytoplasmic stress fibers composed of filamentous actin [37]. Rho activation and actin construction in HSC is therefore required for contraction to occur. RhoA is constitutively active in cultured HSC, and those from injured livers. Its role in cirrhosis is supported by studies in perfused cirrhotic livers that show a decrease in perfusion pressure in the presence of Rho kinase inhibitors [38]. Furthermore, contractile α(alpha)1-adrenoceptors in the intrahepatic microvasculature are coupled to the RhoA/Rho kinase pathway and the RhoA/Rho kinase pathway seems to be involved in the adrenergic regulation of intrahepatic vascular tone [38]. Compared to normal livers, cirrhotic livers require three times the dose of the Rho kinase inhibitor to abolish the response to an α1-adrenoceptor agonist. Therefore, the RhoA/Rho kinase pathway is activated in response to α1-adrenergic stimulation in the intrahepatic microcirculation of cirrhotic animals. On the other hand, it has been recently shown that the vasodilator adenosine is a physiological inhibitor of RhoA and Rho kinase pathway in activated HSC [39].

Decrease in Vasodilaors on the Sinusoidal Level

In addition to increased levels of vasoconstrictors and increased response to vasoconstrictors at the sinusoidal level, production of vasodilators is decreased in the intrahepatic circulation in cirrhosis. The main vasodilator involved in the regulation of the intrahepatic circulation is NO, an endothelial-derived relaxing factor. Recently, hydrogen sulfide, a potent vasodilator, has been proposed as another important vasodilator involved in the regulation of the intrahepatic circulation in cirrhosis.

Nitric Oxide

NO plays a key role in the portal circulation. It is synthesized by a family of three NO synthases (NOS): endothelial NOS (eNOS), neuronal NOS (nNOS), and inducible NOS (iNOS). Among these isoforms, the main synthase in the intrahepatic circulation is eNOS. In cirrhosis, changes in endothelial cells lead to a decrease in eNOS function [3]. NO promotes vasodilatation mainly through activation of soluble guanylyl cyclase (sGC) in contractile cells [2]. Under normal conditions, activated sGC synthesizes cyclic guanosine 3′,5′ monophosphate (cGMP) initiating the cGMP cascade and a sequence of events that culminate with cell relaxation and vasodilation. The vasodilatory effect of NO is normally limited by phosphodiesterases (PDEs) that break down cGMP to its inactive form GMP [40].

Endothelial cells from cirrhotic livers have insufficient NO production. The mechanism leading to reduced NO production by these cells has not been fully elucidated but appears to be multifactorial (Fig. 6.3). Abnormalities in the

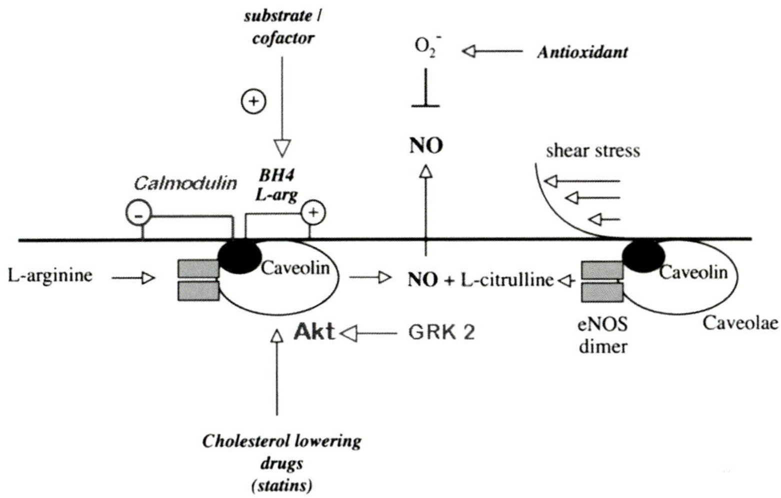

Fig. 6.3 Mechanisms involved in the defective nitric oxide synthesis in cirrhotic livers. Different substrates and cofactors lead to decreased production of nitric oxide, which contributes to increased vascular resistance and a higher number of activated hepatic stellate cells in cirrhosis (see text). Modified figure from Wiest and Groszmann [2]

complex posttranslational regulation of the enzyme that include protein–protein interactions, phosphorylation, and intracellular localization appear to contribute to the defective function in cirrhosis [41–43]. Caveolin and calmodulin are two proteins that regulate NO production. Caveolins are a family of proteins that are involved in receptor-independent endocytosis. The caveolin gene family has three members: CAV1, CAV2, and CAV3, coding for the proteins caveolin-1, caveolin-2 and caveolin-3, respectively. Interaction with caveolin-1 reduces the activity of eNOS. Caveolin-1 expression is increased in the cirrhotic liver and, furthermore, its interaction with eNOS is also increased. This results in decreased activity of eNOS (Fig. 6.4) [41]. On the other hand, the calcium regulatory protein calmodulin dissociates eNOS from caveolin and has been shown to reverse the inhibitory effects of caveolin on eNOS in a model of cirrhosis secondary to bile duct ligation [42].

Another mechanism involved in the regulation of eNOS activity is the Akt pathway [44, 45]. Akt seems to interact with several protein partners, resulting in a number of diverse effects. Akt-dependent eNOS phosphorylation increases its

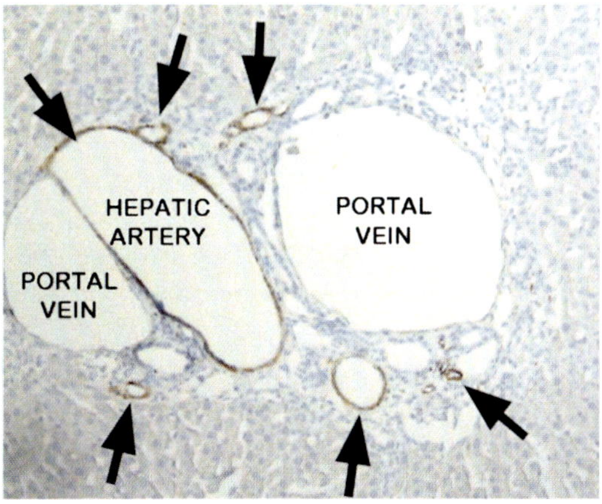

Fig. 6.4 Histological figure of a cirrhotic liver showing neoangiogenesis of arterial vessels (*arrows*) (biopsy stained with elastic-Van Gieson stain, which highlights vessels. Other structural changes of the cirrhotic liver are thus difficult to appreciate). Modified figure from Zipprich et al. [62]

activity. In cirrhosis, Akt-dependent eNOS phosphorylation is decreased (see Fig. 6.4) [44]. This is further supported by studies in animals and in humans showing that simvastatin, which increases Akt-dependent eNOS phosphorylation (and activity), reduces portal pressure (see Fig. 6.3) [45, 46].

G protein-coupled receptor kinases (GRK) are serine/threonine kinases. One of these, GRK2, modulates adrenergic, angiotensin, and endothelin receptors. Recently, it has been shown that GRK2 interacts directly with Akt and that this interaction inhibits its phosphorylation [47], resulting in reduced activation of eNOS and reduced NO production. Since GRK2 is upregulated after liver injury, it would appear to be an important mechanism underlying the defective NO synthesis [48].

Other factors also seem to be involved in the deactivation of eNOS in cirrhosis. Amino acid asymmetric dimethylarginine (ADAM) has been shown to inhibit NO synthesis [49]. Interestingly, bile duct ligated rats showed higher levels of ADAM compared to control rats [50]. Unconjugated pterin cofactor (6R)-l-erythro-5,6,7,8-tetrahydrobiopterin (BH_4), another factor involved in the regulation of NOS activity, also appears to play a role in the endothelial dysfunction in cirrhosis [51].

On the other hand, the response of the liver circulation to NO is impaired. *S*-Nitroso-*N*-acetylpenicillamine (SNAP) is a NO donor that releases NO without undergoing metabolic transformation. The vasodilatation induced by SNAP is impaired in cirrhotic livers [52]. This indicates that, in addition to decreased NO production, there is also decreased response to NO in cirrhotic livers. This decreased response could be caused by increased NO inactivation, dysfunction of the cGMP cascade (an enzymatic system that mediates the NO-induced vasorelaxation) and dysfunction of cGMP-independent mechanisms of NO-induced vasorelaxation [53, 54]. The mechanisms involved in this abnormality are not well understood, but could involve increased degradation of NO before it reaches its targets. Possible mechanisms involved in this degradation are increased oxidative stress and superoxide production, or abnormalities in the downstream signaling pathways of NO. For example, phosphodiesterase-5 is involved in the degradation of NO. Phosphodiesterase-5 expression is increased in cirrhotic livers and leads to increased inactivation of NO in cirrhotic livers [40]. Therefore, deficiency of NO in the cirrhotic liver is a combination of decreased production and increased degradation.

In cirrhotic livers, NO concentrations differ in different sections of the intrahepatic circulation [17]. At the postsinusoidal and sinusoidal levels, the amount of NO is decreased, while it is increased in the presinusoidal area. This explains the lower vascular resistance observed in that area in cirrhotic livers [17].

Due to the central regulatory role of NO in the intrahepatic circulation in cirrhosis, treatments that increase hepatic NO are useful therapeutic target for portal hypertension. Recent studies in experimental animals demonstrate that portal pressure can be reduced by increasing NO bioavailability in the liver circulation, either by transfecting the liver with adenovirus encoding NO synthase or by the administration of a liver-selective NO donor [55–57]. However, such studies still need to be performed in humans.

Hydrogen Sulfide and Homocysteine

Homocysteine is a sulfur-containing amino acid primarily generated from the essential amino acid methionine in a variety of tissues including the liver. Homocysteine is formed upon demethylation of *S*-adenosylmethionine and subsequent hydrolysis of *S*-adenosylhomocysteine. Increased plasma levels of homocysteine due to loss of function, mutation, or heterozygosity of cystathionine-synthase (CBS) and cystathionine-lyase (CSE) are associated with several diseases including cirrhosis [58]. Hyperhomocysteinemia promotes endothelial dysfunction and impairs endothelial-dependent vasodilatation, both in normal and cirrhotic livers [59]. Inhibition of CBS and CSE expression/function is a common finding in patients with chronic liver disorders, leading to hyperhomocysteinemia in patients with cirrhosis [58]. The mechanism of the hyperhomocystenemia-induced impaired vasodilation is not completely understood, but local release of vasoconstrictors triggered by hyperhomocystenemia could be an explanation. In addition to causing homocysteine accumulation, another functional consequence of reduced expression/function of CSE and CBS in the liver is defective generation of H_2S, the end product of homocysteine/l-cysteine metabolism [58, 59]. Hydrogen sulfide (H_2S) is a gaseous neuromodulator that exerts potent vasodilatory effects. In hepatocytes and HSC, H_2S is generated from methionine and l-cysteine by CBS and CSE. Perfusion of cirrhotic livers with H_2S compensates for defective NO production in rodent models of portal hypertension [59]. Homocysteine triggers HSC contraction and this homocysteine-induced contraction is counterbalanced by H_2S suggesting that HSC might be a target for homocysteine and H_2S [59].

Regulation of the Hepatic Arterial Vascular Resistance

The liver has a dual blood supply and the drainage of the hepatic arterial blood into the sinusoids occurs at the beginning of the sinusoidal network (zone 1) [60]. The vascular resistance of the hepatic artery is determined in the presinusoidal area, i.e., in the small hepatic branches before they drain into the sinusoids. Changes in hepatic arterial liver perfusion lead to changes in the sinusoidal and subsequently in the portal venous vascular resistance [18]. In cirrhosis, hepatic arterial vascular resistance is decreased and thus hepatic arterial blood flow is increased [18, 61]. The mechanisms involved in this decreased vascular resistance are not completely identified, although it has been postulated that the mechanism for increased NO levels in the presinusoidal area in cirrhosis also leads to increased NO levels in the hepatic artery [62]. This increased NO level leads to lower vascular resistance of the hepatic artery. On the other hand, it has been shown that the regulation of hepatic arterial flow, and especially the hepatic arterial buffer response, is regulated by adenosine [20]. The vasodilatory response to adenosine is increased in cirrhosis due to a higher expression of the adenosine A1 receptor in hepatic arteries of cirrhotic livers [4]. Both vasodilators, i.e., NO and adenosine, are linked in cirrhosis through the NO-dependent adenosine A1 receptor. Since this receptor leads to increased production of NO, it can be postulated that both adenosine and NO are involved in the lower vascular resistance of hepatic arteries of cirrhotic livers.

Remodeling and Angiogenesis

Sinusoidal Remodeling and Angiogenesis

In addition to liver architectural changes, in cirrhosis the vessels themselves undergo morphological changes. Two complementary processes, angiogenesis, i.e., vascular growth from preexisting vessels, and vasculogenesis, i.e., de novo blood vessel development, are involved in the regulation of vascular development (see Fig. 6.4) [63]. Angiogenesis and sinusoidal remodeling are necessary to supply blood to the newly formed areas of hepatocytes during the regeneration process that takes place during the development of cirrhosis [64]. The formation of these new vessels, including arterio-portal shunts, is one mechanism involved in the development of portal hypertension [63, 65]. Similar to the other changes during the development of fibrosis and cirrhosis, HSC activation also seems to be crucial in the regulation of sinusoidal structural changes. HSC along with endothelial cells migrate to these areas resulting in the formation of new sinusoidal branches [66, 67].

Two different mechanisms seem to be involved in the development of these new vessels and therefore for the new angio-architecture in cirrhosis.

The first is the process of chronic wound healing during the development of cirrhosis. It is characterized by overexpression of several growth factors, cytokines and metalloproteinases (MMPs). Proangiogenic factors such as platelet-derived growth factor (PDGF), transforming growth factor-β(beta)1 (TGF-β1), fibroblast growth factor (FGF), and VEGF, have been shown to be elevated in cirrhosis [67]. These proangiogenic factors are necessary in remodeling and angiogenesis. In addition, increased gene expression of integrins, β-catenin, and ephrins occur in cirrhosis, demonstrating up-regulation of different factors involved in the multifactorial process of angiogenesis and sinusoidal remodeling [64, 67].

Second, neoangiogenesis is stimulated in hepatic tissue by hypoxia. Hypoxia is one of the initial factors leading to morphological and vascular changes in cirrhosis [68]. Capillarization of the sinusoids leads to impairment of oxygen diffusion from sinusoids to hepatocytes (oxygen limitation theory) with consequent up-regulation of proangiogenic pathways [69, 70]. Hypoxic conditions lead to up-regulation of VEGF and angiopoietin I in HSC [71, 72], a process that appears to be mediated by the transcription factor HIF-1α [73].

Recent studies have investigated the effects of inhibiting angiogenesis during the development of cirrhosis and portal hypertension and have demonstrated a beneficial effect both on portal pressure and fibrosis progression [63, 74].

Hepatic Arterial Remodeling and Angiogenesis

The increased need for oxygen in cirrhotic livers is counteracted by increased hepatic arterial blood supply (hepatic arterial buffer response) and also by greater arterial blood flow to the sinusoids [75]. It is speculated that hypoxic conditions could lead to higher concentrations of adenosine, which subsequently leads to hepatic arterial vasodilatation [4]. On the other hand, the increase in proangiogenic factors in cirrhosis could also lead to neoangiogenesis of arterial vessels (see Fig. 6.4). Indeed, the presence of neoangiogenesis of arterial vessels in cirrhosis has been demonstrated in two different animal models [62]. However, the mechanisms that are involved in this arterial neoangiogenesis have been not investigated so far.

Furthermore, it has been shown that the vessel wall of the hepatic artery undergoes morphological changes in cirrhosis as a consequence of the decreased hepatic arterial vascular resistance [62]. This process is called remodeling and the main anatomical change is a decrease in the number of smooth muscle cells [62]. This results in vessels with thinner walls and a larger diameter. Furthermore, due to the decrease in smooth muscle cells the vasoconstrictive properties of the vessels are decreased.

Summary

Portal hypertension is one of the most life-threatening complications of cirrhosis, leading to the development of ascites and esophageal varices. Increased intrahepatic resistance is the initial event in the development of portal hypertension. Anatomical lesions contribute approximately to 70% of the increased intrahepatic vascular resistance. These include regenerative nodules, capillarization of sinusoids due to accumulation of fibrous tissue in the sinusoids, sinusoidal collapse, and hepatocyte enlargement. The remaining 30% represents the dynamic component of the increased intrahepatic vascular resistance. HSCs play a central role in the regulation of sinusoidal resistance. These cells are transformed to a myofibroblast-like cell type with increased constrictive properties. Increased levels of vasoconstrictors and decreased levels of vasodilators lead to HSC constriction and subsequently to an increase in intrahepatic vascular resistance. On the other hand, higher concentrations of vasodilators induce hepatic arterial vasodilatation and a lower vascular resistance of the hepatic artery in cirrhosis. Additionally, vascular architectural changes are present in cirrhosis and recent investigations have focused on the presence of neoangiogenesis and vascular remodeling in the intrahepatic circulation.

References

1. D'Amico G, Garcia-Tsao G, Pagliaro L. Natural history and prognostic indicators of survival in cirrhosis: a systematic review of 118 studies. J Hepatol. 2006;44:217–31.
2. Wiest R, Groszmann RJ. The paradox of nitric oxide in cirrhosis and portal hypertension: too much, not enough. Hepatology. 2002;35:478–91.
3. Gupta TK, Toruner M, Groszmann RJ. Intrahepatic modulation of portal pressure and its role in portal hypertension. Role of nitric oxide. Digestion. 1998;59:413–5.
4. Zipprich A. Hemodynamics in the isolated cirrhotic liver. J Clin Gastroenterol. 2007;41 Suppl 3:S254–8.
5. Pinzani M, Failli P, Ruocco C, Casini A, Milani S, Baldi E, et al. Fat-storing cells as liver-specific pericytes. Spatial dynamics of agonist-stimulated intracellular calcium transients. J Clin Invest. 1992;90: 642–6.

6. Zhang JX, Pegoli Jr W, Clemens MG. Endothelin-1 induces direct constriction of hepatic sinusoids. Am J Physiol. 1994;266:G624–32.
7. Lee CH, Loureiro-Silva MR, Abraldes JG, Iwakiri Y, Haq O, Groszmann RJ. Decreased intrahepatic response to alpha(1)-adrenergic agonists in lipopolysaccharide-treated rats is located in the sinusoidal area and depends on Kupffer cell function. J Gastroenterol Hepatol. 2007;22:893–900.
8. Le Couteur DG, Fraser R, Hilmer S, Rivory LP, McLean AJ. The hepatic sinusoid in aging and cirrhosis: effects on hepatic substrate disposition and drug clearance. Clin Pharmacokinet. 2005;44: 187–200.
9. Burridge K, Wennerberg K. Rho and Rac take center stage. Cell. 2004;116:167–79.
10. Aktories K. Bacterial toxins that target Rho proteins. J Clin Invest. 1997;99:827–9.
11. Amano M, Ito M, Kimura K, Fukata Y, Chihara K, Nakano T, et al. Phosphorylation and activation of myosin by Rho-associated kinase (Rho-kinase). J Biol Chem. 1996;271:20246–9.
12. Nakamura M, Nagano T, Chikama T, Nishida T. Role of the small GTP-binding protein rho in epithelial cell migration in the rabbit cornea. Invest Ophthalmol Vis Sci. 2001;42:941–7.
13. Rockey DC, Weisiger RA. Endothelin induced contractility of stellate cells from normal and cirrhotic rat liver: implications for regulation of portal pressure and resistance. Hepatology. 1996;24:233–40.
14. Mittal MK, Gupta TK, Lee FY, Sieber CC, Groszmann RJ. Nitric oxide modulates hepatic vascular tone in normal rat liver. Am J Physiol. 1994;267:G416–22.
15. Deleve LD, Wang X, Guo Y. Sinusoidal endothelial cells prevent rat stellate cell activation and promote reversion to quiescence. Hepatology. 2008;48: 920–30.
16. Richter S, Vollmar B, Mucke I, Post S, Menger MD. Hepatic arteriolo-portal venular shunting guarantees maintenance of nutritional microvascular supply in hepatic arterial buffer response of rat livers. J Physiol. 2001;531:193–201.
17. Loureiro-Silva MR, Cadelina GW, Groszmann RJ. Deficit in nitric oxide production in cirrhotic rat livers is located in the sinusoidal and postsinusoidal areas. Am J Physiol Gastrointest Liver Physiol. 2003;284: G567–74.
18. Zipprich A, Loureiro-Silva MR, D'Silva I, Groszmann RJ. The role of hepatic arterial flow on portal venous and hepatic venous wedged pressure in the isolated perfused CCl4-cirrhotic liver. Am J Physiol Gastrointest Liver Physiol. 2008;295:G197–202.
19. Richter S, Mucke I, Menger MD, Vollmar B. Impact of intrinsic blood flow regulation in cirrhosis: maintenance of hepatic arterial buffer response. Am J Physiol Gastrointest Liver Physiol. 2000;279:G454–62.
20. Lautt WW, Legare DJ, D'Almeida MS. Adenosine as putative regulator of hepatic arterial flow (the buffer response). Am J Physiol. 1985;248:H331–8.
21. Lautt WW. Mechanism and role of intrinsic regulation of hepatic arterial blood flow: hepatic arterial buffer response. Am J Physiol. 1985;249:G549–56.
22. Nagula S, Jain D, Groszmann RJ, Garcia-Tsao G. Histological-hemodynamic correlation in cirrhosis-a histological classification of the severity of cirrhosis. J Hepatol. 2006;44:111–7.
23. Friedman SL. Mechanisms of hepatic fibrogenesis. Gastroenterology. 2008;134:1655–69.
24. Bataller R, Gasull X, Gines P, Hellemans K, Gorbig MN, Nicolas JM, et al. In vitro and in vivo activation of rat hepatic stellate cells results in de novo expression of L-type voltage-operated calcium channels. Hepatology. 2001;33:956–62.
25. Gasull X, Bataller R, Gines P, Sancho-Bru P, Nicolas JM, Gorbig MN, et al. Human myofibroblastic hepatic stellate cells express Ca(2+)-activated K(+) channels that modulate the effects of endothelin-1 and nitric oxide. J Hepatol. 2001;35:739–48.
26. Laleman W, Van Landeghem L, Severi T, Vander Elst I, Zeegers M, Bisschops R, et al. Both Ca2+ -dependent and -independent pathways are involved in rat hepatic stellate cell contraction and intrahepatic hyperresponsiveness to methoxamine. Am J Physiol Gastrointest Liver Physiol. 2007;292:G556–564.
27. Rockey D. The cellular pathogenesis of portal hypertension: stellate cell contractility, endothelin, and nitric oxide. Hepatology. 1997;25:2–5.
28. Gracia-Sancho J, Lavina B, Rodriguez-Vilarrupla A, Garcia-Caldero H, Bosch J, Garcia-Pagan JC. Enhanced vasoconstrictor prostanoid production by sinusoidal endothelial cells increases portal perfusion pressure in cirrhotic rat livers. J Hepatol. 2007;47:220–7.
29. Graupera M, March S, Engel P, Rodes J, Bosch J, Garcia-Pagan JC. Sinusoidal endothelial COX-1-derived prostanoids modulate the hepatic vascular tone of cirrhotic rat livers. Am J Physiol Gastrointest Liver Physiol. 2005;288:G763–70.
30. Steib CJ, Gerbes AL, Bystron M, Op den Winkel M, Hartl J, Roggel F, et al. Kupffer cell activation in normal and fibrotic livers increases portal pressure via thromboxane A(2). J Hepatol. 2007;47:228–38.
31. Bataller R, Gines P, Nicolas JM, Gorbig MN, Garcia-Ramallo E, Gasull X, et al. Angiotensin II induces contraction and proliferation of human hepatic stellate cells. Gastroenterology. 2000;118:1149–56.
32. Bataller R, Nicolas JM, Ginees P, Gorbig MN, Garcia-Ramallo E, Lario S, et al. Contraction of human hepatic stellate cells activated in culture: a role for voltage-operated calcium channels. J Hepatol. 1998;29:398–408.
33. Bataller R, Sancho-Bru P, Gines P, Lora JM, Al Garawi A, Sole M, et al. Activated human hepatic stellate cells express the renin-angiotensin system and synthesize angiotensin II. Gastroenterology. 2003; 125:117–25.
34. Schepke M, Werner E, Biecker E, Schiedermaier P, Heller J, Neef M, et al. Hemodynamic effects of the

angiotensin II receptor antagonist irbesartan in patients with cirrhosis and portal hypertension. Gastroenterology. 2001;121:389–95.
35. Gonzalez-Abraldes J, Albillos A, Banares R, Del Arbol LR, Moitinho E, Rodriguez C, et al. Randomized comparison of long-term losartan versus propranolol in lowering portal pressure in cirrhosis. Gastroenterology. 2001;121:382–8.
36. Yanase M, Ikeda H, Matsui A, Maekawa H, Noiri E, Tomiya T, et al. Lysophosphatidic acid enhances collagen gel contraction by hepatic stellate cells: association with rho-kinase. Biochem Biophys Res Commun. 2000;277:72–8.
37. Ikeda H, Nagashima K, Yanase M, Tomiya T, Arai M, Inoue Y, et al. Involvement of Rho/Rho kinase pathway in regulation of apoptosis in rat hepatic stellate cells. Am J Physiol Gastrointest Liver Physiol. 2003;285:G880–6.
38. Zhou Q, Hennenberg M, Trebicka J, Jochem K, Leifeld L, Biecker E, et al. Intrahepatic upregulation of RhoA and Rho-kinase signalling contributes to increased hepatic vascular resistance in rats with secondary biliary cirrhosis. Gut. 2006;55:1296–305.
39. Sohail MA, Hashmi AZ, Hakim W, Watanabe A, Zipprich A, Groszmann RJ, et al. Adenosine induces loss of actin stress fibers and inhibits contraction in hepatic stellate cells via Rho inhibition. Hepatology. 2009;49:185–94.
40. Loureiro-Silva MR, Iwakiri Y, Abraldes JG, Haq O, Groszmann RJ. Increased phosphodiesterase-5 expression is involved in the decreased vasodilator response to nitric oxide in cirrhotic rat livers. J Hepatol. 2006;44:886–93.
41. Shah V, Toruner M, Haddad F, Cadelina G, Papapetropoulos A, Choo K, et al. Impaired endothelial nitric oxide synthase activity associated with enhanced caveolin binding in experimental cirrhosis in the rat. Gastroenterology. 1999;117:1222–8.
42. Shah V, Cao S, Hendrickson H, Yao J, Katusic ZS. Regulation of hepatic eNOS by caveolin and calmodulin after bile duct ligation in rats. Am J Physiol Gastrointest Liver Physiol. 2001;280:G1209–16.
43. Shah V. Cellular and molecular basis of portal hypertension. Clin Liver Dis. 2001;5:629–44.
44. Abraldes JG, Rodriguez-Vilarrupla A, Graupera M, Zafra C, Garcia-Caldero H, Garcia-Pagan JC, et al. Simvastatin treatment improves liver sinusoidal endothelial dysfunction in CCl(4) cirrhotic rats. J Hepatol. 2007;46:1040–6.
45. Zafra C, Abraldes JG, Turnes J, Berzigotti A, Fernandez M, Garca-Pagan JC, et al. Simvastatin enhances hepatic nitric oxide production and decreases the hepatic vascular tone in patients with cirrhosis. Gastroenterology. 2004;126:749–55.
46. Abraldes JG, Albillos A, Banares R, Turnes J, Gonzalez R, Garcia-Pagan JC, et al. Simvastatin lowers portal pressure in patients with cirrhosis and portal hypertension: a randomized controlled trial. Gastroenterology. 2009;136:1651–8.
47. Liu S, Premont RT, Kontos CD, Zhu S, Rockey DC. A crucial role for GRK2 in regulation of endothelial cell nitric oxide synthase function in portal hypertension. Nat Med. 2005;11:952–8.
48. Semela D, Langer DA, Shah V. GRK2 makes trouble: a no-NO in portal hypertension. Gastroenterology 2006;130:1001–3; discussion 1003.
49. Tran CT, Leiper JM, Vallance P. The DDAH/ADMA/NOS pathway. Atheroscler Suppl. 2003;4:33–40.
50. Laleman W, Omasta A, Van de Casteele M, Zeegers M, Vander Elst I, Van Landeghem L, et al. A role for asymmetric dimethylarginine in the pathophysiology of portal hypertension in rats with biliary cirrhosis. Hepatology. 2005;42:1382–90.
51. Matei V, Rodriguez-Vilarrupla A, Deulofeu R, Colomer D, Fernandez M, Bosch J, et al. The eNOS cofactor tetrahydrobiopterin improves endothelial dysfunction in livers of rats with CCl4 cirrhosis. Hepatology. 2006;44:44–52.
52. Dudenhoefer AA, Loureiro-Silva MR, Cadelina GW, Gupta T, Groszmann RJ. Bioactivation of nitroglycerin and vasomotor response to nitric oxide are impaired in cirrhotic rat livers. Hepatology. 2002;36:381–5.
53. Gupta TK, Toruner M, Chung MK, Groszmann RJ. Endothelial dysfunction and decreased production of nitric oxide in the intrahepatic microcirculation of cirrhotic rats. Hepatology. 1998;28:926–31.
54. Iwakiri Y, Groszmann RJ. Vascular endothelial dysfunction in cirrhosis. J Hepatol. 2007;46:927–34.
55. Loureiro-Silva MR, Cadelina GW, Iwakiri Y, Groszmann RJ. A liver-specific nitric oxide donor improves the intra-hepatic vascular response to both portal blood flow increase and methoxamine in cirrhotic rats. J Hepatol. 2003;39:940–6.
56. Fiorucci S, Antonelli E, Brancaleone V, Sanpaolo L, Orlandi S, Distrutti E, et al. NCX-1000, a nitric oxide-releasing derivative of ursodeoxycholic acid, ameliorates portal hypertension and lowers norepinephrine-induced intrahepatic resistance in the isolated and perfused rat liver. J Hepatol. 2003;39:932–9.
57. Shah V, Chen AF, Cao S, Hendrickson H, Weiler D, Smith L, et al. Gene transfer of recombinant endothelial nitric oxide synthase to liver in vivo and in vitro. Am J Physiol Gastrointest Liver Physiol. 2000;279:G1023–30.
58. Robert K, Nehme J, Bourdon E, Pivert G, Friguet B, Delcayre C, et al. Cystathionine beta synthase deficiency promotes oxidative stress, fibrosis, and steatosis in mice liver. Gastroenterology. 2005;128:1405–15.
59. Fiorucci S, Antonelli E, Mencarelli A, Orlandi S, Renga B, Rizzo G, et al. The third gas: H2S regulates perfusion pressure in both the isolated and perfused normal rat liver and in cirrhosis. Hepatology. 2005;42:539–48.
60. Ekataksin W, Kaneda K. Liver microvascular architecture: an insight into the pathophysiology of portal hypertension. Semin Liver Dis. 1999;19:359–82.

61. Kleber G, Steudel N, Behrmann C, Zipprich A, Hubner G, Lotterer E, et al. Hepatic arterial flow volume and reserve in patients with cirrhosis: use of intra-arterial Doppler and adenosine infusion. Gastroenterology. 1999;116:906–14.
62. Zipprich A, Loureiro-Silva MR, Jain D, D'Silva I, Groszmann RJ. Nitric oxide and vascular remodeling modulate hepatic arterial vascular resistance in the isolated perfused cirrhotic rat liver. J Hepatol. 2008;49:739–45.
63. Mejias M, Garcia-Pras E, Tiani C, Miquel R, Bosch J, Fernandez M. Beneficial effects of sorafenib on splanchnic, intrahepatic, and portocollateral circulations in portal hypertensive and cirrhotic rats. Hepatology. 2009;49:1245–56.
64. Semela D, Das A, Langer D, Kang N, Leof E, Shah V. Platelet-derived growth factor signaling through ephrin-b2 regulates hepatic vascular structure and function. Gastroenterology. 2008;135:671–9.
65. Angermayr B, Fernandez M, Mejias M, Gracia-Sancho J, Garcia-Pagan JC, Bosch J. NAD(P)H oxidase modulates angiogenesis and the development of portosystemic collaterals and splanchnic hyperaemia in portal hypertensive rats. Gut. 2007;56:560–4.
66. Lee JS, Semela D, Iredale J, Shah VH. Sinusoidal remodeling and angiogenesis: a new function for the liver-specific pericyte? Hepatology. 2007;45:817–25.
67. Fernandez M, Semela D, Bruix J, Colle I, Pinzani M, Bosch J. Angiogenesis in liver disease. J Hepatol. 2009;50:604–20.
68. Medina J, Arroyo AG, Sanchez-Madrid F, Moreno-Otero R. Angiogenesis in chronic inflammatory liver disease. Hepatology. 2004;39:1185–95.
69. Hickey PL, Angus PW, McLean A, Morgan DJ. Oxygen supplementation restores theophylline clearance to normal in cirrhotic rats. Gastroenterology. 1995;1995:1504–9.
70. Bozova S, Elpek GO. Hypoxia-inducible factor-1alpha expression in experimental cirrhosis: correlation with vascular endothelial growth factor expression and angiogenesis. APMIS. 2007;115:795–801.
71. Corpechot C, Barbu V, Wendum D, Kinnman N, Rey C, Poupon R, et al. Hypoxia-induced VEGF and collagen I expressions are associated with angiogenesis and fibrogenesis in experimental cirrhosis. Hepatology. 2002;35:1010–21.
72. Rosmorduc O, Wendum D, Corpechot C, Galy B, Sebbagh N, Raleigh J, et al. Hepatocellular hypoxia-induced vascular endothelial growth factor expression and angiogenesis in experimental biliary cirrhosis. Am J Pathol. 1999;155:1065–73.
73. Mottet D, Dumont V, Deccache Y, Demazy C, Ninane N, Raes M, et al. Regulation of hypoxia-inducible factor-1alpha protein level during hypoxic conditions by the phosphatidylinositol 3-kinase/Akt/glycogen synthase kinase 3beta pathway in HepG2 cells. J Biol Chem. 2003;278:31277–85.
74. Tugues S, Fernandez-Varo G, Munoz-Luque J, Ros J, Arroyo V, Rodes J, et al. Antiangiogenic treatment with sunitinib ameliorates inflammatory infiltrate, fibrosis, and portal pressure in cirrhotic rats. Hepatology. 2007;46:1919–26.
75. Mucke I, Richter S, Menger MD, Vollmar B. Significance of hepatic arterial responsiveness for adequate tissue oxygenation upon portal vein occlusion in cirrhotic livers. Int J Colorectal Dis. 2000;15:335–41.

Portal Hypertension: Extrahepatic Mechanisms

7

Jaime Bosch and Juan G. Abraldes

Abstract

The primary event leading to portal hypertension in liver cirrhosis is increased hepatic resistance. However, portal hypertension induces marked alterations in the systemic and splanchnic circulation that result in an increase in portal blood inflow that maintains and aggravates portal hypertension. These include a decrease in systemic vascular resistance, arterial hypotension, increased cardiac output, and plasma volume expansion and are collectively known as the hyperdynamic circulatory state. This chapter provides an overview of the contribution of splanchnic and systemic circulatory abnormalities to the pathogenesis of portal hypertension.

Keywords

Portal hypertension • Vasodilatation • Hyperdynamic circulation

Introduction

Portal hypertension is a frequent clinical syndrome. It is most commonly caused by chronic liver disease, which is relevant since its complications, gastrointestinal bleeding, ascites, renal dysfunction, bacterial infections, and hepatic encephalopathy represent the main cause for liver-related deaths and for liver transplantation worldwide. Cirrhosis of the liver (viral, toxic, metabolic, genetic, or autoimmune) is the most common cause of portal hypertension, followed by hepatic schistosomiasis. Other liver diseases (vascular, granulomatous, tumoral, and idiopathic) and prehepatic portal vein obstruction are responsible for the so-called "non-cirrhotic portal hypertension," which accounts for only 10% of cases.

Portal hypertension is characterized by a pathological increase in portal venous pressure, which results in an increased pressure gradient between the portal vein and the inferior vena cava (the portal pressure gradient, or PPG, which represents the liver portal perfusion pressure). In patients with cirrhosis, the PPG is usually determined indirectly by measuring the hepatic venous pressure gradient (HVPG). Normal values of HVPG are 1–5 mmHg; thus values of 6 mmHg and above are indicative of portal hypertension.

J. Bosch (✉)
Hepatic Hemodynamic Laboratory, Liver Unit, Hospital Clinic-Idibaps, University of Barcelona and Centro de Investigación Biomédica de Enfermedades Hepáticas y Digestivas (Ciberehd), Barcelona, Spain
e-mail: jbosch@clinic.ub.es

L.D. DeLeve and G. Garcia-Tsao (eds.), *Vascular Liver Disease: Mechanisms and Management*,
DOI 10.1007/978-1-4419-8327-5_7, © Springer Science+Business Media, LLC 2011

However, for portal hypertension to become associated with clinical consequences, the HVPG has to increase above critical thresholds, which define what is known as clinically significant portal hypertension. The threshold for the formation of varices is 10 mmHg, and that for variceal bleeding is 12 mmHg, which is also that required for ascites formation and renal dysfunction in most studies [1]. This concept is of key importance, because it provides the rationale and the targets in the prevention and treatment of the complications of portal hypertension [1].

As in any vascular system, the PPG is determined by the interaction of two factors, blood flow (Q) and the vascular resistance that opposes that flow (R), which are described by Ohm's law in Eq. (1):

$$\mathrm{PPG} = \mathrm{Q} \times \mathrm{R}. \quad (1)$$

In established portal hypertension, Q represents the entire blood flow through the portal vein and the portal-systemic collaterals, which is equivalent to the sum of blood flow from splanchnic organs draining into the portal system. Portal-collateral blood flow is thus equivalent to the portal venous inflow [2]. In turn, R is the sum of the vascular resistance of the hepatic circulation and that of the portal-systemic collaterals.

It is evident from the above equation that the PPG may increase due to an increment in vascular resistance, to an increased flow, or to a combination of both factors. The liver is the main site of resistance to portal blood flow but the liver itself has no active role in regulating portal inflow; this function is provided by resistance vessels at the splanchnic arteriolar level. Hence, the normal liver is a passive recipient of fluctuating amounts of blood flow that, due to its large and distensible vascular network, can encompass a wide range of portal blood flow with minimal effect on pressure in the portal system [3]. Thus, in clinical situations, portal hypertension is always initiated by an increased vascular resistance. However, once portal hypertension develops, a series of mechanisms lead to an increase in portal venous inflow that contributes to perpetuate and aggravate portal hypertension.

This chapter deals with the extrahepatic mechanisms involved in the pathogenesis of portal hypertension. For practical purposes, these will be divided to (a) mechanisms leading to increased splanchnic blood inflow and (b) mechanisms involved in collateral formation and the regulation of collateral vascular tone.

The Increase in Portal Blood Inflow

Chronic portal hypertension is associated with a marked increase in splanchnic blood inflow [2, 4, 5]. The ensuing increase in portal-collateral blood flow maintains and aggravates portal hypertension despite the formation of an extensive network of portal-systemic collaterals. Its importance in the pathophysiology of portal hypertension and its complications is well established, to the point that it is the target of most pharmacological therapies for portal hypertension, from vasopressin and its derivatives, to nonselective beta-blockers [6]. This increase in portal venous inflow occurs in portal hypertension of any etiology, and is so pronounced that it represents the major component of the hyperkinetic syndrome, characterized by an increased cardiac index and plasma volume and reduced peripheral vascular resistance [2, 4, 5, 7]. Thus, while the intrahepatic circulation in cirrhosis exhibits an increased vascular tone (see Chap. 6), the splanchnic circulation has a pronounced vasorelaxation.

Splanchnic arteriolar vasodilation is the initial factor leading to the increase in portal blood inflow. At least three mechanisms are thought to contribute to vasodilatation in portal hypertension: (1) increased concentration of systemic vasodilators, (2) increased endothelial production of local vasodilators, and (3) decreased vascular responsiveness to endogenous vasoconstrictors. The latter mechanism is probably due to the effect of the first two components. Additionally, a recent line of evidence suggests that vascular remodeling and VEGF-dependent angiogenesis is required to maintain a sustained increase in portal blood inflow [8].

Circulatory Vasodilators

Glucagon

Initial studies focused on circulating mediators that would be increased due to a deficient removal by the cirrhotic liver because of a deteriorated liver function and/or portosystemic shunting [9]. Glucagon is probably the humoral vasodilator for which there is the most evidence supporting a role in promoting splanchnic hyperemia in portal hypertension [10–13]. Many studies have demonstrated that plasma glucagon levels are elevated in cirrhosis. Hyperglucagonemia results, in part, from decreased hepatic clearance but, more importantly, from an increased secretion by pancreatic alpha cells [14]. The support for a role of glucagon in modulating splanchnic blood flow comes from studies showing that normalization of circulating glucagon levels partially reverses the increased splanchnic blood flow, and this can be prevented by a concomitant glucagon infusion [10, 12]. However, some studies have shown no correlation between glucagon levels and splanchnic blood flow, thus calling into question a major role for hyperglucagonemia in portal hypertension. Glucagon release is clearly implicated in postprandial hyperemia, which in patients with cirrhosis is associated with marked increases in portal pressure [15]. Collectively, these data provide the rationale for the use of somatostatin and octreotide in the treatment of patients with portal hypertension [16], although it was recently demonstrated that these drugs promote vasoconstriction by mechanisms independent of glucagon inhibition [17].

Endocannabinoids

In rats and in patients with advanced cirrhosis, there is an increase in the production of the endogenous cannabinoid anandamide by monocytes [18, 19], and the specific blockade of the peripheral cannabinoid receptor CB1 attenuates the hyperdynamic circulation [18, 19] and decreases portal pressure [18]. In addition, resistance mesenteric arteries from cirrhotic rats exhibit an increased vasodilatory response to anandamide related to an overexpression of CB1 receptor. This represents a local mesenteric phenomenon, because it does not occur in other peripheral vessels. It has been postulated that cannabinoids act through an increase in nitric oxide (NO) production [18], but recent data do not support this contention [19, 20]. The mechanisms that would induce anandamide production are not clear, but could be related to the frequent endotoxemia observed in cirrhosis [21].

Several other circulating vasodilators, such as calcitonin gene-related peptide (CGRP) [22], adrenomedullin [23, 24], and urotensin [25], have also been linked to the pathogenesis of vasodilatation in portal hypertension, but evidence is still scarce.

Local Vasodilators

Nitric Oxide

The role of NO in portal hypertension was initially suggested by Vallance and Moncada [26]. Several lines of evidence have since confirmed the central role of NO in the development of the hyperdynamic circulation [27, 28]. On the one hand, patients with cirrhosis have increased levels of nitrites and nitrates [29], the degradation products of NO. In experimental animals, it was demonstrated that NO production is increased in the splanchnic vascular bed of portal hypertensive rats, and this accounts for the hyporesponsiveness to vasoconstrictors characteristic of portal hypertension [30]. Furthermore, inhibition of NO production reduces portal pressure and portosystemic shunting and prevents (though not completely) the development of hyperdynamic circulation [27, 28, 31, 32]. This latter finding, together with the fact that a double eNOS/iNOS knock-out mice still develops the hyperdynamic circulation after the induction of portal hypertension [33], suggests that NO is the principal, but not the only, mediator of vasodilatation.

A number of molecular studies have characterized the mechanisms leading to increased NO production in portal hypertension. At odds with the original hypothesis, which suggested that endotoxemia present in cirrhosis would upregulate the *inducible* nitric oxide synthase (iNOS) [26], overwhelming data suggest that increased NO in portal hypertension is mainly mediated by *endothelial* nitric oxide synthase (eNOS) [34]. Recent data suggest that *neuronal* nitric oxide syntase (nNOS) activation could also have a role in the increased NO production that occurs in portal hypertension [35], but this role would be far outweighed by that of eNOS [36].

The most powerful stimulus for eNOS up-regulation is shear stress [37]. Indeed, shear stress is increased in portal hypertension once the hyperdynamic circulation is established. Furthermore, the superior mesenteric vascular bed from portal hypertensive rats shows enhanced production of NO in response to shear stress [30]. Bacterial translocation also contributes to increased NO production in advanced cirrhosis, but the mechanism involves up-regulation of eNOS, not iNOS [38, 39]. Finally, portosystemic shunting, per se, can induce NO-mediated vasodilation [40, 41]. However, sequential studies in the portal vein ligated model have shown that eNOS activation occurs before any of these three mechanisms are present [42, 43]. This indicates, on the one hand, that increased eNOS production is a primary factor in the development of vasodilation and, on the other hand, that mechanisms different from the above-mentioned activate eNOS in the very early phases of portal hypertension. Recent data indicate that this initial eNOS up-regulation occurs at the microcirculation of the intestinal mucosa, and that it is secondary to VEGF up-regulation [44], raising the possibility that the first stimulus that upregulates eNOS is intestinal hypoxia, secondary to congestion or to superior mesenteric artery reflex vasoconstriction in response to increased portal pressure [43]. In keeping with these findings, it was recently demonstrated that blocking VEGF action from the onset of portal hypertension markedly attenuates the development of the hyperdynamic circulation and decreases portal blood inflow by 50% [8] (Fig. 7.1). Whether these mechanisms account for the development of the hyperdynamic circulation in human cirrhosis needs to be confirmed.

Molecular studies have shown that, in the early stages of portal hypertension, increased eNOS activity is detected prior to the increase in eNOS expression. This is due to activation of eNOS at the posttranslational level, mediated by increased Akt-dependent eNOS phosphorylation [43, 45]. In more advanced stages of portal hypertension, NO production increases both due to an increase in eNOS expression [38] and an increase

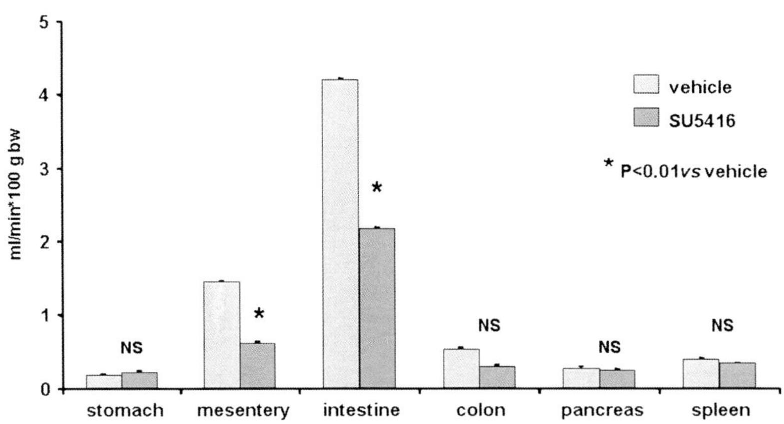

Fig. 7.1 Effects of the inhibition of VEGF signaling on splanchnic blood flow in a model of prehepatic portal hypertension. The administration of SU5416, an inhibitor of VEGF receptor 2 activity, results in a marked reduction in mesenteric and intestinal blood flow. This suggests that VEGF activation contributes to the increase in splanchnic inflow observed in portal hypertension (constructed with data from Fernandez et al. [8])

in eNOS activity related to changes at the posttranslational level. This latter mechanism involves an increased interaction of eNOS with the molecular chaperone Hsp90 [46]. It has also been shown that bacterial translocation activates eNOS through a TNF-alpha-mediated increase in tetrahydrobiopterin (BH_4) [38, 39], an essential cofactor of eNOS. Taken together, these studies show that different mechanisms upregulate eNOS in portal hypertension, and that the relative importance of these mechanisms varies along the course of the syndrome.

In summary, in striking contrast to what occurs in the intrahepatic circulation, in which there is a deficit in NO production, in the splanchnic circulation there is an increase in NO production [34]. Therefore, pharmacological therapies aimed at manipulating NO production should be formulated cautiously, taking into account the opposing roles of NO in the splanchnic and in the hepatic vascular beds. What can be a "friend" by reducing the liver vascular tone (i.e., supplementing NO by means of NO donors) may be a "foe" by aggravating the hyperkinetic syndrome and causing systemic hypotension [47]. Because of this, liver-specific or splanchnic-specific agents are being investigated [48–51].

Additionally, it is important to note that the primary defect is the increase in intrahepatic resistance, and splanchnic vasodilation is a secondary alteration. Furthermore, the severity of the hyperdynamic circulation closely correlates with the resistance to portal blood flow [44] (Fig. 7.2). Therefore, it is likely that the hyperkinetic

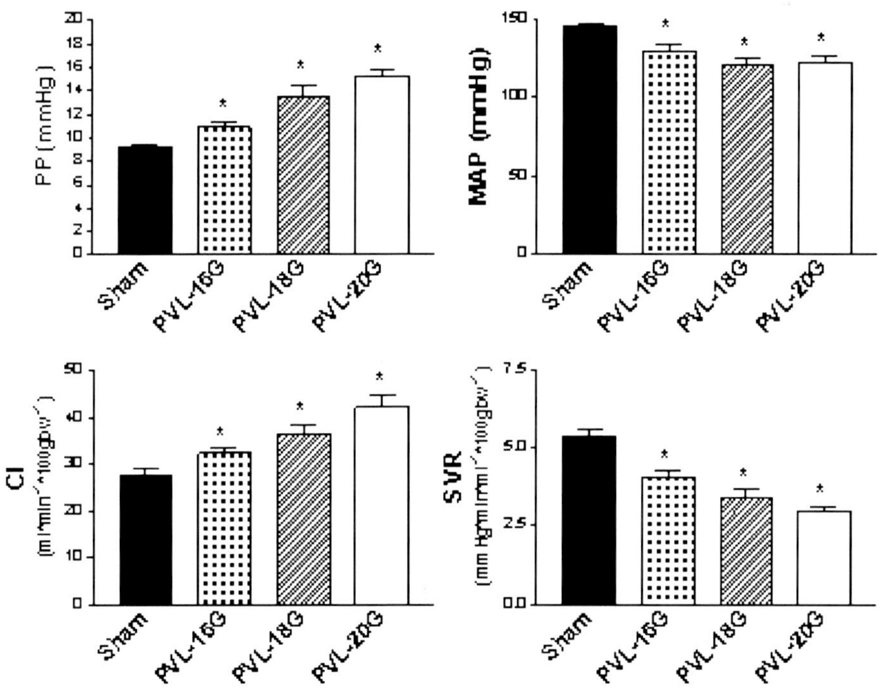

Fig. 7.2 The degree of hyperdynamic circulation is proportional to the degree of increased portal vein resistance: Portal vein ligation (PVL) performed using different needles of increasing caliber (16- (16G), 18- (18G), and 20-gauge (20G)) produces rats with different degrees of increased portal resistance and portal pressure (PP). The decrease in mean arterial pressure (MAP) and systemic vascular resistance (SVR) and the increase in cardiac index (CI) are proportional to the degree of portal vein stenosis (constructed with data from Abraldes et al. [44]

syndrome might be, at least partly, reversed by attenuating the increase in hepatic resistance.

Prostacyclin

Another local vasodilator that has been linked to splanchnic hyperemia in portal hypertension is prostacyclin [52, 53], but the available evidence is less extensive than that for NO. Systemic and splanchnic production of prostacyclin is increased in portal hypertension as a consequence of an increased expression of COX-1 and COX-2 [54]. Blocking either of the two isoforms increases the response of the splanchnic vasculature to vasoconstrictors, but the effect of COX-2 blockade is more intense [54]. Furthermore, COX blockade has been shown to attenuate the hyperdynamic circulation in portal hypertension [55, 56].

Carbon Monoxide

Carbon monoxide (CO) is an end product of the heme oxygenase (HO) pathway, which seems to play an important role in the regulation of vascular resistance in several vascular beds, including mesenteric arteries [57]. CO is generated in endothelial and smooth muscle layers of arterial vessels and, similar to NO, induces vasodilation through stimulation of soluble guanylyl cyclase (sGC) in vascular smooth muscle cells. Several studies have demonstrated that the inducible isoform of HO (HO-1) is upregulated in the systemic and splanchnic circulation of portal hypertensive animals, contributing to vasodilation and the hyperdynamic circulatory state [58–60].

Plasma Volume Expansion and the Hyperkinetic Syndrome

Splanchnic vasodilatation is characteristically associated with peripheral vasodilatation and a systemic hyperkinetic syndrome, characterized by reduced arterial pressure and peripheral resistance, and increased plasma volume and cardiac output. The pathophysiological mechanisms involved in peripheral vasodilatation are similar to those previously discussed for splanchnic vasodilatation. Peripheral vasodilatation plays a major role in the activation of endogenous neurohumoral systems leading to sodium retention and expansion of the plasma volume that is followed by the increase in cardiac index [61, 62], which contributes to aggravate portal hypertension. This provides the rationale for using a low sodium diet and/or diuretics in the treatment of portal hypertension [63]. These abnormalities also contribute to the development of other complications of portal hypertension, such as ascites and the hepatorenal syndrome [7].

Collateral Resistance

The development of collaterals in portal hypertension is the key event that leads to severe complications such as variceal bleeding and hepatic encephalopathy. Collaterals develop as a consequence of the pressure increase in the portal system, theoretically allowing the decompression of the portal territory to vascular beds of low pressure. However, this decompression does not occur because in parallel with the development of collaterals, an increase in portal blood inflow maintains portal hypertension [2, 4, 5].

Collateral formation results in part from the opening and dilation of preformed vascular channels but also from active, VEGF-dependent angiogenesis (Fig. 7.3). In this regard, recent studies have shown that VEGF expression increases in the intestine and mesentery of rats with prehepatic portal hypertension and that early VEGF blockade leads to a 50% reduction in collateral development in this model [8, 64]. Collateral formation has also been shown to be NO-dependent [65], raising the possibility that VEGF acts upstream of NO in the collateralization process. Additionally, studies have shown that local NADPH-dependent oxidative stress in the splanchnic circulation [66], PDGF [67, 68], and apelin signaling [69] contribute to the development and stabilization of collaterals. Further clarification is required regarding interactions and the relative importance among these mediators in the development and maintenance of portosystemic collaterals.

Since in advanced portal hypertension as much as 90% of portal blood flow could be shunted through portosystemic collaterals, changes in collateral resistance can modify portal pressure.

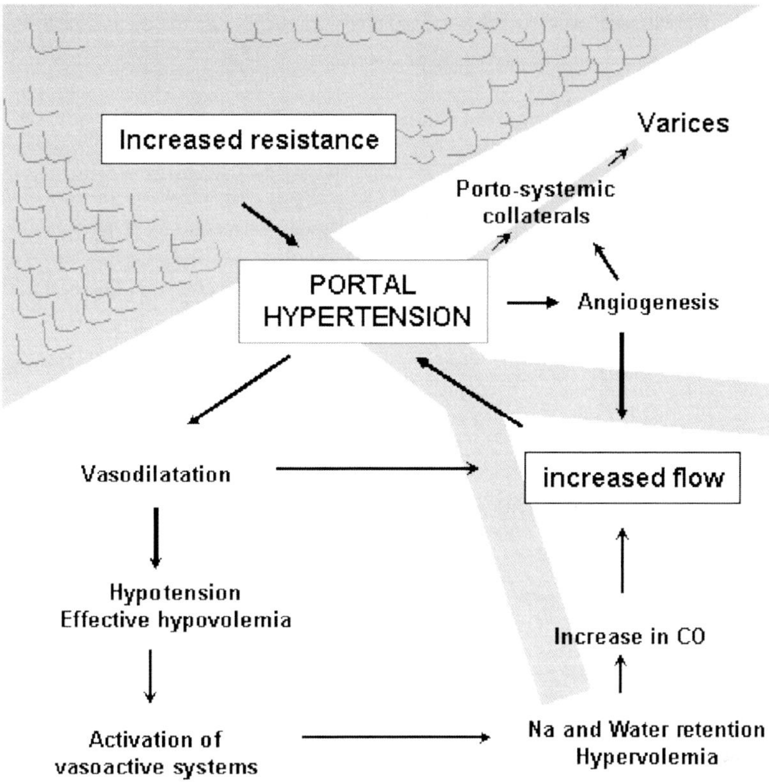

Fig. 7.3 The increase in hepatic resistance leads to an increase in portal pressure. This leads to a cascade of disturbances in the splanchnic and systemic circulation characterized by vasodilation, sodium and water retention, and plasma volume expansion, which play a major role in the pathogenesis of ascites and hepatorenal syndrome. Additionally, these alterations, together with an increase in angiogenesis, lead to an increase in portal blood inflow that maintains and aggravates portal hypertension. Another characteristic feature is the development of portosystemic collaterals, which are responsible for complications such as variceal bleeding and hepatic encephalopathy (*CO* cardiac output)

A number of studies performed in a model in which the collateral bed is perfused in situ have demonstrated that these vessels have functional receptors for vasopressin, endothelin, serotonin, and alpha and beta-adrenergic receptors, and respond to NO with vasodilation [70, 71].

Conclusions

Though the primary event leading to portal hypertension in cirrhosis is increased hepatic resistance, portal hypertension induces marked alterations in the systemic and splanchnic circulation, characterized by a decrease in systemic vascular resistance, arterial hypotension, increased cardiac output, and plasma volume expansion, known as the hyperdynamic circulatory state. This leads to an increase in portal blood inflow that maintains and aggravates portal hypertension (see Fig. 7.3).

References

1. Bosch J, Abraldes JG, Berzigotti A, et al. The clinical use of HVPG measurements in chronic liver disease. Nat Rev Gastroenterol Hepatol. 2009;6:576–82.
2. Vorobioff J, Bredfeldt JE, Groszmann RJ. Increased blood flow through the portal system in cirrhotic rats. Gastroenterology. 1984;87:1120–3.
3. Witte CL, Tobin GR, Clark DS, et al. Relationship of splanchnic blood flow and portal venous resistance to

elevated portal pressure in the dog. Gut. 1976;17:122–6.
4. Groszmann RJ, Vorobioff J, Riley E. Splanchnic hemodynamics in portal-hypertensive rats: measurement with gamma-labeled microspheres. Am J Physiol. 1982;242:G156–60.
5. Vorobioff J, Bredfeldt J, Groszmann RJ, et al. Hyperdynamic circulation in a portal hypertensive rat model: a primary factor for maintenance of chronic portal hypertension. Am J Physiol. 1983;244:G52–6.
6. Bosch J, Abraldes JG, Berzigotti A, et al. Portal hypertension and gastrointestinal bleeding. Semin Liver Dis. 2008;28:3–25.
7. Groszmann RJ. Hyperdynamic circulation of liver disease 40 years later: pathophysiology and clinical consequences. Hepatology. 1994;20:1359–63.
8. Fernandez M, Mejias M, Angermayr B, et al. Inhibition of VEGF receptor-2 decreases the development of hyperdynamic splanchnic circulation and portal-systemic collateral vessels in portal hypertensive rats. J Hepatol. 2005;43:98–103.
9. Benoit JN, Barrowman JA, Harper SL, et al. Role of humoral factors in the intestinal hyperemia associated with chronic portal hypertension. Am J Physiol. 1984;247:G486–93.
10. Kravetz D, Bosch J, Arderiu MT, et al. Effects of somatostatin on splanchnic hemodynamics and plasma glucagon in portal hypertensive rats. Am J Physiol. 1988;254:G322–8.
11. Silva G, Navasa M, Bosch J, et al. Hemodynamic effects of glucagon in portal hypertension. Hepatology. 1990;11:668–73.
12. Pizcueta MP, Garcia-Pagan JC, Fernandez M, et al. Glucagon hinders the effects of somatostatin on portal hypertension. A study in rats with partial portal vein ligation. Gastroenterology. 1991;101:1710–5.
13. Benoit JN, Granger DN. Splanchnic hemodynamics in chronic portal hypertension. Semin Liver Dis. 1986;6:287–98.
14. Gomis R, Fernandez-Alvarez J, Pizcueta P, et al. Impaired function of pancreatic islets from rats with portal hypertension resulting from cirrhosis and partial portal vein ligation. Hepatology. 1994;19:1257–61.
15. Albillos A, Rossi I, Iborra J, et al. Octreotide prevents postprandial splanchnic hyperemia in patients with portal hypertension. J Hepatol. 1994;21:88–94.
16. Abraldes JG, Bosch J. Somatostatin and analogues in portal hypertension. Hepatology. 2002;35:1305–12.
17. Wiest R, Tsai MH, Groszmann RJ. Octreotide potentiates PKC-dependent vasoconstrictors in portal-hypertensive and control rats. Gastroenterology. 2001; 120:975–83.
18. Batkai S, Jarai Z, Wagner JA, et al. Endocannabinoids acting at vascular CB1 receptors mediate the vasodilated state in advanced liver cirrhosis. Nat Med. 2001;7:827–32.
19. Ros J, Claria J, To-Figueras J, et al. Endogenous cannabinoids: a new system involved in the homeostasis of arterial pressure in experimental cirrhosis in the rat. Gastroenterology. 2002;122:85–93.
20. Domenicali M, Ros J, Fernandez-Varo G, et al. Increased anandamide induced relaxation in mesenteric arteries of cirrhotic rats: role of cannabinoid and vanilloid receptors. Gut. 2005;54:522–7.
21. Varga K, Wagner JA, Bridgen DT, et al. Platelet- and macrophage-derived endogenous cannabinoids are involved in endotoxin-induced hypotension. FASEB J. 1998;12:1035–44.
22. Hori N, Okanoue T. SYKK. Role of calcitonin gene-related peptide in the vascular system on the development of the hyperdynamic circulation in conscious cirrhotic rats. Hepatology. 1997;1999(26):1111–9.
23. Fernandez-Rodriguez CM, Prada IR, Prieto J, et al. Circulating adrenomedullin in cirrhosis: relationship to hyperdynamic circulation. J Hepatol. 1998;29:250–6.
24. Genesca J, Gonzalez A, Catalan R, et al. Adrenomedullin, a vasodilator peptide implicated in hemodynamic alterations of liver cirrhosis: relationship to nitric oxide. Dig Dis Sci. 1999;44:372–6.
25. Trebicka J, Leifeld L, Hennenberg M, et al. Hemodynamic effects of urotensin II and its specific receptor antagonist palosuran in cirrhotic rats. Hepatology. 2008;47:1264–76.
26. Vallance P, Moncada S. Hyperdynamic circulation in cirrhosis: a role for nitric oxide? Lancet. 1991;337:776.
27. Pizcueta P, Piqué JM, Fernández M, et al. Modulation of the hyperdynamic circulation of cirrhotic rats by nitric oxide inhibition. Gastroenterology. 1992;103: 1909–15.
28. Pizcueta MP, Piqué JM, Bosch J, et al. Effects of inhibiting nitric oxide biosynthesis on the systemic and splanchnic circulation of rats with portal hypertension. Br J Pharmacol. 1992;105:105–84.
29. Guarner C, Soriano G, Tomas A, et al. Increased serum nitrite and nitrate levels in patients with cirrhosis: relationship to endotoxemia. Hepatology. 1993;18: 1139–43.
30. Hori N, Wiest R, Groszmann RJ. Enhanced release of nitric oxide in response to changes in flow and shear stress in the superior mesenteric arteries of portal hypertensive rats. Hepatology. 1998;28:1467–73.
31. Lee FY, Colombato LA, Albillos A, et al. Administration of N omega-nitro-l-arginine ameliorates portal-systemic shunting in portal-hypertensive rats. Gastroenterology. 1993;105:1464–70.
32. García-Pagán JC, Fernandez M, Bernadich C, et al. Effects of continued nitric oxide inhibition on the development of the portal hypertnesive syndrome following portal vein stenosis in the rat. Am J Physiol. 1994;30:984–90.
33. Iwakiri Y, Cadelina G, Sessa WC, et al. Mice with targeted deletion of eNOS develop hyperdynamic circulation associated with portal hypertension. Am J Physiol Gastrointest Liver Physiol. 2002;283: G1074–81.
34. Wiest R, Groszmann RJ. The paradox of nitric oxide in cirrhosis and portal hypertension: too much, not enough. Hepatology. 2002;35:478–91.
35. Jurzik L, Froh M, Straub RH, et al. Up-regulation of nNOS and associated increase in nitrergic vasodilation

in superior mesenteric arteries in pre-hepatic portal hypertension. J Hepatol. 2005;43:258–65.
36. Kwon SY, Groszmann RJ, Iwakiri Y. Increased neuronal nitric oxide synthase interaction with soluble guanylate cyclase contributes to the splanchnic arterial vasodilation in portal hypertensive rats. Hepatol Res. 2007;37:58–67.
37. Sessa WC. eNOS at a glance. J Cell Sci. 2004;117:2427–9.
38. Wiest R, Das S, Cadelina G, et al. Bacterial translocation in cirrhotic rats stimulates eNOS-derived NO production and impairs mesenteric vascular contractility. J Clin Invest. 1999;104:1223–33.
39. Wiest R, Cadelina G, Milstien S, et al. Bacterial translocation up-regulates GTP-cyclohydrolase I in mesenteric vasculature of cirrhotic rats. Hepatology. 2003;38:1508–15.
40. Bernadich C, Bandi JC, Piera C, et al. Circulatory effects of graded diversion of portal blood flow to the systemic circulation in rats: role of nitric oxide. Hepatology. 1997;26:262–7.
41. Bandi JC, Fernandez M, Bernadich C, et al. Hyperkinetic circulation and decreased sensitivity to vasoconstrictors following portacaval shunt in the rat. Effects of chronic nitric oxide inhibition. J Hepatol. 1999;31:719–24.
42. Wiest R, Shah V, Sessa WC, et al. NO overproduction by eNOS precedes hyperdynamic splanchnic circulation in portal hypertensive rats. Am J Physiol. 1999;276:G1043–51.
43. Tsai MH, Iwakiri Y, Cadelina G, et al. Mesenteric vasoconstriction triggers nitric oxide overproduction in the superior mesenteric artery of portal hypertensive rats. Gastroenterology. 2003;125:1452–61.
44. Abraldes JG, Iwakiri Y, Loureiro-Silva M, et al. Mild increases in portal pressure upregulate vascular endothelial growth factor and endothelial nitric oxide synthase in the intestinal microcirculatory bed, leading to a hyperdynamic state. Am J Physiol Gastrointest Liver Physiol. 2006;290:G980–7.
45. Iwakiri Y, Tsai MH, McCabe TJ, et al. Phosphorylation of eNOS initiates excessive NO production in early phases of portal hypertension. Am J Physiol Heart Circ Physiol. 2002;282:H2084–90.
46. Shah V, Wiest R, Garcia-Cardena G, et al. Hsp90 regulation of endothelial nitric oxide synthase contributes to vascular control in portal hypertension. Am J Physiol. 1999;277:G463–8.
47. Groszmann RJ. Beta-adrenergic blockers and nitrovasodilators for the treatment of portal hypertension: the good, the bad, the ugly. Gastroenterology. 1997;113:1794–7.
48. Loureiro-Silva MR, Cadelina GW, Iwakiri Y, et al. A liver-specific nitric oxide donor improves the intrahepatic vascular response to both portal blood flow increase and methoxamine in cirrhotic rats. J Hepatol. 2003;39:940–6.
49. Fiorucci S, Antonelli E, Brancaleone V, et al. NCX-1000, a nitric oxide-releasing derivative of ursodeoxycholic acid, ameliorates portal hypertension and lowers norepinephrine-induced intrahepatic resistance in the isolated and perfused rat liver. J Hepatol. 2003;39:932–9.
50. Abraldes JG, Rodriguez-Vilarrupla A, Graupera M, et al. Simvastatin treatment improves liver sinusoidal endothelial dysfunction in CCl4 cirrhotic rats. J Hepatol. 2007;46:1040–6.
51. Abraldes JG, Albillos A, Banares R, et al. Simvastatin lowers portal pressure in patients with cirrhosis and portal hypertension: a randomized controlled trial. Gastroenterology. 2009;136:1651–8.
52. Guarner C, Soriano G, Such J, et al. Systemic prostacyclin in cirrhotic patients. Relationship with portal hypertension and changes after intestinal decontamination [see comments]. Gastroenterology. 1992;102:303–9.
53. Sitzmann JV, Bulkley GB. Role of prostacyclin in the splanchnic hyperemia contributing to portal hypertension. Ann Surg. 1989;209:322–7.
54. Potenza MA, Botrugno OA, De Salvia MA, et al. Endothelial COX-1 and -2 differentially affect reactivity of MVB in portal hypertensive rats. Am J Physiol Gastrointest Liver Physiol. 2002;283:G587–94.
55. Fernandez M, Garcia-Pagan JC, Casadevall M, et al. Acute and chronic cyclooxygenase blockade in portal hypertensive rats. Influence on nitric oxide biosynthesis. Gastroenterology. 1996;110:1529–35.
56. Bruix J, Bosch J, Kravetz D, et al. Effects of prostaglandin inhibition on systemic and hepatic hemodynamics in patients with cirrhosis of the liver. Gastroenterology. 1985;88:430–5.
57. Naik JS, O'Donaughy TL, Walker BR. Endogenous carbon monoxide is an endothelial-derived vasodilator factor in the mesenteric circulation. Am J Physiol Heart Circ Physiol. 2003;284:H838–45.
58. Chen YC, Gines P, Yang J, et al. Increased vascular heme oxygenase-1 expression contributes to arterial vasodilation in experimental cirrhosis in rats. Hepatology. 2004;39:1075–87.
59. Fernandez M, Lambrecht RW, Bonkovsky HL. Increased heme oxygenase activity in splanchnic organs from portal hypertensive rats: role in modulating mesenteric vascular reactivity. J Hepatol. 2001;34:812–7.
60. Angermayr B, Mejias M, Gracia-Sancho J, et al. Heme oxygenase attenuates oxidative stress and inflammation, and increases VEGF expression in portal hypertensive rats. J Hepatol. 2006;44:1033–9.
61. Albillos A, Colombato LA, Groszmann RJ. Vasodilatation and sodium retention in prehepatic portal hypertension [see comments]. Gastroenterology. 1992;102:931–5.
62. Colombato LA, Albillos A, Groszmann RJ. The role of central blood volume in the development of sodium retention in portal hypertensive rats. Gastroenterology. 1996;110:193–8.
63. Garcia-Pagan JC, Salmeron JM, Feu F, et al. Effects of low-sodium diet and spironolactone on portal

pressure in patients with compensated cirrhosis. Hepatology. 1994;19:1095–9.
64. Fernandez M, Vizzutti F, Garcia-Pagan JC, et al. Anti-VEGF receptor-2 monoclonal antibody prevents portal-systemic collateral vessel formation in portal hypertensive mice. Gastroenterology. 2004;126:886–94.
65. Sieber CC, Sumanovski LT, Stumm M, et al. In vivo angiogenesis in normal and portal hypertensive rats: role of basic fibroblast growth factor and nitric oxide. J Hepatol. 2001;34:644–50.
66. Angermayr B, Fernandez M, Mejias M, et al. NAD(P)H oxidase modulates angiogenesis and the development of portosystemic collaterals and splanchnic hyperaemia in portal hypertensive rats. Gut. 2006;56(4):560–4.
67. Fernandez M, Mejias M, Garcia-Pras E, et al. Reversal of portal hypertension and hyperdynamic splanchnic circulation by combined vascular endothelial growth factor and platelet-derived growth factor blockade in rats. Hepatology. 2007;46:1208–17.
68. Mejias M, Garcia-Pras E, Tiani C, et al. Beneficial effects of sorafenib on splanchnic, intrahepatic, and portocollateral circulations in portal hypertensive and cirrhotic rats. Hepatology. 2009;49:1245–56.
69. Tiani C, Garcia-Pras E, Mejias M, et al. Apelin signaling modulates splanchnic angiogenesis and portosystemic collateral vessel formation in rats with portal hypertension. J Hepatol. 2009;50:296–305.
70. Mosca P, Lee FY, Kaumann AJ, et al. Pharmacology of portal-systemic collaterals in portal hypertensive rats: role of endothelium. Am J Physiol. 1992;263:G544–50.
71. Chan CC, Wang SS, Lee FY, et al. Endothelin-1 induces vasoconstriction on portal-systemic collaterals of portal hypertensive rats. Hepatology. 2001;33:816–20.

Part II

Management

8 Histological Diagnosis

Dhanpat Jain and A. Brian West

Abstract

The vascular system of the liver is composed of four major components: the portal venous system, the hepatic venous system, the hepatic arterial (HA) system, and the hepatic sinusoids. Functionally, they are all connected, and disorders of one often secondarily involve others. Besides various hypercoagulable states that are a common risk factor for many of these disorders, a variety of congenital and inherited disorders, infections, drugs, and toxins can involve different components of the liver vasculature. Alterations in hepatic blood flow can have a significant impact on the architecture and function of the liver. The effects of reduced blood flow on the liver are varied and depend on many factors. Critical ischemic injury results in hepatocyte necrosis of varying extent, while subcritical chronic ischemia merely causes attenuation of hepatocytes and atrophy of the hepatic parenchyma. Involvement of the biliary tree can mimic a primary biliary disorder. In many of these disorders the clinical setting is distinct, while in others the histology is diagnostic, and some others require a careful clinicopathological correlation to arrive at a correct diagnosis. This chapter describes the pathology of various vascular disorders of the liver and also discusses a practical approach to pathologic diagnosis.

Keywords

Liver • Vascular disease • Pathology • Ischemia

Introduction

The vascular system of the liver is composed of four major components: the portal venous system, the hepatic venous system, the hepatic arterial (HA) system, and the hepatic sinusoids. As summarized in Table 8.1, different disease processes can affect each of these components. Functionally, they are all connected, and disorders of one often secondarily involve others. The liver receives about one third of the cardiac output via the hepatic artery (HA), which supplies only one third of the blood flow to the liver, the rest coming from the portal vein (PV). Alterations in hepatic blood flow can have a significant impact

A.B. West (✉)
Department of Pathology, Yale University School of Medicine, New Haven, CT, USA
e-mail: brian.west@yale.edu

L.D. DeLeve and G. Garcia-Tsao (eds.), *Vascular Liver Disease: Mechanisms and Management*, DOI 10.1007/978-1-4419-8327-5_8,

on the architecture and function of the liver, although its dual blood supply tends to protect it from severe injury caused by isolated obstruction of either HA or PV. This forms the basis of the "dual-hit" theory of vascular injury proposed by Ian Wanless [1]. The effects of reduced blood flow on the liver are varied and depend on many factors. Critical ischemic injury results in hepatocyte necrosis of varying extent, while subcritical chronic ischemia merely causes attenuation of hepatocytes and atrophy of the hepatic parenchyma [2]. In such situations, regeneration of the better perfused regions may result in compensatory hyperplasia and nodularity, sometimes to the extent of mimicking cirrhosis or a tumor.

An often-neglected component of vascular injury to the liver is its effect on the biliary tree, sometimes mimicking a primary biliary disorder. Hepatic blood vessels are frequently involved secondarily in other primary hepatic disorders, such as primary biliary cirrhosis, alcoholic liver disease, sarcoidosis, and infections. In such conditions, the diagnosis of the primary disorder is often obvious, and although the vascular changes may have functional consequences, they have little clinical or diagnostic significance. Also, involvement of one component of the vascular system may result in secondary involvement of the others, e.g., stasis and back pressure in the PV in cases of Budd–Chiari syndrome (HV thrombosis) may result in PV thrombosis [3]. Similarly, thrombosis of the HA is not infrequent in cases of PV thrombosis. Hypercoagulable states, listed in Table 8.1, are a common risk factor for thrombosis in several different components of the vascular system. These vascular disorders of the liver are

Table 8.1 Etiologic classification of various disorders affecting the liver vasculature as per the predominant vessel-type involved

I. Portal vein thrombosis
1. Local risk factors
i. Cancer (any intraabdominal organ)
ii. Focal inflammatory lesions
a. Neonatal omphalitis, umbilical catheterization
b. Diverticulitis, appendicitis, pylephlebitis
c. Pancreatitis
d. Crohn's disease, ulcerative colitis
e. Cytomegalovirus hepatitis
f. Cholecystitis
g. Duodenal ulcer
iii. Injury to portal venous system
a. Splenectomy
b. Colectomy, gastrectomy
c. Liver transplantation
d. Abdominal trauma
e. Surgical portosystemic shunting, TIPS
iv. Cirrhosis
2. Systems risk factors
i. Myeloproliferative disorders
ii. Antiphospholipid syndrome
iii. Paroxysmal nocturnal hemoglobinuria
iv. Behcet's disease
v. Coagulation factor abnormalities
a. Factor V Leiden
b. Protein C deficiency
c. Protein S deficiency
d. Factor II mutation
e. Antithrombin deficiency
vi. Hyperhomocysteinemia
vii. Recent pregnancy
viii. Oral contraceptive pill use
ix. TT677 MTH FR genotype
II. Disorders of small portal vein branches
1. Idiopathic portal hypertension/NCPF/hepatoportal sclerosis
2. HIV-associated hepatoportal sclerosis
3. Drug/toxin associated
i. Arsenic
ii. Drugs
4. Infections
i. Schistosomiasis
ii. HIV-associated hepatoportal sclerosis
5. Coagulation disorders
6. Immunologic disorders
III. Disorders of the main hepatic vein/inferior vena cava (IVC) (Budd–Chiari syndrome)
1. Primary
i. Membranous obstruction or web of IVC
ii. Tumors (HCC, RCC)
iii. Thrombosis and phlebitis
a. Coagulation disorders
b. Myeloproliferative disorders
c. Paroxymal nocturnal hemoglobinuria
iv. Pregnancy, postpartum
v. Oral contraceptive pills
vi. Idiopathic

(continued)

Table 8.1 (continued)

2. Secondary
i. Hydatid cyst
ii. Amebic abscess
iii. Tuberculosis
iv. Aspergillosis
v. Tumors
IV. Disorders of terminal hepatic veins and sinusoids (SOS)
1. Bone marrow transplant
2. Radiation
3. Toxins
i. Pyrrolizidine alkaloids
4. Drugs
i. Cyclophosphamide
ii. Azathioprine
iii. 6-Mercaptopurine
iv. 6-Thioguanine
v. Dicarbazine
vi. Oxaliplatin
vii. Urethane
5. Coagulation disorders
V. Disorders of hepatic artery
1. Thrombosis and aneurysm
2. Accidental ligation or trauma
3. Vasculitis
4. Foam cell arteriopathy (posttransplant)
VI. Disorders of small and medium size HA
1. Thrombosis
2. Vasculitis
3. DIC and microangiopathy
4. Eclampsia of pregnancy
5. Amyloidosis
6. Diabetic microangiopathy
VII. Disorders of sinusoids
1. Infiltration or obstruction of sinusoids
i. Stellate cell hyperplasia
ii. Extramedullary hematopoiesis
iii. Amyloidosis
iv. Sickle cell disease
2. Sinusoidal dilatation
i. Venous outflow obstruction
ii. Drugs and toxins
a. Oral contraceptive pills
b. Vinyl chloride
c. Heroin use
iii. Infections
a. Bacillary angiomatosis
iv. Paraneoplastic
a. Renal cell carcinoma
VIII. Other miscellaneous disorders
1. Cardiac failure and pericarditis
2. Nodular regenerative hyperplasia
i. Hematologic malignancies
ii. Collagen vascular disorders
iii. Chemotherapy
iv. Vasculitis
v. Renal transplantation
3. Hereditary hemorrhagic telangiectasia
4. Intrahepatic arteriovenous shunts

categorized here according to the predominant vascular unit and the caliber of the vessels involved, although it should be recognized that these features are not as sharply demarcated functionally, clinically, or pathologically.

Disorders of the Portal Venous (PV) System

Disorders of the Main PVs

The portal vasculature is commonly involved secondarily in many hepatic disorders, e.g., cirrhosis from any cause, sarcoidosis, autoimmune hepatitis, primary biliary cirrhosis, thorotrast, or heavy metal toxicity. As discussed more extensively in Chap. 12, obstruction of the main PV results from thrombosis, congenital atresia, tumors, or extrinsic compression, of which thrombosis is the most common (Table 8.1) [4–6]. PV thrombosis may result from local causes (30%) or be secondary to systemic factors (70%) [7]. Malignant tumors in the PV territory, even without direct invasion of the PV, and cirrhosis are the most common local risk factors [8, 9]. In young individuals in the absence of cancer or cirrhosis, PV thrombosis may be the initial manifestation of an underlying myeloproliferative disorder [7].

As described in Chap. 12, acute and chronic PV thrombosis differ in their clinical presentation and management and are considered as separate disorders, although they represent successive stages of the same disease process with common risk factors [4].

PV thrombosis of recent origin (acute PV thrombosis) is readily identified on gross and microscopic examination of explants or at autopsy (see Fig. 8.1a). With time thrombi may undergo resolution, and eventually all that may remain may be an eccentric plaque or patch of intimal fibrosis, best appreciated with elastic tissue stains. In long-standing cases, the vein may be replaced by a fibrous cord and be difficult to identify. Following acute PV thrombosis, multiple small- or medium-sized collaterals develop in the region of the hilum, often referred to as "cavernous transformation of the PV" (see Fig. 8.1c) [10]. The collaterals start to form as early as 6 days after acute PV occlusion, but take about 5 weeks to develop fully. They are best demonstrated on angiographic or other imaging studies, and may extend along the main PV and its right and left branches into the liver. They are seldom present in biopsies and the full spectrum of changes is appreciated only at transplantation, resection, or autopsy.

It has been shown that thrombosis of the main PV may result in atrophy of the right lobe and the left lateral segment, while segment IV and the caudate lobe undergo hypertrophy (see Fig. 8.1b) [11]. This is believed to be secondary to decreased peripheral perfusion and preserved central perfusion due to collaterals. The histological changes in the hepatic parenchyma are often subtle and

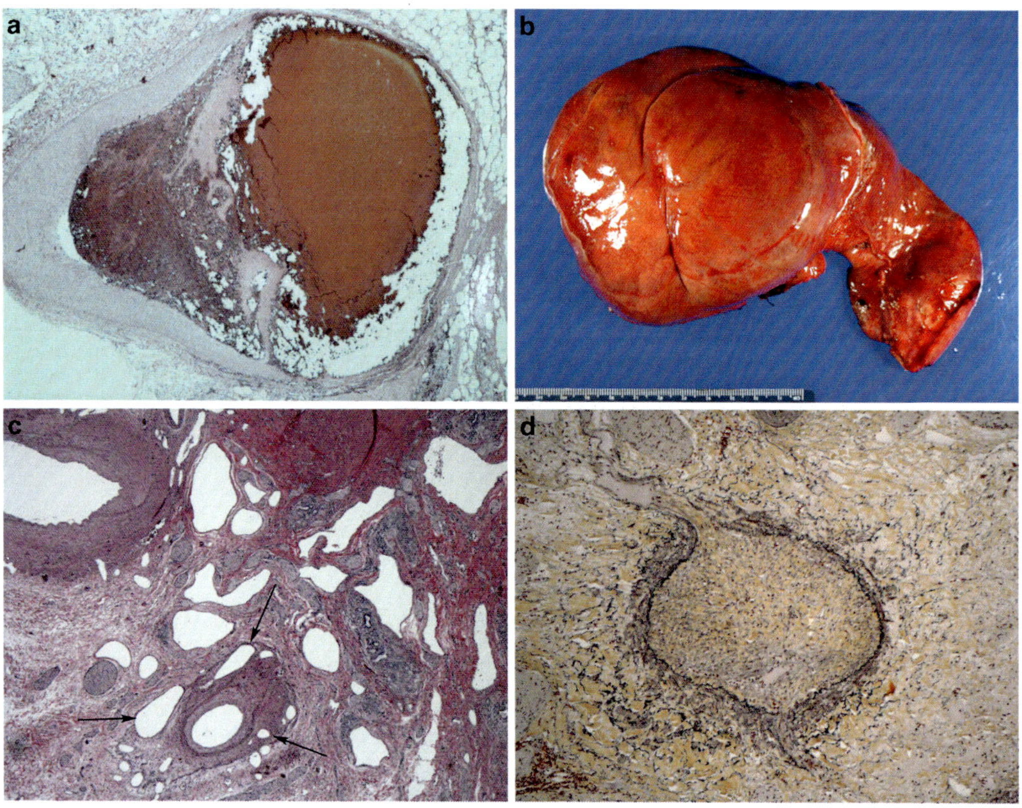

Fig. 8.1 Portal vein thrombosis. (**a**) A large portal vein branch near the hilum contains a recent nonocclusive thrombus. Early organization of the thrombus is evident even at this low magnification. (**b**) A case of portal vein thrombosis showing massive hypertrophy of the segment 4 and caudate lobe. (**c**) Sections of the same case from the hilum showing multiple dilated vascular channels (cavernous transformation). Multiple collaterals that are part of this cavernous transformation are seen even in the wall of a partly occluded branch of the thrombosed portal vein (*arrows*). (**d**) A smaller portal vein branch is completely occluded by an organized thrombus. The outlines of the vessel are readily appreciated in this elastic tissue stain

secondary, and the role of biopsy is mainly to exclude cirrhosis or any comorbidities. There may be increased hepatocyte apoptosis, although in many cases the liver histology appears normal. Sometimes a combination of atrophy and hypertrophy may be seen, which may be best appreciated on imaging studies or gross examination, rather than histology. In cases without cirrhosis or significant architectural distortion, the portal areas are relatively easily identified and changes in PV branches are easy to observe. The smaller branches in portal tracts may show intimal sclerosis or at times complete obliteration (see Fig. 8.1d). In cases where the lobular architecture is distorted, distinguishing between HV tributaries and PV branches may be extremely difficult and connective tissue stains and step-sections may be needed. The connective tissue stains may also show the location of the obliterated PV.

In some cases, the smaller PV branches and adjacent sinusoids may appear dilated, the distended venules almost bulging through the limiting plate into the parenchyma, similar to changes seen in cases of idiopathic portal hypertension (IPH) discussed later. Hepatic artery thrombosis or hepatic vein thrombosis may accompany PV thrombosis in some cases [1].

Pylephlebitis

Pylephlebitis, a dreaded complication of appendicitis, diverticulitis, chronic inflammatory bowel disease (IBD), and pancreatitis in the preantibiotic era, is now rare [12]. Bacterial infection in suppurative appendicitis, acute diverticulitis, active IBD, or pancreatitis involves the veins draining these organs, and the infection is transmitted via the PV to the liver where it leads to septic portal thrombophlebitis, formation of liver abscesses, and sometimes PV thrombosis. The possibility of pylephlebitis should be considered if phlebitis is observed in appendectomy or colectomy specimens removed because of acute appendicitis or diverticulitis, and especially if there is evidence of bacterial involvement of the vessels.

Disorders of the Small- and Medium-Sized PV Branches

Hepatoportal Sclerosis

Sclerosis or obstruction of small- and medium-sized PVs may lead to portal hypertension in the absence of cirrhosis. This disorder has been variously called IPH, noncirrhotic portal fibrosis (NCPF), obliterative portal venopathy, and hepatoportal sclerosis, the choice of term largely depending upon regional preferences around the world and the perceived pathophysiology of the disease [13, 14]. It is characterized pathologically by dense portal fibrosis and obliteration of small- or medium-sized branches of the PV, although the thrombosis or obstruction may not always be demonstrated. The overall histology in these cases remains variable, patchy, and often subtle.

Grossly, the liver is noncirrhotic and may appear normal or somewhat small. Atrophy and compensatory hypertrophy may sometimes result in patchy nodularity, especially near the hepatic hilum, referred to as "partial nodular transformation" [15, 16]. Regeneration and atrophy may also lead to disproportionate sizes of the two lobes. The main PV and its larger branches may appear dilated.

Microscopically, the portal tracts appear normal or enlarged due to dense fibrosis, and in some cases the profiles of the enlarged portal tracts appear distinctly rounded (see Fig. 8.2a). The PV branches may be thickened with sclerosis and luminal narrowing or be completely obliterated (see Fig. 8.2b). Organized thrombi may be seen in some, whereas others are replaced by multiple dilated thin-walled smaller venules. The sinusoids may be dilated secondary to portal hypertension. Sometimes the dilated portal venules appear juxtaposed to the limiting plate without any intervening portal connective tissue, and there may be dilatation of immediately adjacent sinusoids (see Fig. 8.2c). This appearance is often referred to as "herniation" of the portal venules into the hepatic lobules, and many different morphologic patterns of this phenomenon have been

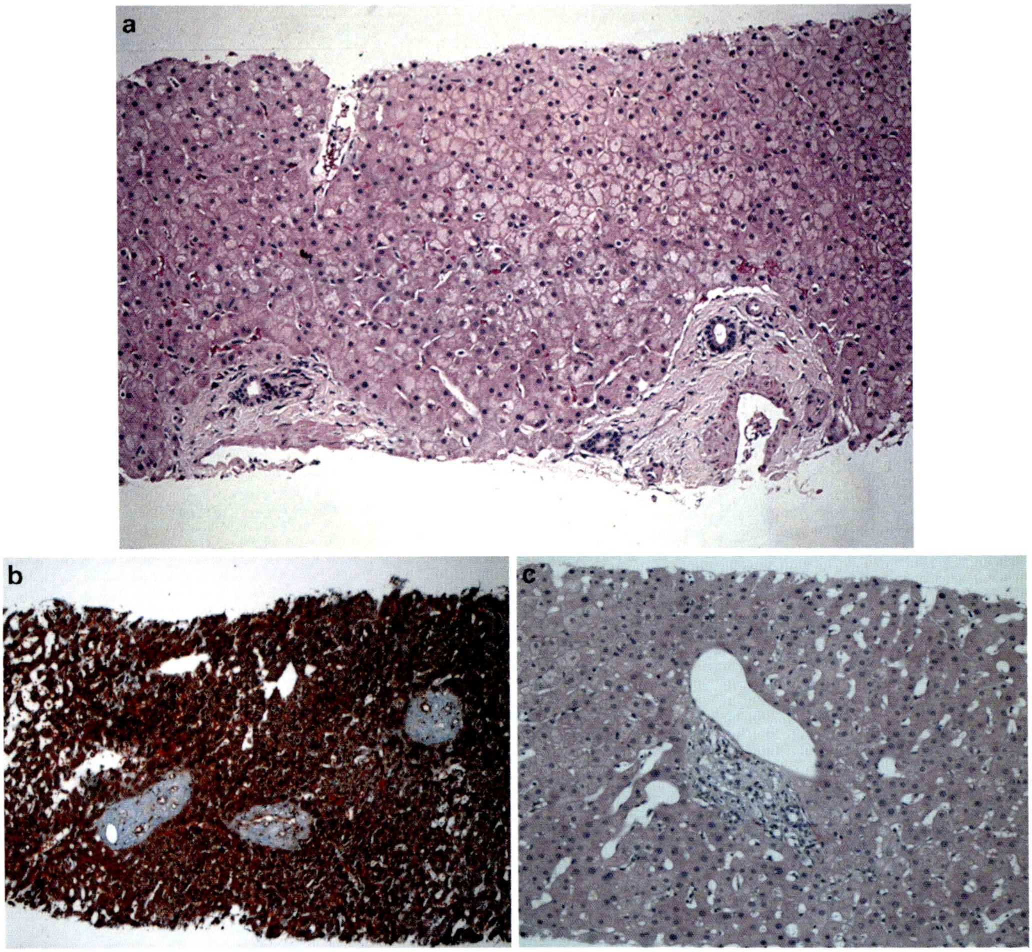

Fig. 8.2 Hepatoportal sclerosis. (**a**) The portal tracts are enlarged and somewhat rounded. The portal vein branches show thickening and sclerosis. The hepatic parenchyma appears normal. (**b**) Trichrome stain showing rounded profiles of the portal tracts, sclerosis of some portal veins, and total absence of a portal vein in some of the tracts. (**c**) A markedly dilated portal vein branch is juxtaposed to the limiting plate (herniation of the portal vein), and nearby sinusoids are focally dilated

described [17]. The portal lymphatics may also increase in number [18]. In the absence of any other comorbidities, portal tracts generally lack inflammation. The hepatic lobules and architecture most often appear normal; however, thin fibrous septa or portal-to-portal bridging fibrosis with some regeneration and suggestion of nodularity may sometimes be seen [19, 20]. In such cases, the appearance can be identical to incomplete septal cirrhosis or the so-called "regressed cirrhosis." In hepatoportal sclerosis associated with exposure to vinyl chloride, perisinusoidal fibrosis and increased numbers of perisinusoidal Kupffer cells may be seen.

HIV-Associated Hepatoportal Sclerosis

Cases of hepatoportal sclerosis associated with HIV infection show similar features and are attributed to treatment with HAART [21, 22].

Schistosomiasis

Hepatic involvement in schistosomiasis results in obstruction of small portal venules and, if extensive, leads to noncirrhotic portal hypertension [23]. The adult worms live in the mesenteric veins, and the eggs, which have a chitinous shell

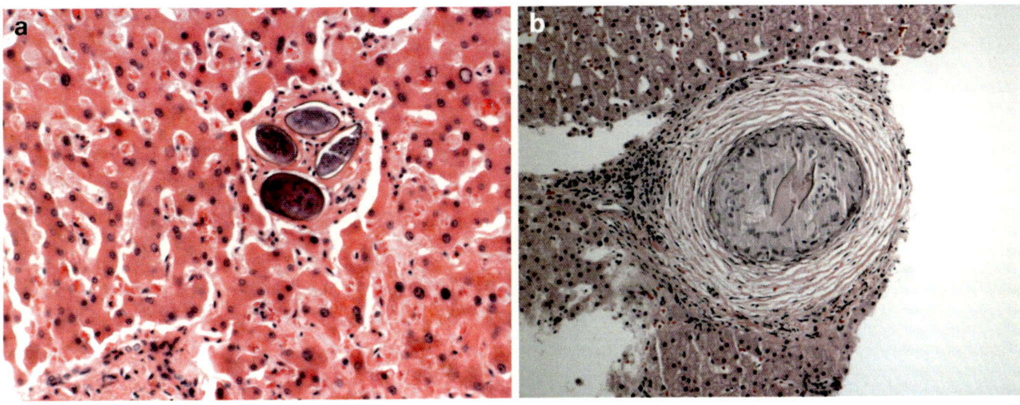

Fig. 8.3 Schistosomiasis. (**a**) Multiple eggs with preserved morphology are present in the portal tract without any associated fibrosis or inflammation. The patient did not have portal hypertension and this was an incidental finding. (**b**) A poorly preserved schistosome egg is present in this portal tract, within an epithelioid granuloma and surrounded by a rim of fibrosis. The patient presented with portal hypertension

with a single spine, are carried by the bloodstream into the PV and its branches in the triads, eliciting variable amounts and patterns of inflammation (including eosinophil-rich infiltrates), fibrosis, and granulomas (Fig. 8.3). Classical descriptions of advanced disease in the liver refer to the concentrically thickened, fibrotic PVs at autopsy as "pipestem fibrosis" because of the similarity of the damaged tracts to the stems of white clay tobacco pipes [23]. The commonest species that involve the liver are *Schistosoma mansoni, S. japonicum,* and *S. hematobium*. The eggs may be well preserved, in which case identification of the position of the spine helps in the identification of the species (*S. mansoni,* lateral; *S. japonicum* lateral but minute; *S. hematobium,* terminal); however, not infrequently the morphology of the eggs is poorly preserved, and they appear as empty wrinkled barely recognizable structures (see Fig. 8.3b). Calcification of the eggs or deposition of pigment is not uncommon.

Disorders of the Hepatic Venous System

Obstruction of the HV can occur at any level from the opening of the inferior vena cava (IVC) into the right atrium, IVC, major HV, sublobular veins, or terminal hepatic venules (central veins). Most of the gross and histological changes in the liver are identical irrespective of the level of venous outflow obstruction, and without clinical correlation it may be impossible to distinguish amongst the various causes based on pathology, especially on needle biopsies. By international consensus Budd–Chiari syndrome (BCS) is used as an eponym for hepatic venous outflow obstruction independent of the level or mechanism of obstruction [4]. Venous outflow obstruction secondary to cardiac conditions or sinusoidal obstruction syndrome is excluded from this definition. Various underlying etiologies are listed in Table 8.1.

Obstruction of the IVC and Main HV (Budd–Chiari Syndrome)

As discussed more extensively in Chap. 13, BCS may result from obstruction of the IVC downstream of the liver or obstruction of the main hepatic veins (HVs) [4]. Obstruction of the veins may result from thrombus, tumor, or extrinsic compression and may involve a short or long segment of the vein [24]. BCS is considered primary when it occurs due to primary venous disease and secondary when due to extrinsic compression or a lesion outside the vein. Thrombosis of the HV or IVC remains the most common cause of BCS.

As the caudate lobe drains into the IVC separately through multiple small veins and the inferior HV, it frequently escapes the effects of venous obstruction due to thrombi occluding the openings of right and left HVs [25]. In such a situation, the caudate lobe may undergo massive compensatory hypertrophy and can be clinically and grossly mistaken for a neoplasm. Caudate lobe hypertrophy will not occur if the obstruction is in the IVC.

In cases of acute BCS, the liver is enlarged and congested. The congestion is most marked in the pericentral sinusoids and accentuation of these vascular markings due to congestion and hemorrhage results in the so-called "nutmeg liver" (see Fig. 8.4a). Microscopically, the changes vary depending on the extent and severity of obstruction. Early on, or in milder cases, the changes may be limited to dilatation of central veins and perivenular sinusoids. Later, frank hemorrhage in the centrizonal area with erythrocyte extravasation into the space of Disse and the hepatocyte cords, and hemorrhagic necrosis become evident (see Fig. 8.4b & c). Thrombi may be seen in hepatic venules. As the process becomes subacute to chronic, organization of thrombi, gradual resolution of hemorrhage, accumulation of hemosiderin-laden macrophages, and progressive fibrosis are noted. The fibrosis has a unique pattern early on and is predominantly pericentral, often with obliteration of the central veins (see Fig. 8.4d) [1]. The fibrosis spreads from the central areas towards the portal regions in a manner different from postnecrotic cirrhosis

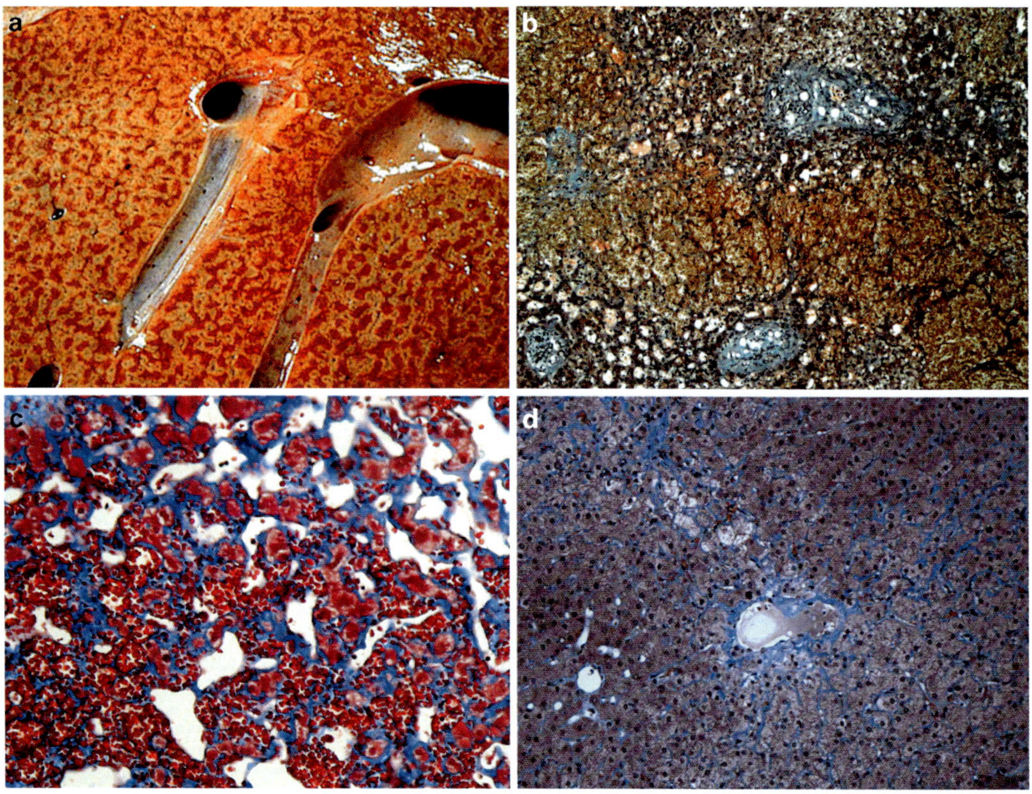

Fig. 8.4 Hepatic venous outflow obstruction. (**a**) Gross photograph showing "nutmeg liver" due to passive venous congestion in a patient with right-sided heart failure. (**b**) Centrizonal hemorrhagic necrosis in a case of acute Budd–Chiari syndrome (trichrome stain). (**c**) Red cell extravasation into the hepatocyte cords forming so-called "red blood-cell trabecular lesion" (trichrome stain). (**d**) Delicate pericentral "stellate" scarring in the liver (trichrome stain). The patient was subsequently found to have pulmonary hypertension and right-sided heart failure

and is often referred to as "reverse cirrhosis." Eventually the process may progress to cirrhosis, and advanced cirrhosis from chronic venous outflow obstruction is difficult to differentiate from cirrhosis of other causes, especially on needle biopsies [3]. Other factors that may adversely affect microscopic interpretation include patchy and heterogenous involvement of the liver, and the presence of concomitant PV thrombosis which occurs in 10–20% of cases [26]. Even in the rat model of BCS, marked reduction in PV branches is noted after 6 weeks of HV ligation. This is accompanied by a compensatory decrease in portal blood flow and lobar atrophy. Moreover, BCS-like features can be seen in localized areas in the liver around space occupying lesions (tumors, cysts, or abscesses) due to compression of branches of the HVs.

BCS may also result from membranes or webs in the suprahepatic portion of the IVC [27]. To judge from the frequency of reported cases, the incidence of this entity, which commonly affects children, is higher in Japan, India, and South Africa than in Europe and America. It has been suggested that the webs are the residua of ancient thrombi that formed secondary to portal sepsis or infection early in life. However, their presence in twins argues for a congenital malformation, and some patients have associated congenital abnormalities, further supporting this notion [28]. There is an increased incidence of hepatocellular carcinoma in this group, perhaps related to the prevalence of hepatitis B infection in regions where webs are common.

Heart Failure and Cardiac Sclerosis

Hepatic venous outflow obstruction may also result from increased back pressure secondary to heart failure or constrictive pericarditis [29]. Apart from lack of a mechanical obstruction in the IVC or HVs, the gross and histological changes are identical to BCS of other etiologies, and may show similar acute and chronic phases (see Fig. 8.4d). In general, the changes of cardiac sclerosis tend to develop insidiously and mimic chronic changes of BCS. Typically, they are patchy and heterogenous, and even in cases with portal hypertension and severe fibrosis, cirrhosis with typical rounded regenerative nodules is seldom seen. Some cases show a combination of congestive hepatopathy due to right heart failure and hepatic ischemia secondary to a failing left heart [30]. In advanced stages, the increased resistance to flow is also reflected in the PV system, which develops portal hypertensive changes. The PV branches may show intimal thickening and fibrosis. In some cases, even bile duct injury and ductular proliferation may be seen, simulating a primary biliary disorder, both histologically and clinically [31].

Disorders of the Sublobular HVs and Terminal Hepatic Venules

Obstruction of the smaller tributaries of the hepatic venous system (sublobular HVs and central veins or terminal hepatic venules) has variously been termed obliterative hepatic venopathy, veno-occlusive disease, and sinusoidal obstruction syndrome. It may result from thrombosis, phlebitis, extrinsic compression, or toxic injury. As discussed more extensively in Chap. 2, veno-occlusive disease was originally described in Jamaica where plants containing toxic pyrrolizidine alkaloids were used to make bush tea [32]. Subsequently, similar histological changes were described following radiation injury to the liver associated with chemotherapy. In current practice, most cases result from myeloablative therapy used in preparation for hematopoietic stem cell transplantation. It is now recognized that occlusion of the central vein is not an essential component of the disorder and that damage to the perivenular sinusoidal endothelium is the key event: hence the term "sinusoidal obstruction syndrome (SOS)" is now preferred [33]. Similar to other vascular disorders, the changes can be patchy and severity may vary.

The histological findings due to various causes are identical. The earliest changes appear around 7–10 days of cytoreductive therapy in bone marrow transplant patients. Early stages tend to show marked dilatation of pericentral sinusoids and central veins, subendothelial edema, and extravasation of red cells into the space of Disse (see Fig. 8.5a, b). The endothelial lining of central veins and adjacent sinusoids is disrupted and sometimes fibrin may be seen occluding the central vein (Fig. 8.5c). Stains for elastic tissue and fibrin highlight these findings. Within 10–14 days of onset of the injury, activated stellate cells lay down extracellular matrix in the subendothelial and perisinusoidal spaces (sinusoidal fibrosis). The lumens of central veins may become narrowed by expansion of the subendothelial region. At this time, macrophages move in and start cleaning up the debris. Subsequently, fibrosis leads to obliteration of central veins with extension of fibrous strands into the pericentral area in a stellate manner. In mild cases or with patchy involvement, the changes may resolve completely. When fibrosis develops, the pattern resembles cardiac sclerosis. Portal changes similar to venous outflow obstruction with bile ductular proliferation may also be seen [31]. Based on autopsy data, 20–30% of cases remain asymptomatic, and the clinical severity depends upon the extent of liver involvement and of occlusion of central veins. About 45% patients with mild to moderate SOS, and 25% patients with severe SOS, do not have occlusion of central veins [34]. The strongest predictors of clinical severity are pericentral hepatocytic necrosis, sinusoidal fibrosis, eccentric thickening of the subendothelial zone of the venules, phlebosclerosis, and overall extent of venular narrowing.

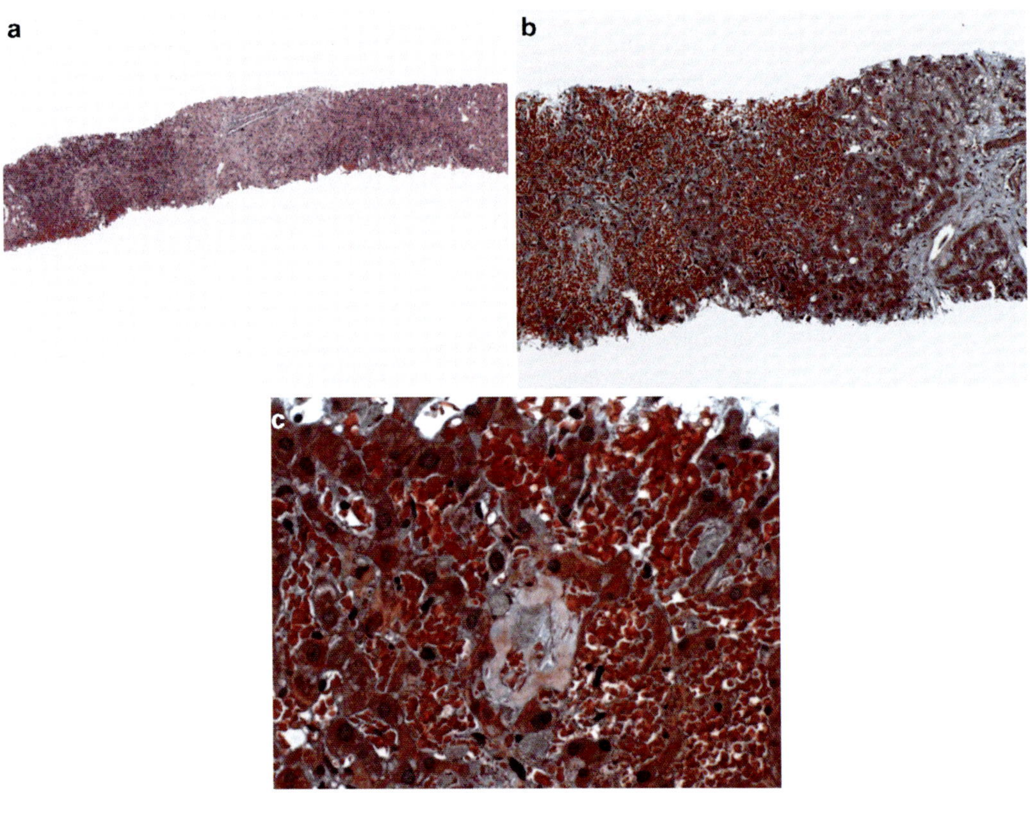

Fig. 8.5 Sinusoidal obstruction syndrome in a patient following stem cell transplantation. (**a**) Extensive centrizonal hemorrhagic necrosis. (**b**) Medium power shows lack of fibrosis at this stage and highlights the centrizonal hemorrhage (trichrome stain). (**c**) Centrilobular region with occlusion of the central vein by a fibrin thrombus, severe sinusoidal congestion, and red cell extravasation into the hepatocyte cords

Disorders of the Sinusoidal System

Infiltrative and Obstructive Lesions of the Sinusoids

Compromise of sinusoidal function may result from infiltration of the lumen or the space of Disse by abnormal cell populations (e.g., posttransplant lymphoproliferative disorder, extramedullary hematopoiesis, sickle cells, lymphomas, Langerhans cell histiocytosis, macrophages) or by extracellular material such as amyloid (see Fig. 8.6a–c) [35–37]. While this may remain asymptomatic, as is usually the case with extramedullary hematopoiesis, some infiltrates may rarely result in functional sinusoidal obstruction and portal hypertension. Sinusoids may become clogged by sickling red cells in cases of sickle cell disease during a crisis (Fig. 8.6d) [38]: this may result in ischemic hepatic necrosis or areas of hepatic atrophy with compensatory regenerative changes. Other changes in the liver seen in patients with sickle cell disease include Kupffer cell hyperplasia, hepatic siderosis, and rarely erythrophagocytosis. It should be recognized that in some of the conditions mentioned here, splenomegaly occurs due to involvement by the primary disease, rather than portal hypertension.

Sinusoidal Dilatation

Sinusoidal dilatation is a frequent finding in liver biopsies and often represents a nonspecific change or an artifact due to biopsy procedure,

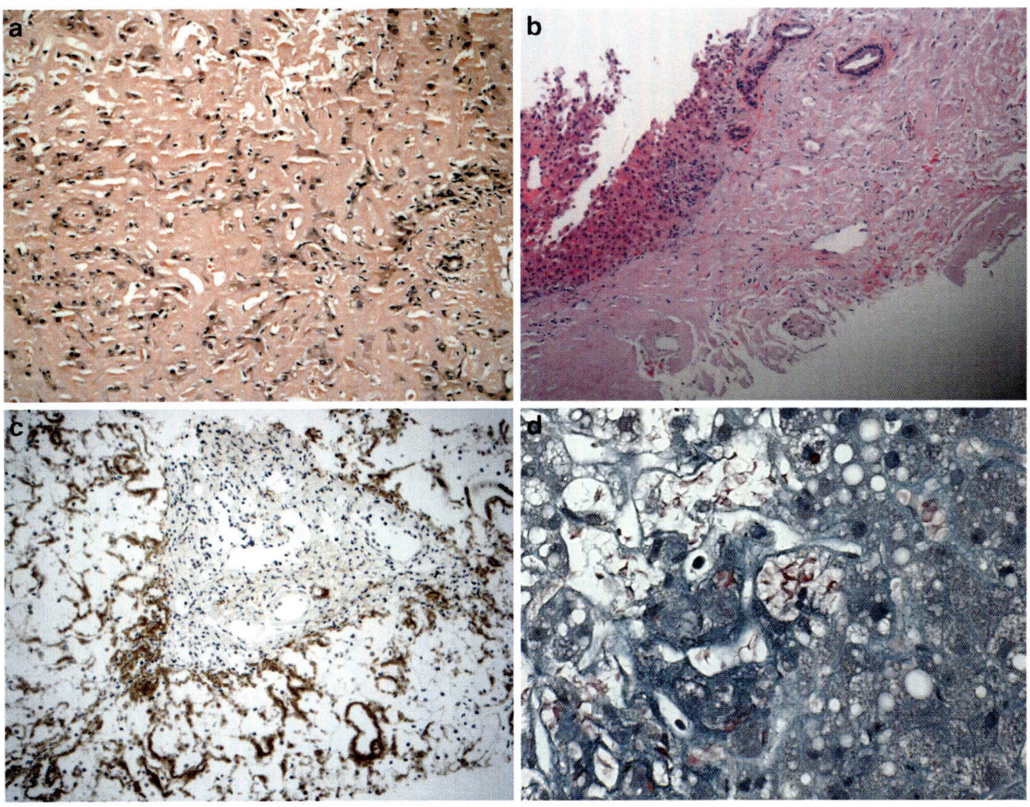

Fig. 8.6 (**a**) Sinusoidal amyloidosis causing near total effacement of the hepatic sinusoids. (**b**) Vascular amyloidosis with extensive amyloid deposition in portal vessels and portal tract stroma. Note the complete lack of sinusoidal amyloid. (**c**) Immunostain for amyloid A protein (AA) showing staining in the sinusoids. (**d**) Dilated sinusoids obstructed by sickled red cells in a patient in sickle cell crisis (Trichrome stain)

tissue handling, or tissue processing. Although a perivenular distribution may indicate venous outflow obstruction, the only way to differentiate artifact from a pathologic state is to look for a consistent pattern and other associated findings that are more definitive. Sometimes this is nearly impossible. Sinusoidal dilatation is an important histological feature in cases of venous outflow obstruction from different causes. It may also be seen in patients on long-term oral contraceptive use, when it is often associated with a minor elevation in aminotransferases [39]. However, it has been reported in association with a wide variety of other conditions, including congenital syphilis, vinyl chloride exposure, hypervitaminosis A, heroin toxicity, renal transplantation, extramedullary hematopoiesis, thrombocytopenic purpura, and renal cell carcinoma [36, 40, 41].

Peliosis Hepatitis

Peliosis hepatitis is characterized by dilated blood-filled spaces in the liver parenchyma that may be localized or diffuse (see Fig. 8.7a, b) [42, 43]. It occurs most commonly in association with various hepatocytic neoplasms, although it may also be seen as an isolated finding. Other causes of peliosis include various hematologic malignancies, conditions causing cachexia, and exposure to drugs or toxins, such as anabolic steroids, tamoxifen, corticosteroids, methotrexate, vinyl chloride, arsenic, and thorotrast [44]. The lesions are often detected incidentally on gross examination or microscopy. Rarely, peliosis is diagnosed following hemoperitoneum due to rupture of the lesions [45]. Grossly, the lesions may be difficult to appreciate as they are generally

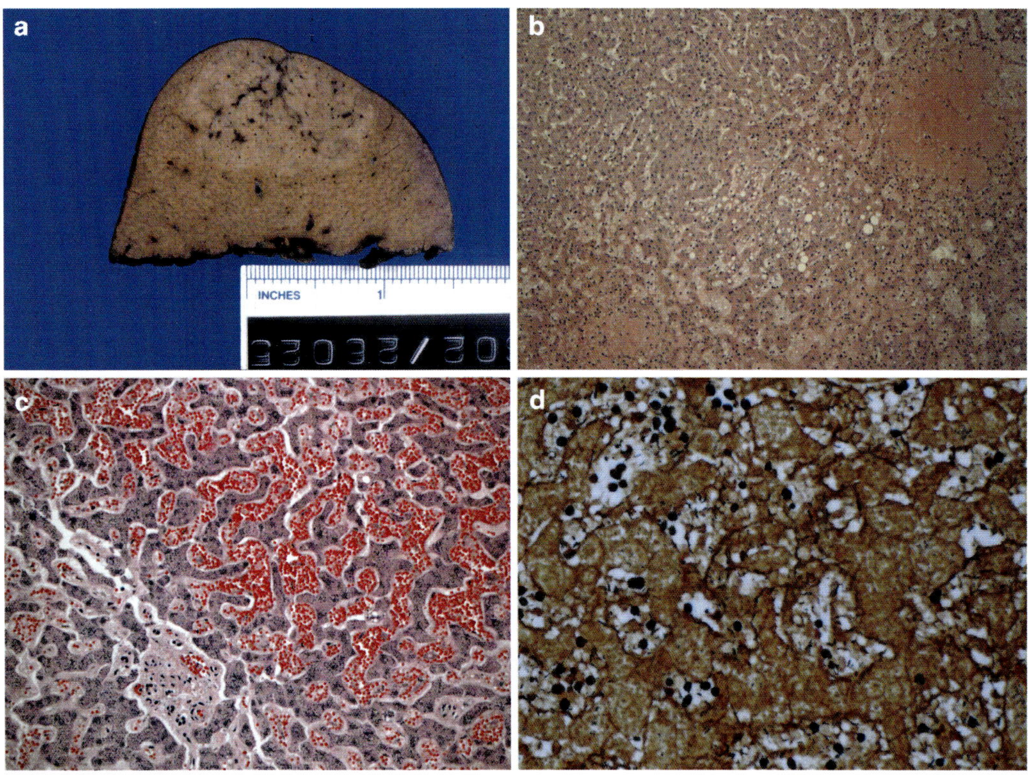

Fig. 8.7 (**a**) Peliosis hepatis in a 45-year-old female taking oral contraceptives and with no other underlying disease. The lesion is the ill-defined area of pallor, speckled with dark areas of congestion and hemorrhage. (**b**) Microscopy shows dilated blood-filled spaces that mostly lack a well-defined endothelial lining. (**c**) Bacillary angiomatosis with markedly distended sinusoids filled with red cells. (**d**) Warthin–Starry stain shows numerous small black-staining bacilli consistent with *Bartonella* species

small, and when large they appear as areas of congestion or blood-filled spaces. In early stages, the blood-filled spaces lack an endothelial lining, but on long standing may develop one.

Bacillary Angiomatosis

Bacillary angiomatosis is a bacterial infection of the sinusoidal endothelium, usually caused by organisms of the genus *Bartonella*. It occurs almost exclusively in severely immunocompromised individuals [46]. The organisms may be visualized both in the endothelial cells and extracellularly with the use of a silver stain such as a Warthin–Starry (see Fig. 8.7d). However, they may be absent or difficult to detect in some cases, especially following treatment. Associated with sinusoidal endothelial injury, there is sinusoidal dilatation with extravasation of red cells into the space of Disse, localized breakdown of hepatocyte cords and swelling of the sinusoidal spaces to form the blood-filled lacunae typical of peliosis (see Fig. 8.7c).

Disorders of the HA System

Disorders of the Main HA

Interruption of HA flow in a normal liver, even due to complete obstruction of the main HA secondary to thrombosis or accidental ligation, does not result in a fatal outcome, and may even go completely unnoticed [47, 48]. This is largely due to significant arterial collaterals and adequacy of the portal circulation to perfuse the liver. In the transplanted liver, the rich arterial collateral circulation is disrupted and the HA is the sole source of arterial blood to the liver and the biliary tree. Thus, in this setting HA obstruction may result in severe consequences, including infarction, perihilar necrosis, fulminant hepatic failure, bile leakage, biliary tract necrosis and sepsis [49]. In an already compromised liver, even mildly impaired HA circulation may have significant consequences. The etiology of HA occlusion includes thrombosis due to hypercoagulable states, accidental ligation, posttransplant complications including chronic vascular rejection, vasculitis, and extrinsic compression. Rare examples of fatal HA dissection presenting with pain in the abdomen and liver transaminase abnormalities have also been described [50].

Disorders of Small Branches of the HA

Involvement of the small branches of the HA system is seen with various vasculitides, disseminated intravascular coagulation (DIC), and other microangiopathies, amyloidosis, diabetic microangiopathy, and eclampsia of pregnancy [51]. Disorders of these vessels may lead to ischemic injury of the liver and biliary tree depending upon the extent and severity of the involvement. They are discussed below under each specific disorder.

Vasculitis and Microangiopathy

Vasculitis, when it involves the liver, is usually part of a systemic disorder, and isolated hepatic involvement is rare. The manifestations depend upon the extent and caliber of the involved vessels [52]. Disorders affecting medium or large caliber vessels may result in ischemic necrosis or infarcts, as occur in polyarteritis nodosa or Wegener's granulomatosis [53–57]. In polyarteritis nodosa, the HA or its branches may show thrombosis or aneurysmal dilation, sometimes with hemorrhage or hematoma formation. These findings are best demonstrated on imaging studies. Histology shows segmental necrotizing inflammation and fibrinoid necrosis of the muscular wall of medium-sized arteries (Fig. 8.8). In healed lesions, fragmentation of the elastic lamina and scarring are the only identifiable findings; these should be sought in stains for elastin and other connective tissues. The consequences of vasculitis may be seen as hepatic ischemia, localized infarction, or bile duct necrosis. We have seen one case in which vasculitis affecting the vasa recta of large bile ducts in the hilum of the liver caused focal ischemic scarring and stenosis of the ducts, mimicking primary sclerosing

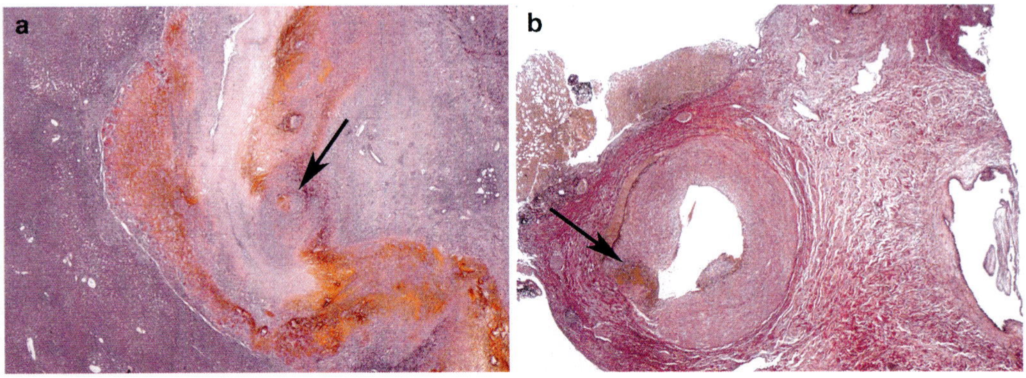

Fig. 8.8 Polyarteritis nodosa. (**a**) Necrosis of a large intrahepatic bile duct has caused a bile leak. An artery in a portal area shows necrosis as well (*arrow*). (**b**) A medium-sized artery near the hilum shows focal segmental arteritis with fibrinoid necrosis (*arrow*) (elastin tissue stain)

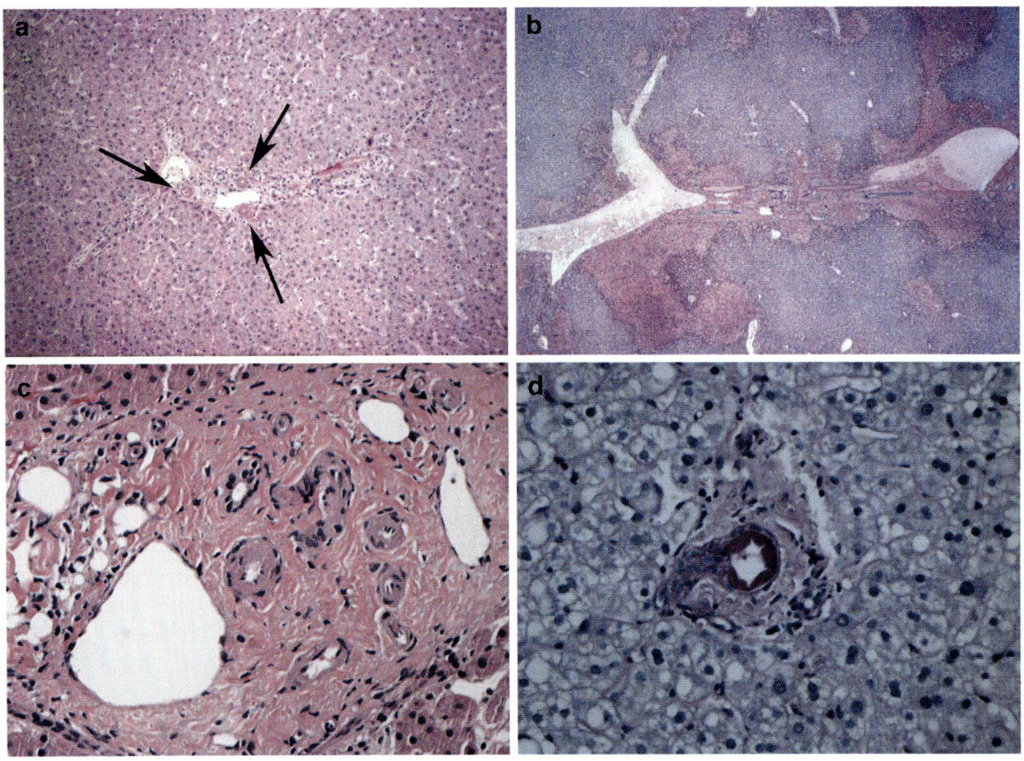

Fig. 8.9 (**a**) Multiple fibrin thrombi (*arrows*) in hepatic artery branches in small portal tracts in a case of disseminated intravascular coagulation. (**b**) Coagulative necrosis of periportal hepatocytes with multiple fibrin thrombi in small portal vessels. The fibrin thrombi are not visible at this magnification. (**c**) Thickened hepatic arterioles with hyaline arteriolosclerosis in a portal tract of a patient with diabetes mellitus (H&E stain). (**d**) Small hepatic arteriole showing intramural deposition of PAS-positive material similar to diabetic hyaline arteriolosclerosis elsewhere (PAS stain)

cholangitis. DIC and microangiopathy may result in ischemia due to fibrin thrombi deposition in small vessels and necrosis of periportal hepatocytes (see Fig. 8.9a, b) [51]. Similar changes have been described in patients with pregnancy-associated eclampsia [58] (Fig. 8.9).

Diabetic Microangiopathy and Diabetic Hepatosclerosis

Similar to other organs, the hepatic arterioles in the liver may also show microangiopathy [59–62]. The arterioles in portal tracts show variable amount of wall thickening due to deposition of basement membrane-like material that can be highlighted by a PAS, laminin, or collagen IV stain (see Fig. 8.9c, d). Most of these patients have severe complications of diabetes and evidence of microangiopathy in other organs, notably kidneys. The microangiopathy may result in bile duct ischemia, typically manifested by elevation of alkaline phosphatase, although the bile ducts histologically tend to appear normal. Some cases may show elevations of aminotransferases or cholestasis. There may be associated deposition of thick collagen in the perisinusoidal space (sinusoidal fibrosis), often referred to as diabetic hepatosclerosis. This finding is often overshadowed on histology by coexisting nonalcoholic steatohepatitis. In an autopsy study, once steatohepatitis was excluded, 19 (12%) of the remaining 159 liver specimens showed diabetic hepatosclerosis [59].

Miscellaneous Lesions with Underlying Vascular Pathology

Nodular Regenerative Hyperplasia (NRH)

NRH is characterized by areas of parenchymal hypertrophy separated by intervening areas of atrophy giving a nodular appearance to the liver, both grossly and microscopically (see Fig. 8.10a, b and e) [63, 64]. The precise mechanisms underlying NRH are poorly understood and are likely to be multifactorial, however, it is believed to be caused by altered microvascular structure and blood flow [2]. Compromise of randomly distributed small vessels results in atrophy of the discrete areas of parenchyma they supply, while intervening areas with normal blood supply undergo compensatory hypertrophy. NRH occurs in association with numerous disorders (see Table 8.1). Grossly, the liver shows varying degrees of nodularity and in extreme cases mimics cirrhosis. Microscopically, the nodular architecture may be evident at low magnification on H&E stains but is best appreciated with a reticulin stain (see Fig. 8.10d). Most importantly, the nodules are not separated by fibrosis, but by attenuated parenchyma, as is easily shown with a trichrome stain (see Fig. 8.10c). In the nodules, hepatocytes appear hypertrophic, whereas in the intervening areas they are attenuated. The histological changes in some cases can be striking, while in many cases they are subtle and easily overlooked on needle biopsy (see Fig. 8.10e).

Hepatic Infarcts

Hepatic infarcts result from obstruction of the HA, the PV, or their branches (see Fig. 8.11a) [65–67], occurring particularly when the vascular supply of both the PV and the HA is compromised. They are also seen in patients with toxemia of pregnancy and in liver transplants. Iatrogenic infarcts may be found in the adjacent parenchyma following chemoembolization of hepatic tumors. Microscopically, they are represented by well-demarcated areas of coagulative necrosis (see Fig. 8.11b) that with time become surrounded by a zone of inflammation, and are gradually replaced by fibrosis. Small areas of coagulative ischemic necrosis are not infrequently seen in cirrhotic nodules.

Zahn infarcts also need mention here as they are not true infarcts, but may be grossly confused for one [66]. Grossly, these appear as well-demarcated subcapsular wedge-shaped areas of congested liver. Histologically, there is hepatic cord atrophy associated with sinusoidal congestion, but no necrosis. Initially there is no fibrosis; however, on long standing scarring may occur. The underlying etiology is most often obstruction to local PV flow with back pressure from the hepatic venous system resulting in congestion.

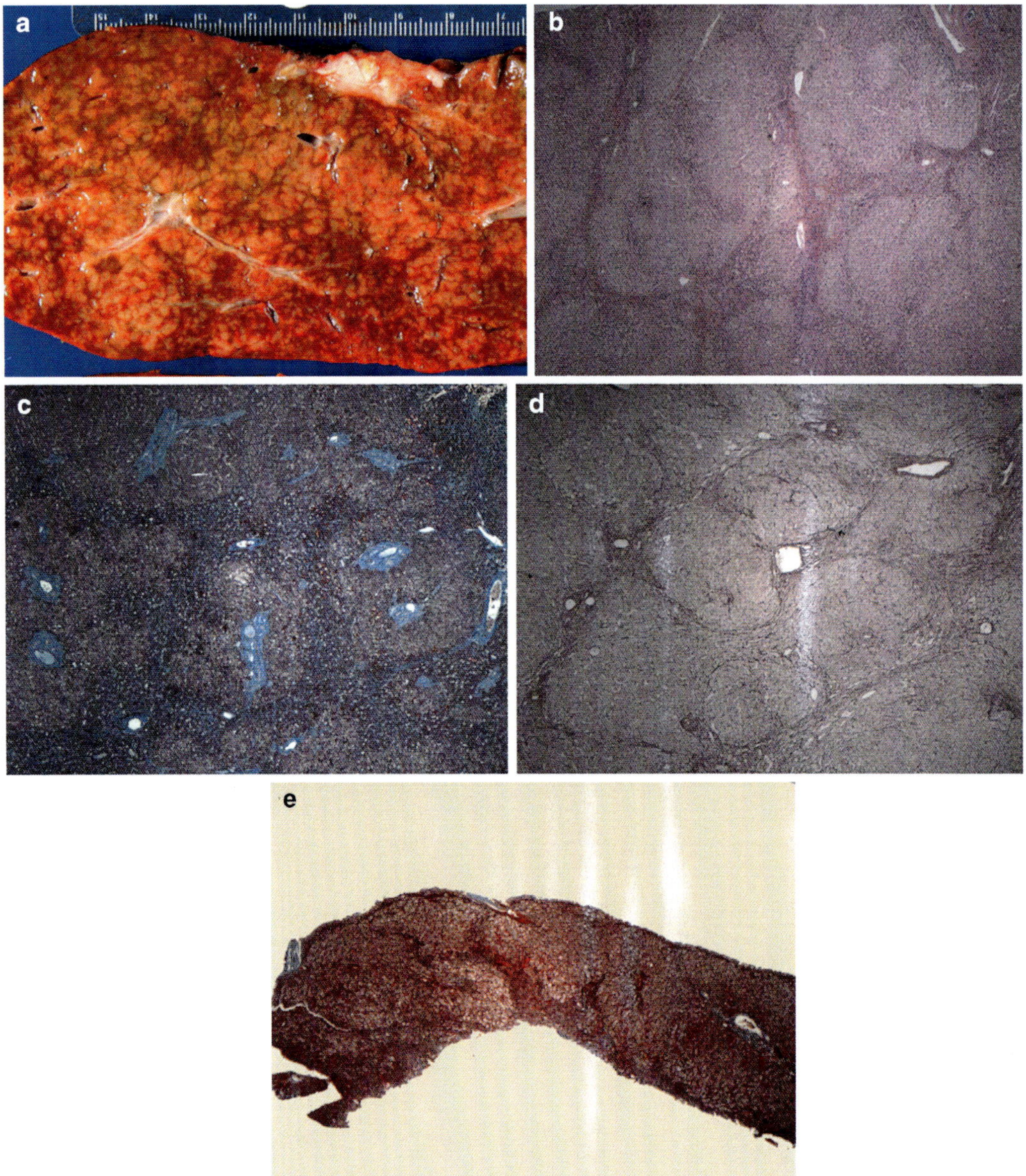

Fig. 8.10 Nodular regenerative hyperplasia. (**a**) Diffuse nodularity of NRH is present in this case of hemorrhagic hereditary telangiectasia. Cases that truly resemble cirrhosis grossly are rare in practice. (**b**) Low magnification photomicrograph from the same case showing nodular areas of regeneration mimicking cirrhotic nodules. (**c**) Trichrome stain shows a lack of fibrosis separating the nodules, while (**d**) the reticulin stain clearly outlines the regenerative nodules with thickened hepatic cords separated by atrophic areas. (**e**) Needle biopsy of the liver from a patient with a renal transplant showing obvious features of nodular regenerative hyperplasia (trichrome stain). However, in many cases these findings can be very subtle and difficult to appreciate in needle biopsies

Ischemic Hepatitis

Hepatic ischemia, most commonly resulting from severe hypoperfusion secondary to cardiac failure or shock, may clinically mimic viral hepatitis and is often referred to as "ischemic hepatitis" [68–69]. Histologically, there is often coagulative necrosis of hepatocytes in zone 3 that may extend

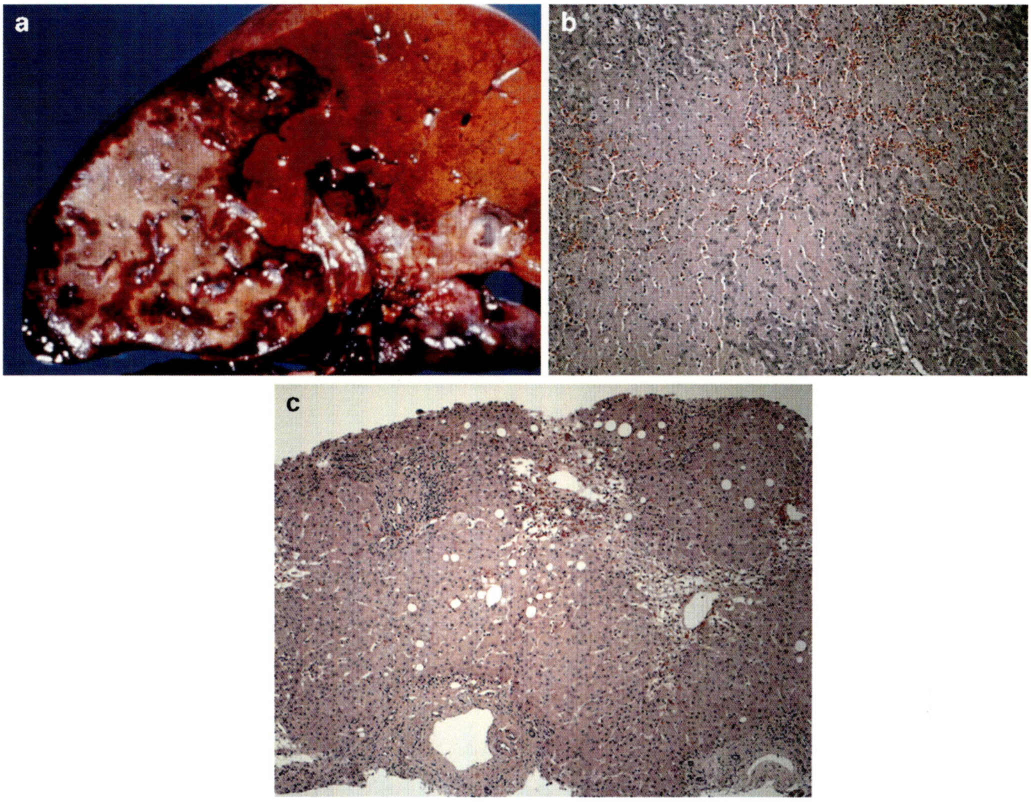

Fig. 8.11 (**a**) Liver infarct in the form of a well-demarcated area of pale parenchyma. (**b**) Photomicrograph of an infarct showing an area of parenchymal coagulative necrosis. (**c**) Liver biopsy from a patient with heart failure complicated by fulminant hepatic failure and showing extensive hepatocyte necrosis and drop out in pericentral areas (ischemic hepatitis)

to zone 2 in severe cases, along with increased apoptosis (see Fig. 8.11c). Rarely, patients may present with fulminant hepatic failure.

Ischemic Cholangitis

Since bile ducts obtain their vascular supply from branches of the HA, disorders of the splanchnic circulation frequently involve the biliary tree [70]. However, vascular disorders of the portal and hepatic venous systems may also affect the biliary system [31]. The bile ducts may be involved in systemic vasculitides such as polyarteritis nodosa, systemic lupus erythematosus, Henoch-Schonlein purpura, and giant cell arteritis and in other stenosing or occlusive conditions such as vascular amyloidosis, atherosclerotic vascular disease, and diabetic microangiopathy. Bile duct injury may result in necrosis, rupture, cholangitis, or stricture. Collaterals in PV thrombosis result in varices in the bile ducts [71].

Hereditary Hemorrhagic Telangiectasia

The majority of individuals with hereditary hemorrhagic telangiectasia (Osler–Weber–Rendu syndrome) have vascular malformations in the liver, although only a few become symptomatic from these, usually late in adult life. The clinical manifestations may vary from high-output heart failure to portal hypertension, biliary disease, or NRH (see Fig. 8.10a) [72, 73]. The vascular malformations, when visible, are best appreciated on the external surface of the liver, rather than on

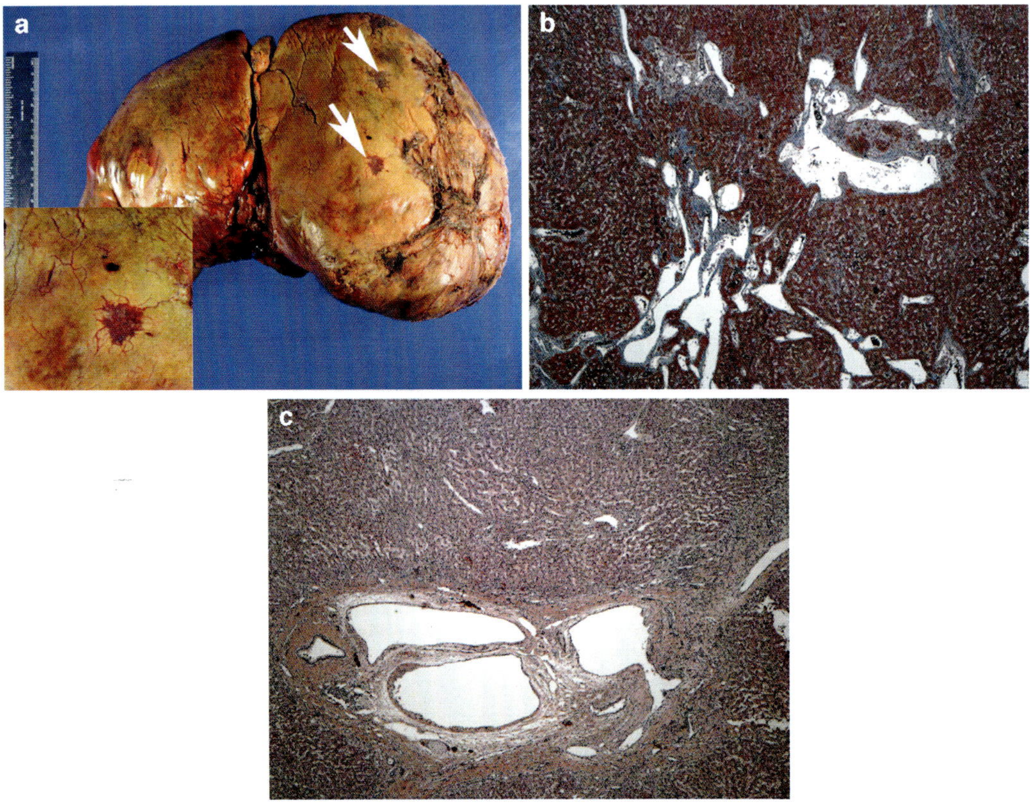

Fig. 8.12 Hereditary hemorrhagic telangiectasia. (**a**) A gross specimen of liver showing multiple "spider-like" telangiectatic vessels (*arrows*) seen on the surface. (**b**) Microscopy reveals a bizarre arrangement of dilated portal vascular channels and hepatic sinusoids (trichrome stain). (**c**) Markedly dilated hepatic artery and portal veins with irregularly thinned walls in a medium-sized portal tract

the cut surface (see Fig. 8.12a). The malformations consist of varying sized telangiectatic portal tract vessels that may "herniate" through the limiting plates into the hepatic lobules and sinusoids (see Fig. 8.12b, c). The vessels are irregularly shaped, dilated, and with walls of varying thickness. Sometimes biliary ischemia, spontaneous or procedure related, may lead to biliary necrosis. Bile duct strictures, dilatation, or cysts may also form; however, these are better seen on imaging studies. Extensive blood shunting (arteriovenous, arterioportal, and/or portovenous) may occur and is also best demonstrated with imaging studies or painstaking resin casts of hepatic vasculature of livers obtained at autopsy. Vascular shunting and perfusion disparity in parts of the liver often lead to NRH. Some cases may also show development of focal nodular hyperplasia as a result of perfusion abnormalities (see Fig. 8.10a). Some cases may show cirrhosis, most likely due to other causes (e.g., alcohol) [74].

The Role of the Liver Biopsy in the Evaluation of Vascular Disorders

When evaluating the liver for vascular disorders there are certain advantages to having wedge biopsies, principally because they provide more tissue for examination. Wedge biopsies have their own limitations, however, and in routine clinical practice one is more often provided with a percutaneous or a transjugular core biopsy. The clinical findings and settings are distinct in many conditions, e.g., in bone marrow transplant-related SOS, such that the histological diagnosis is straightforward. In some cases, the histological findings are characteristic and easily identified, e.g., schistosomiasis or amyloidosis. However, in many cases one is faced with a difficult differential diagnosis and few histological findings, and in these circumstances arriving at a diagnosis will depend upon close clinicopathological correlation. The needle biopsy may appear normal in such cases or show only nonspecific changes secondary to altered blood flow. The changes often include varying combinations of increased apoptosis, atrophy, compensatory hyperplasia, or biliary abnormalities. Critical hepatic ischemia can result in a variable extent of necrosis, while subcritical chronic ischemia merely results in atrophy of hepatic parenchyma that is difficult to evaluate on liver biopsy. Vascular changes in the smaller portal tracts are often subtle and easily missed. If, in the presence of clinical portal hypertension, the biopsy appears near normal, hepatoportal sclerosis, PV thrombosis, and NRH should be considered. Also, one should recognize that, as mentioned above, the liver biopsy can appear entirely normal in these conditions. Sometimes elevation of alkaline phosphatase and biliary changes may mislead one to consider a primary biliary disorder, while changes may be secondary to a vascular disorder. Occasionally, the diagnosis of cardiac failure and congestive hepatopathy may be first suggested by subtle perivascular fibrosis and/or sinusoidal congestion on a liver biopsy. In summary, one should consider the following situations in clinical practice:

1. Clinically obvious portal hypertension with minimal or no changes in the liver, consider hepatoportal sclerosis, extrahepatic PV obstruction (EHPVO), or NRH.
2. Clinical and imaging features suggestive of cirrhosis with biopsy lacking fibrosis, consider NRH.
3. Subtle pericentral fibrosis with or without pericentral sinusoidal dilatation or hepatocyte atrophy, consider cardiac failure.
4. Sinusoidal dilatation may be indicative of disorders other than venous outflow obstruction (e.g., long-term oral contraceptive use) and careful evaluation of the differential diagnosis may lead to important clinical findings.
5. An often-neglected component of vascular injury to the liver is the effect on the biliary tree, which may mimic a primary biliary disorder.

References

1. Tanaka M, Wanless IR. Pathology of the liver in Budd-Chiari syndrome: portal vein thrombosis and the histogenesis of veno-centric cirrhosis, veno-portal cirrhosis, and large regenerative nodules. Hepatology. 1998 Feb;27(2):488–96.
2. Shimamatsu K, Wanless IR. Role of ischemia in causing apoptosis, atrophy, and nodular hyperplasia in human liver. Hepatology. 1997 Aug;26(2):343–50.
3. Wanless IR, Liu JJ, Butany J. Role of thrombosis in the pathogenesis of congestive hepatic fibrosis (cardiac cirrhosis). Hepatology. 1995 May;21(5):1232–7.
4. DeLeve LD, Valla DC, Garcia-Tsao G. Vascular disorders of the liver. Hepatology. 2009 May;49(5): 1729–64.
5. De Gaetano AM, Gui B, Macis G, Manfredi R, Di Stasi C. Congenital absence of the portal vein associated with focal nodular hyperplasia in the liver in an adult woman: imaging and review of the literature. Abdom Imaging. 2004 Jul-Aug;29(4):455–9.
6. Janssen HL, Wijnhoud A, Haagsma EB, van Uum SH, van Nieuwkerk CM, Adang RP, et al. Extrahepatic portal vein thrombosis: aetiology and determinants of survival. Gut. 2001 Nov;49(5):720–4.
7. Denninger MH, Chait Y, Casadevall N, Hillaire S, Guillin MC, Bezeaud A, et al. Cause of portal or hepatic venous thrombosis in adults: the role of multiple concurrent factors. Hepatology. 2000 Mar;31(3): 587–91.
8. Tublin ME, Dodd 3rd GD, Baron RL. Benign and malignant portal vein thrombosis: differentiation by CT characteristics. AJR Am J Roentgenol. 1997 Mar;168(3):719–23.
9. Okuda K, Ohnishi K, Kimura K, Matsutani S, Sumida M, Goto N, et al. Incidence of portal vein thrombosis in liver cirrhosis. An angiographic study in 708 patients. Gastroenterology. 1985 Aug;89(2):279–86.
10. De Gaetano AM, Lafortune M, Patriquin H, De Franco A, Aubin B, Paradis K. Cavernous transformation of the portal vein: patterns of intrahepatic and splanchnic collateral circulation detected with Doppler sonography. AJR Am J Roentgenol. 1995 Nov;165(5): 1151–5.
11. Vilgrain V, Condat B, Bureau C, Hakime A, Plessier A, Cazals-Hatem D, et al. Atrophy-hypertrophy complex in patients with cavernous transformation of the portal vein: CT evaluation. Radiology. 2006 Oct;241(1):149–55.

12. Plemmons RM, Dooley DP, Longfield RN. Septic thrombophlebitis of the portal vein (pylephlebitis): diagnosis and management in the modern era. Clin Infect Dis. 1995 Nov;21(5):1114–20.
13. Ibarrola C, Colina F. Clinicopathological features of nine cases of non-cirrhotic portal hypertension: current definitions and criteria are inadequate. Histopathology. 2003 Mar;42(3):251–64.
14. Sarin SK, Kapoor D. Non-cirrhotic portal fibrosis: current concepts and management. J Gastroenterol Hepatol. 2002 May;17(5):526–34.
15. Terayama N, Terada T, Hoso M, Nakanuma Y. Partial nodular transformation of the liver with portal vein thrombosis. A report of two autopsy cases. J Clin Gastroenterol. 1995 Jan;20(1):71–6.
16. Wanless IR, Lentz JS, Roberts EA. Partial nodular transformation of liver in an adult with persistent ductus venosus. Review with hypothesis on pathogenesis. Arch Pathol Lab Med. 1985 May;109(5):427–32.
17. Ludwig J, Hashimoto E, Obata H, Baldus WP. Idiopathic portal hypertension; a histopathological study of 26 Japanese cases. Histopathology. 1993 Mar;22(3):227–34.
18. Oikawa H, Masuda T, Sato S, Yashima A, Suzuki K, Satodate R. Changes in lymph vessels and portal veins in the portal tract of patients with idiopathic portal hypertension: a morphometric study. Hepatology. 1998 Jun;27(6):1607–10.
19. Nakanuma Y, Hoso M, Sasaki M, Terada T, Katayanagi K, Nonomura A, et al. Histopathology of the liver in non-cirrhotic portal hypertension of unknown aetiology. Histopathology. 1996 Mar;28(3):195–204.
20. Bernard PH, Le Bail B, Cransac M, Barcina MG, Carles J, Balabaud C, et al. Progression from idiopathic portal hypertension to incomplete septal cirrhosis with liver failure requiring liver transplantation. J Hepatol. 1995 Apr;22(4):495–9.
21. Buckley JA, Hutchins GM. Association of hepatic veno-occlusive disease with the acquired immunodeficiency syndrome. Mod Pathol. 1995 May;8(4):398–401.
22. Schiano TD, Kotler DP, Ferran E, Fiel MI. Hepatoportal sclerosis as a cause of noncirrhotic portal hypertension in patients with HIV. Am J Gastroenterol. 2007 Nov;102(11):2536–40.
23. Silva LM, Ribeiro-Dos-Santos R, Soares MB, Andrade ZA. Characterization of the vascular changes in schistosomal portal (pipestem) fibrosis of mice. Acta Trop. 2006 Apr;98(1):34–42.
24. Orloff MJ, Daily PO, Orloff SL, Girard B, Orloff MS. A 27-year experience with surgical treatment of Budd-Chiari syndrome. Ann Surg. 2000 Sep;232(3):340–52.
25. Miller WJ, Federle MP, Straub WH, Davis PL. Budd-Chiari syndrome: imaging with pathologic correlation. Abdom Imaging. 1993 Fall;18(4):329–35.
26. Wanless IR, Peterson P, Das A, Boitnott JK, Moore GW, Bernier V. Hepatic vascular disease and portal hypertension in polycythemia vera and agnogenic myeloid metaplasia: a clinicopathological study of 145 patients examined at autopsy. Hepatology. 1990 Nov;12(5):1166–74.
27. Okuda K. Obliterative hepatocavopathy-inferior vena cava thrombosis at its hepatic portion. Hepatobiliary Pancreat Dis Int. 2002 Nov;1(4):499–509.
28. Riemens SC, Haagsma EB, Kok T, Gouw AS, van der Jagt EJ. Familial occurrence of membranous obstruction of the inferior vena cava: arguments in favor of a congenital etiology. J Hepatol. 1995 Apr;22(4):404–9.
29. Arcidi Jr JM, Moore GW, Hutchins GM. Hepatic morphology in cardiac dysfunction: a clinicopathologic study of 1000 subjects at autopsy. Am J Pathol. 1981 Aug;104(2):159–66.
30. Lefkowitch JH, Mendez L. Morphologic features of hepatic injury in cardiac disease and shock. J Hepatol. 1986;2(3):313–27.
31. Kakar S, Batts KP, Poterucha JJ, Burgart LJ. Histological changes mimicking biliary disease in liver biopsies with venous outflow impairment. Mod Pathol. 2004 Jul;17(7):874–8.
32. Ridker PM, McDermott WV. Comfrey herb tea and hepatic veno-occlusive disease. Lancet. 1989 Mar 25;1(8639):657–8.
33. DeLeve LD, Shulman HM, McDonald GB. Toxic injury to hepatic sinusoids: sinusoidal obstruction syndrome (veno-occlusive disease). Semin Liver Dis. 2002 Feb;22(1):27–42.
34. Shulman HM, Fisher LB, Schoch HG, Henne KW, McDonald GB. Veno-occlusive disease of the liver after marrow transplantation: histological correlates of clinical signs and symptoms. Hepatology. 1994 May;19(5):1171–81.
35. Bioulac-Sage P, Quinton A, Saric J, Grimaud JA, Mourey MS, Balabaud C. Chance discovery of hepatic fibrosis in patient with asymptomatic hypervitaminosis A. Arch Pathol Lab Med. 1988 May;112(5):505–9.
36. Bruguera M, Aranguibel F, Ros E, Rodes J. Incidence and clinical significance of sinusoidal dilatation in liver biopsies. Gastroenterology. 1978 Sep;75(3):474–8.
37. Chopra S, Rubinow A, Koff RS, Cohen AS. Hepatic amyloidosis. A histopathologic analysis of primary (AL) and secondary (AA) forms. Am J Pathol. 1984 May;115(2):186–93.
38. Charlotte F, Bachir D, Nenert M, Mavier P, Galacteros F, Dhumeaux D, et al. Vascular lesions of the liver in sickle cell disease. A clinicopathological study in 26 living patients. Arch Pathol Lab Med. 1995 Jan;119(1):46–52.
39. Oligny LL, Lough J. Hepatic sinusoidal ectasia. Hum Pathol. 1992 Aug;23(8):953–6.
40. Kakar S, Kamath PS, Burgart LJ. Sinusoidal dilatation and congestion in liver biopsy: is it always due to venous outflow impairment? Arch Pathol Lab Med. 2004 Aug;128(8):901–4.
41. Aoyagi T, Mori I, Ueyama Y, Tamaoki N. Sinusoidal dilatation of the liver as a paraneoplastic manifestation of renal cell carcinoma. Hum Pathol. 1989 Dec;20(12):1193–7.
42. Tzirogiannis KN, Papadimas GK, Kondyli VG, Kourentzi KT, Demonakou MD, Kyriakou LG, et al. Peliosis hepatis: microscopic and macroscopic type,

time pattern, and correlation with liver cell apoptosis in a model of toxic liver injury. Dig Dis Sci. 2006 Nov;51(11):1998–2006.
43. Wold LE, Ludwig J. Peliosis Hepatis: Two Morphologic variants? Human Pathology. 1981;12: 388–9.
44. Fine KD, Solano M, Polter DE, Tillery GW. Malignant histiocytosis in a patient presenting with hepatic dysfunction and peliosis hepatis. Am J Gastroenterol. 1995 Mar;90(3):485–8.
45. Khadilkar UN, Prabhu S, Sharma D. Peliosis hepatis presenting as hemoperitoneum. Indian J Med Sci. 2008 Jun;62(6):236–7.
46. Steeper TA, Rosenstein H, Weiser J, Inampudi S, Snover DC. Bacillary epithelioid angiomatosis involving the liver, spleen, and skin in an AIDS patient with concurrent Kaposi's sarcoma. Am J Clin Pathol. 1992 May;97(5):713–8.
47. Brittain RS, Marchioro TL, Hermann G, Waddell WR, Starzl TE. Accidental Hepatic Artery Ligation in Humans. Am J Surg. 1964 Jun;107:822–32.
48. Zhao JC, Lu SC, Yan LN, Li B, Wen TF, Zeng Y, et al. Incidence and treatment of hepatic artery complications after orthotopic liver transplantation. World J Gastroenterol. 2003 Dec;9(12):2853–5.
49. Valente JF, Alonso MH, Weber FL, Hanto DW. Late hepatic artery thrombosis in liver allograft recipients is associated with intrahepatic biliary necrosis. Transplantation. 1996 Jan 15;61(1):61–5.
50. Takeda H, Matsunaga N, Sakamoto I, Obata S, Nakamura S, Hayashi K. Spontaneous dissection of the celiac and hepatic arteries treated by transcatheter embolization. AJR Am J Roentgenol. 1995 Nov; 165(5):1288–9.
51. Shimamura K, Oka K, Nakazawa M, Kojima M. Distribution patterns of microthrombi in disseminated intravascular coagulation. Arch Pathol Lab Med. 1983 Oct;107(10):543–7.
52. Matsumoto T, Yoshimine T, Shimouchi K, Shiotu H, Kuwabara N, Fukuda Y, et al. The liver in systemic lupus erythematosus: pathologic analysis of 52 cases and review of Japanese Autopsy Registry Data. Hum Pathol. 1992 Oct;23(10):1151–8.
53. Parangi S, Oz MC, Blume RS, Bixon R, Laffey KJ, Perzin KH, et al. Hepatobiliary complications of polyarteritis nodosa. Arch Surg. 1991 Jul;126(7): 909–12.
54. Heneghan MA, Feeley KM, DeFaoite N, Little MP, O'Gorman TA. Granulomatous liver disease and giant-cell arteritis. Dig Dis Sci. 1998 Sep;43(9): 2164–7.
55. Goritsas CP, Repanti M, Papadaki E, Lazarou N, Andonopoulos AP. Intrahepatic bile duct injury and nodular regenerative hyperplasia of the liver in a patient with polyarteritis nodosa. J Hepatol. 1997 Mar;26(3):727–30.
56. Boissy C, Bernard E, Chazal M, Fuzibet JG, Michiels JF, Saint-Paul MC. Wegener's granulomatosis disclosed by hepato-splenic involvement. Gastroenterol Clin Biol. 1997;21(8–9):633–5.
57. Rousselet MC, Kettani S, Rohmer V, Saint-Andre JP. A case of temporal arteritis with intrahepatic arterial involvement. Pathol Res Pract. 1989 Sep;185(3): 329–31.
58. Rolfes DB, Ishak KG. Liver disease in pregnancy. Histopathology. 1986 Jun;10(6):555–70.
59. Chen G, Brunt EM. Diabetic hepatosclerosis: a 10-year autopsy series. Liver Int. 2009 Aug;29(7):1044–50.
60. Bernuau D, Guillot R, Durand AM, Raoux N, Gabreau T, Passa P, et al. Ultrastructural aspects of the liver perisinusoidal space in diabetic patients with and without microangiopathy. Diabetes. 1982 Dec;31(12):1061–7.
61. Harrison SA, Brunt EM, Goodman ZD, Di Bisceglie AM. Diabetic hepatosclerosis: diabetic microangiopathy of the liver. Arch Pathol Lab Med. 2006 Jan;130(1):27–32.
62. Hudacko RM, Sciancalepore JP, Fyfe BS. Diabetic microangiopathy in the liver: an autopsy study of incidence and association with other diabetic complications. Am J Clin Pathol. 2009 Oct;132(4):494–9.
63. Degott C, Capron JP, Bettan L, Molas G, Bernuau D, Potet F, et al. Myeloid metaplasia, perisinusoidal fibrosis, and nodular regenerative hyperplasia of the liver. Liver. 1985 Oct;5(5):276–81.
64. Arvanitaki M, Adler M. Nodular regenerative hyperplasia of the liver. A review of 14 cases. Hepatogastroenterology. 2001 Sep-Oct;48(41):1425–9.
65. Schuler JG, Filtzer HS, Rogoff P. Liver infarct after sigmoid resection: an unusual case of mesenteric ischemia. Surgery. 1993 Sep;114(3):607–12.
66. Matsumoto T, Kuwabara N, Abe H, Fukuda Y, Suyama M, Fujii D, et al. Zahn infarct of the liver resulting from occlusive phlebitis in portal vein radicles. Am J Gastroenterol. 1992 Mar;87(3):365–8.
67. Saegusa M, Takano Y, Okudaira M. Human hepatic infarction: histopathological and postmortem angiological studies. Liver. 1993 Oct;13(5):239–45.
68. Seeto RK, Fenn B, Rockey DC. Ischemic hepatitis: clinical presentation and pathogenesis. Am J Med. 2000 Aug 1;109(2):109–13.
69. Bynum TE, Boitnott JK, Maddrey WC. Ischemic hepatitis. Dig Dis Sci. 1979 Feb;24(2):129–35.
70. Batts KP. Ischemic cholangitis. Mayo Clin Proc. 1998 Apr;73(4):380–5.
71. Condat B, Vilgrain V, Asselah T, O'Toole D, Rufat P, Zappa M, et al. Portal cavernoma-associated cholangiopathy: a clinical and MR cholangiography coupled with MR portography imaging study. Hepatology. 2003 Jun;37(6):1302–8.
72. Garcia-Tsao G. Liver involvement in hereditary hemorrhagic telangiectasia (HHT).[see comment]. Journal of Hepatology. 2007;46(3):499–507.
73. Garcia-Tsao G, Korzenik JR, Young L, Henderson KJ, Jain D, Byrd B, et al. Liver disease in patients with hereditary hemorrhagic telangiectasia. N Engl J Med. 2000 Sep 28;343(13):931–6.
74. Martini GA. The liver in hereditary haemorrhagic teleangiectasia: an inborn error of vascular structure with multiple manifestations: a reappraisal. Gut. 1978 Jun;19(6):531–7.

Radiological Diagnosis

9

Christopher G. Roth and Donald G. Mitchell

Abstract

Imaging lends itself to the evaluation of vascular liver diseases because of the ability of many imaging modalities to directly visualize the vessels and the secondary parenchymal findings. The most commonly employed imaging modalities in the setting of vascular liver disease include ultrasound (US), computed tomography (CT), magnetic resonance imaging (MRI), and catheter angiography (CA). Each modality possesses unique utility for interrogating hepatic vessels and demonstrating associated parenchymal abnormalities.

The US, CT, and MRI are all used as noninvasive methods to image the hepatic vasculature and parenchyma. US is the most operator-dependent modality, harnessing sound waves, which are used to document vessel patency and grade stenoses and screen the liver parenchyma. US is best suited for targeted assessment of the hepatic vessels for patency or stenosis, such as transjugular intrahepatic portosystemic shunt (TIPS) evaluation, and post-transplant portal venous and/or hepatic arterial assessment, also providing an overview of the hepatic parenchyma. MRI exploits a strong magnetic field to yield images of the liver and hepatic vessels with or without the benefit of intravenous gadolinium. MRI requires more time, cost and attention to technical demands, but generates images of the vessels and liver parenchyma with exquisite tissue contrast. The combination of sensitivity to vascular structures and solid tissue recommends its use for transplant complications, assessment of the liver in cirrhosis and portal hypertension, and other diffuse liver diseases, such as Budd-Chiari syndrome (BCS). CT employs ionizing radiation to generate high-resolution images of the abdomen rapidly, relying on iodinated contrast to evaluate blood vessels. CT is the most easily acquired, versatile modality, capable of rapidly acquiring images of all of the hepatic vessels (following contrast administration) and the liver parenchyma, but lacks the tissue contrast of MRI. CT has the same applications as MRI, for the most part, relying on MRI to solve difficult or equivocal cases.

C.G. Roth (✉)
Department of Radiology, Thomas Jefferson University Hospital, Philadelphia, PA 19102, USA
e-mail: Christopher.Roth@jefferson.edu

L.D. DeLeve and G. Garcia-Tsao (eds.), *Vascular Liver Disease: Mechanisms and Management*,
DOI 10.1007/978-1-4419-8327-5_9,

The CA is generally reserved for cases potentially involving intervention, such as TIPS, angioplasty, or embolization procedures. Direct access to the vascular system is achieved with placement of specialized catheters into the relevant vascular anatomy through which iodinated contrast is administered to visualize the vessels. Interventional devices or embolization material are directed through the catheter to perform therapeutic procedures.

Keywords
Ultrasound • Computed tomography • Magnetic resonance imaging • Catheter angiography • Transjugular intrahepatic portosystemic shunt • Portal hypertension • Budd-Chiari Syndrome • Portal venous thrombosis

Introduction

Various imaging modalities visualize the hepatic vasculature, including ultrasound (US), computed tomography (CT), magnetic resonance imaging (MRI), and catheter angiography (CA). The choice of imaging modality depends on the clinical circumstances and objective, since each modality has advantages and limitations. Metrics include patient safety based on invasiveness and risk of complications, patient safety based on ionizing radiation and/or radiofrequency energy deposition, spatial resolution, temporal resolution, tissue contrast, physiologic capabilities, anatomic coverage and cost (Table 9.1).

Ultrasound is a focused examination based on sound waves and is dependent on the skill of the operator – usually a technologist (at least in the US). A "probe" sends sound waves that reverberate at "acoustic interfaces" that are subsequently received by the probe. The information received by the probe represents the sum of the acoustic interfaces encountered by all of the sound waves interrogating the region of interest. This information is usually displayed in "gray-scale" format (or B mode), rendering an anatomic image with brighter shades representing greater attenuation of sound waves or a higher density of acoustic interfaces. Gray-scale images may be supplemented with color (or power) Doppler information, which superimposes flow, or motion, information on to the anatomic data encoded with specific colors assigned to specific motion direction with intensity proportional to magnitude. Velocity values are obtained at

Table 9.1 Attributes of various imaging modalities

	Invasiveness	Radiation/RF safety	Spatial resolution
US	–	–	++
CT	IV access	Ionizing radiation	+++
MRI	IV access	–	++
CA	Vascular access	Ionizing radiation	++++
	Temporal resolution	Tissue contrast	Anatomic coverage
US	++++	+	+
CT	++	++	++++
MRI	+++	++++	++
CA	+++	+	++
	Physiologic assessment	Cost	
US	Velocity, directionality	$$	
CT	Only anatomy/structure	$$$	
MRI	Directionality and velocity time prohibitive	$$$$	
CA	Pressure gradient assessment	$$$$	

locations specified by the operator (solved by the system using the Doppler equation).

Liver echotexture is generally monotonous, or homogeneous, and becomes coarse and heterogeneous as chronic liver disease evolves and inflammation and fibrosis interrupt the normal hepatic architecture. Parenchymal perfusion changes are usually assessed with CT and MRI; and while US contrast agents exist, they are still investigational.

CT relies less on operator skill and more on hardware specifications and protocol parameters. The process of acquiring images involves spinning an X-ray tube circularly around the gantry, sending X-ray photons through the patient – who is passing through the gantry – into the X-ray detector system on the other side. X-rays not attenuated – or blocked – by the patient constitute the information received by the detectors, which is ultimately processed into CT images. The end result is a 3-D volume map of electron density, which dictates the ability to attenuate X-rays. In-plane resolution is excellent; slice resolution is dependent on technical parameters, such as pitch and the number of detector units. Better slice resolution improves image quality and facilitates 3-D reformatting.

CT imaging of vascular structures requires contrast enhancement, otherwise vascular structures are isodense to surrounding tissues and cannot be discriminated from the background. Following the intravenous administration of iodinated contrast material, CT arteriographic (CTA) image acquisition begins when contrast reaches the celiac axis and hepatic arteries – generally approximately 20 s later. Accurate timing prevents simultaneous enhancement of adjacent parenchyma and/or venous structures and isolates the arteries for optimal visualization. Newer CT systems employ an automated system to detect the arrival of contrast to a predesignated region of interest, which triggers the acquisition of CTA images.

Portal venous imaging is less technically demanding and less enhancement-specific. Over time, the contrast bolus gradually disperses and adjacent structures become relatively more enhanced. Therefore, contrast between the portal vein and surrounding structures is less marked compared with CTA.

Normal liver parenchyma exhibits a predictable temporal enhancement pattern as a function of its dual blood supply. During the arterial phase, the liver enhances mildly, commensurate with the hepatic arterial smaller contribution (approximately 20%). Enhancement peaks during the portal phase, when the portal vein perfuses the hepatic parenchyma. Because most contrast agents are extracellular agents, liver parenchyma remains enhanced thereafter, since contrast persists in the interstitium.

MRI takes advantage of the predictable behavior of protons in a strong magnetic field, avoiding ionizing radiation. Radiofrequency waves are sent to the region of interest and protons emit radiofrequency energy back to a receiver coil – or antenna – which is processed by the MRI system into images. Tissue contrast can isolate different proton species from one another (i.e., water vs. lipid) and can manipulate a virtually infinite number of parameters. In addition to selectively highlighting different proton species, MRI is able to isolate motion or vascular flow (i.e., time-of-flight) without requiring intravenous contrast.

Contrast enhancement using gadolinium will supplement the unenhanced images and is more robust compared with CT. However, enhancement kinetics are the same, and the liver enhancement pattern is identical to CT.

Contrast angiography is generally reserved for interventional procedures, such as transjugular intrahepatic portosystemic shunt (TIPS) procedures, vascular angioplasty procedures, and ablative embolization procedures. Vascular access is requisite and imaging involves rapid radiographic image acquisition during/following the administration of radioopaque iodinated contrast material. Because CA is essentially exclusively therapeutic, further discussion is beyond the scope of this review.

Normal and Variant Anatomy

Hepatic vascular anatomy encompasses three distinct systems: the hepatic arterial system (arising from the celiac axis), the portal venous system, and the hepatic veins. Inflow is shared by the portal venous system, accounting for 75–80% of hepatic blood supply, and the hepatic arterial system, accounting for the rest. Outflow is via the hepatic veins into the inferior vena cava (IVC).

The relevance of understanding normal hepatic vascular anatomy is most apparent when screening prior to LT and when anticipating abdominal surgery (to identify potential anomalous anatomy complicating surgery) or transarterial chemoembolization. Classic – or standard – celiac anatomy is observed in approximately 50% of patients (see Fig. 9.1) [1–6]. Standard celiac anatomy is defined by the presence of three branch vessels. Following the origin of the first branch, the left gastric artery (LGA), the vessel divides into the splenic artery (SA) and common hepatic artery (CHA). The CHA bifurcates into the gastroduodenal artery (GDA) and proper hepatic artery (PHA). The PHA subsequently bifurcates into the right hepatic artery (RHA) and left hepatic artery (LHA). Common variants include an accessory or aberrant RHA arising from the superior mesenteric artery (SMA) and an accessory or aberrant LHA arising from the LGA (Table 9.2).

CT angiography (CTA) and MR angiography (MRA) are most commonly employed to delineate the mesenteric arterial anatomy. Both involve the intravenous administration of contrast material with accurate timing for the arrival of contrast into the abdominal aorta. The outcome is a structural rendering of the arterial system for depicting anatomy and generating multiplanar reformatted and volume-rendered images (Fig. 9.1).

The portal vein represents the confluence of the superior mesenteric and splenic veins, continuing into the porta hepatis to supply the liver (Fig. 9.2). Within a few centimeters more centrally within the liver, the main portal vein typically measures 8 mm and divides into the right portal vein (RPV) and left portal vein (LPV). The RPV bifurcates into anterior and posterior branches, which subsequently divide into superior and inferior branches. The LPV courses horizontally to the left, curves anteriorly sending branches to the lateral segment and ultimately terminating in superior and inferior branches to the medial segment.

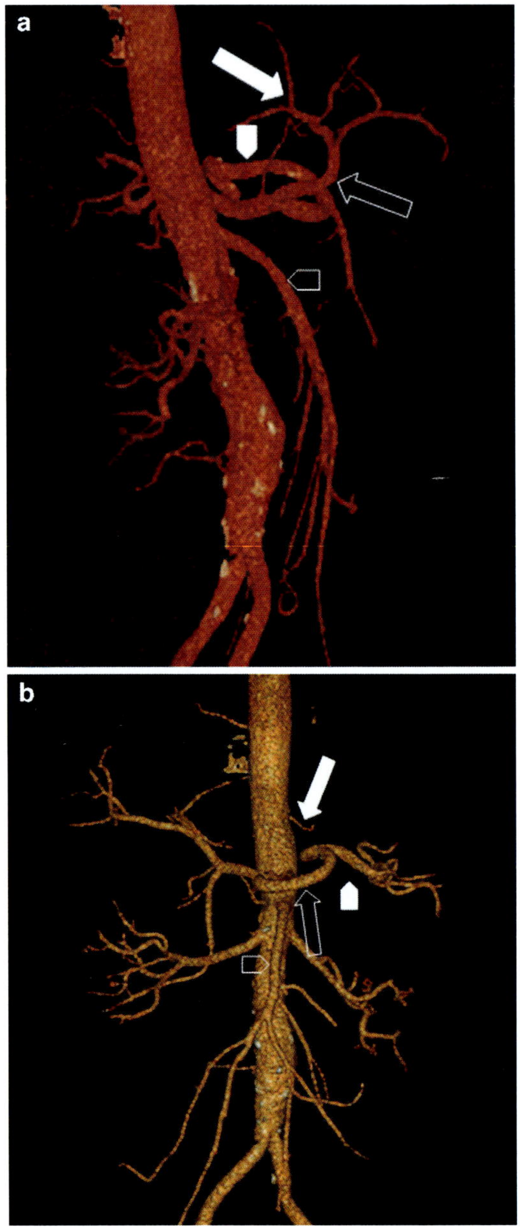

Fig. 9.1 Normal celiac anatomy. Volume-rendered sagittally-oriented (**a**) and coronally-oriented (**b**) images depict standard celiac anatomy. The left gastric origin arises first, coursing superiorly (*arrow*), after which the vessel bifurcates into splenic (*arrowhead*) and common hepatic (*open arrow*) arteries. Note the lack of accessory or replaced hepatic arteries arising from the superior mesenteric artery (*open arrowhead*)

The hepatic vasculature is routinely insonated during abdominal US examinations. Because of the relatively deep location of portions of the liver and hepatic vasculature, a 2–5 MHz sector or curved array transducer with relatively high acoustic penetration is favored. Characteristic images of the central hepatic vessels are routinely included. An axial image through the porta hepatis shows the circular, anechoic (black) structures

Table 9.2 Celiac axis variant anatomy

Hepatic trunk arising from CHA (approximately 80%)
Replaced RHA arising from SMA (<10%)
Accessory LHA arising from LGA (<10%)
Hepatic trunk arising from SMA
Replaced RHA and accessory LHA
Replaced LHA and accessory RHA
Accessory LHA and RHA

CHA common hepatic artery; *LHA* left hepatic artery; *LGA* left gastric artery; *RHA* right hepatic artery; *SMA* superior mesenteric artery

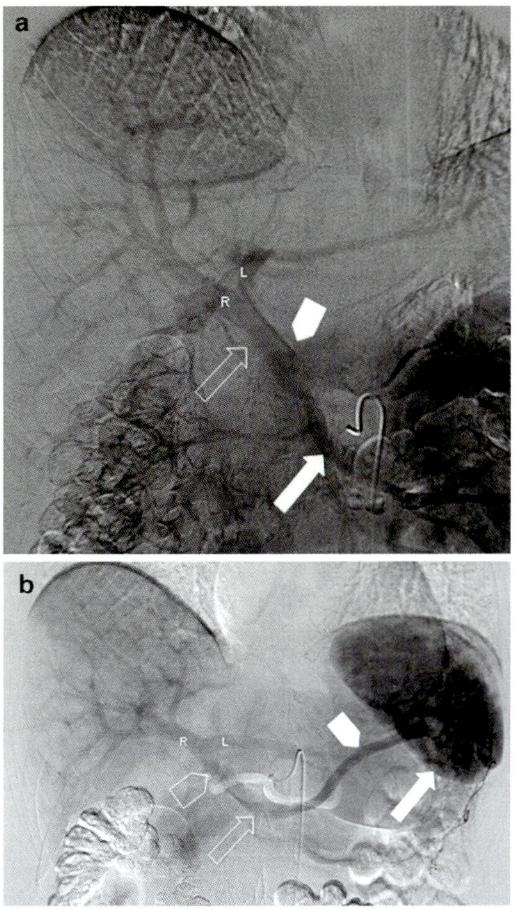

Fig. 9.2 Portal venous anatomy. The delayed image following injection of the SMA (**a**) shows the superior mesenteric vein (*arrow*) with the approximate site of the splenic venous confluence (*arrowhead*) constituting the main portal vein (*open arrow*), which branches within the liver into the right (R) and left (L) main portal veins. The delayed image following injection of the celiac axis (**b**) reveals dense opacification of the spleen (*arrow*) with opacification of the splenic vein (*arrowhead*) and the approximate anastomosis with the SMV (*open arrow*) draining into the main portal vein (*open arrowhead*). The main portal vein branches promptly into right (R) and left (L) main portal veins

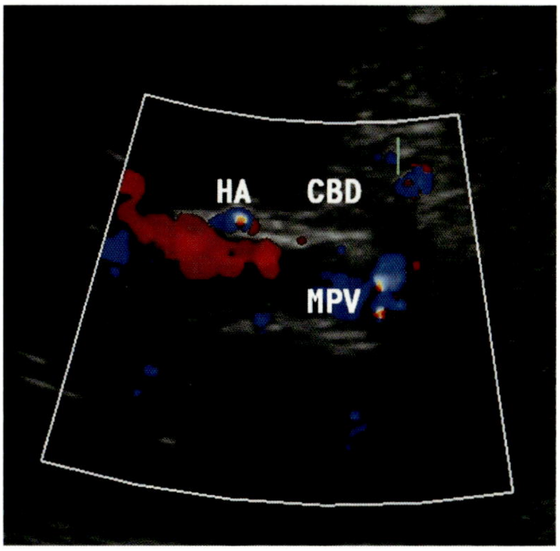

Fig. 9.3 Ultrasound of the porta hepatis. Color Doppler US image through the porta hepatis shows the hepatic artery and common bile duct anterior to the main portal vein. The common bile duct remains anechoic due to the absence of continuous flow

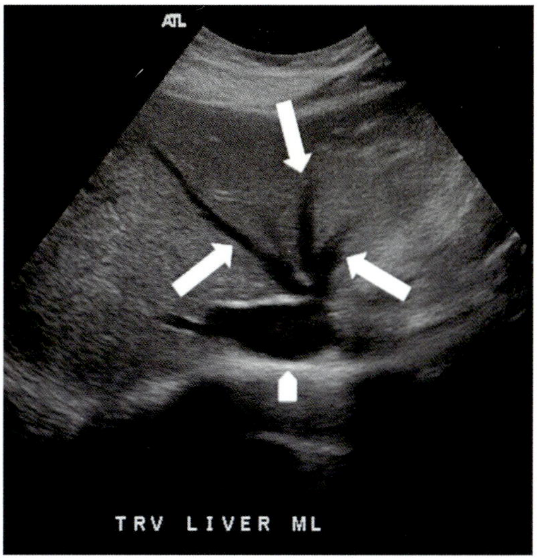

Fig. 9.4 "Moose" or "playboy bunny" sign. Axial ultrasound image through the hepatic venous confluence simulates the appearance of a moose with antlers (*arrows*) or a "playboy bunny" corresponding to the hepatic veins with the IVC representing the head (*arrowhead*)

corresponding to the HA, PV, and common bile duct. Only the common bile duct remains anechoic with color Doppler (Fig. 9.3). A more cephalad image through the liver at the confluence of the hepatic veins simulates both a moose or a "playboy bunny" (Fig. 9.4).

The main portal vein measures 10 ± 2 mm [7] with flow directed toward the liver (hepatopedal), averaging 20–30 cm/s. Portal flow is continuous, with no pulsations as commonly observed in other vessels (Fig. 9.5a). HA arterial flow demonstrates characteristics of flow to a low-resistance arterial bed, with a broad systolic upstroke and relatively high diastolic flow (Fig. 9.5b). The HVs merge at or immediately proximal to the IVC and the proximity to the heart explains the flow pattern reflecting nearby right atrial activity. Right atrial contraction induces retrograde flow in the HVs, constituting the first phase of the triphasic HV waveform. Subsequent rapid right atrial filling triggers rapid antegrade flow in the HVs – the second phase of the waveform. As the right atrium fills and antegrade flow begins to slow, the opening of the tricuspid valve accelerates HV antegrade flow – the third phase (Fig. 9.5c).

Portal venous anatomic variants are less common than celiac arterial anomalies and include congenital absence of major portal venous

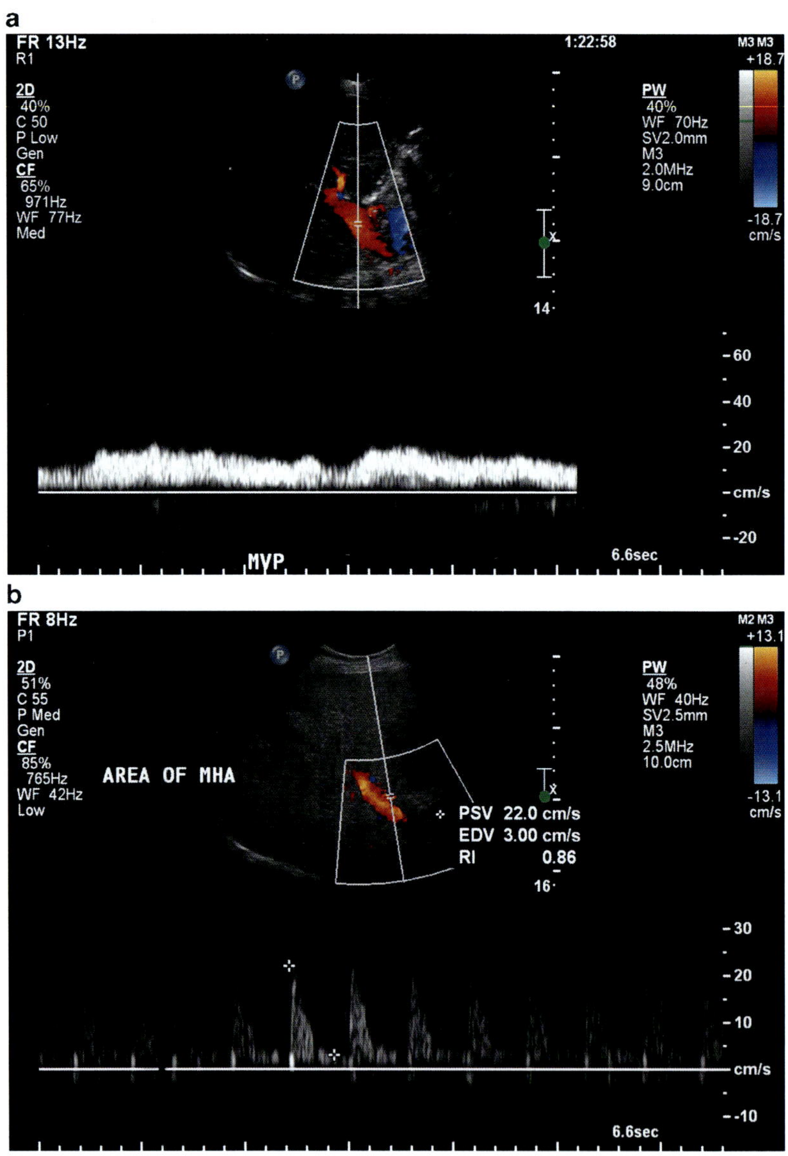

Fig. 9.5 Portal venous, hepatic arterial, and hepatic venous Doppler waveforms. Pulsed Doppler waveforms reveal continuous hepatopetal flow in the portal vein (**a**), pulsatile flow with a sharp systolic upstroke in the hepatic artery (**b**) and triphasic flow in the middle hepatic vein (**c**)

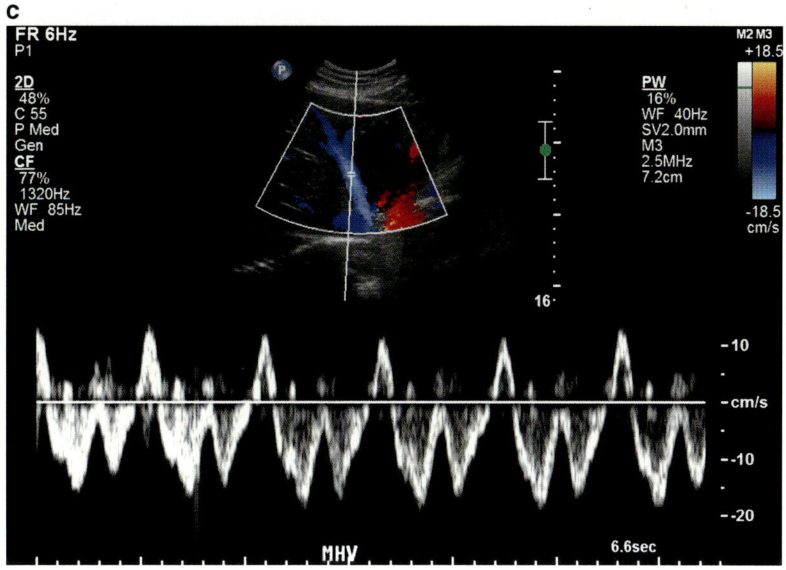

Fig. 9.5 (continued)

branches and anomalous branching patterns [8]. The prepancreatic portal vein is the most common congenital portal venous anomaly; other anomalies include agenesis of the portal vein and portal venous branches. Variation in the normal portal venous branching pattern encompasses a variety of branching patterns and may occur up to 30–40% of the time [9]. Common branching anomalies include portal venous trifurcation, separate origin for the RPV as the first branch of the main portal vein and separate branches for segmental RPV vessels.

Postliver Transplant Vascular Complications

The liver is the second most commonly transplanted organ after the kidney. Liver transplantation (LT) involves grafting either a cadaveric liver (orthotopic liver transplant – OLT) or a portion of a living donor liver (living donor liver transplant – LDLT). Both techniques involve multiple vascular anastomoses including HA, PV and proximal and distal IVC anastomoses.

Hepatic artery thrombosis (HAT) – the leading vascular complication – occurs in up to 9% of patients [10–12]. HAT often presents within 4 weeks with graft failure, biliary stricturing or leak (due to ischemia), or liver abscess or sepsis (arising from infarcted parenchyma). HAT demands urgent surgical intervention with revascularization techniques or retransplantation. Lack of enhancement of the HA constitutes HAT on CTA and MRA images [13–16]. Lack of Doppler flow suggests the diagnosis on US [17]. Because the biliary system receives blood supply solely from the arterial system, biliary strictures form, reflected by segmental narrowing of bile ducts with upstream dilatation. Liver infarcts and/or abscesses develop in perfusion-deprived liver tissue. Liver infarcts often respect anatomic boundaries and conform to a segmental shape [18, 19], exhibiting a lack of enhancement and signs of parenchymal edema, best visualized on MRI images (Fig. 9.6). Abscesses have a variable appearance, depending on the phase of evolution [20]. As tissue necrosis and liquefaction progress, clusters of small abscess cavities begin to coalesce, ultimately forming a larger multiseptated abscess cavity (Fig. 9.7).

HA stenosis (HAS) usually arises at the anastomosis and appears as a relatively narrowed segment compared with larger caliber proximal and

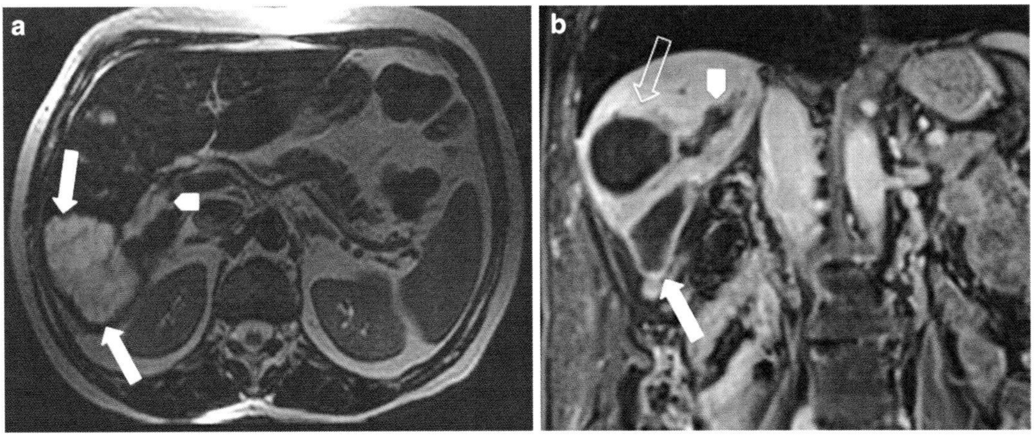

Fig. 9.6 Liver infarct. (**a**) Axial T2-weighted MR image shows a peripheral, wedge-shaped lesion (*arrows*) with absent enhancement on the coronal enhanced MR image (**b**) corresponding to an infarct subtended by a hyperintense, nonenhancing portal venous branch (*arrowhead*). The large hypointense lesion on the enhanced image is a simple cyst (*open arrow*)

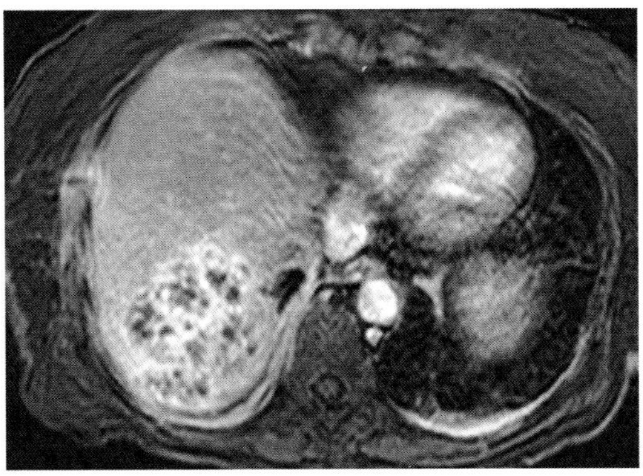

Fig. 9.7 Pyogenic liver abscess complicating a liver infarct. Axial enhanced MR image through the dome of the liver reveals a large complex multiloculated cystic lesion, typical of a pyogenic abscess

distal segments (Fig. 9.8). HAS has a prevalence of approximately 5% [21, 22] and leads to similar complications, albeit evolving at a slower rate. Other arterial complications, including pseudoaneurysms and arteriovenous fistulae, occur in less than 5% of cases [23, 24]. Pseudoaneurysms preferentially form at the anastomotic site or at the ligated GDA site (see Fig. 9.8) [25, 26]. As saccular outpouchings from the parent vessel, pseudoaneurysms assume roughly spherical morphology with evidence of central enhancement or flow and variable peripheral thrombus. Intraparenchymal AVFs and pseudoaneurysms complicate biopsy, biliary interventions and other procedures.

Portal venous complications occur in less than 5% of patients and include PV thrombosis (PVT) and PV stenosis (PVS) [27, 28]. These complications risk graft failure and portal hypertension. Lack of PV enhancement with concomitant arterial parenchymal enhancement on CT and MR images reflects PVT (see Fig. 9.9). PV thrombus usually appears hypoechoic (occasionally hyperechoic) on gray-scale US images, with absent color Doppler flow (Fig. 9.9).

While PVS potentially progresses to PVT and graft failure, the diagnosis is less straightforward. Turbulent flow – often signifying stenosis in native vessels – is generated by surgical factors, including recipient-donor PV size mismatch. A relatively larger recipient PV anastomosed to a smaller donor PV results in pseudostenosis with turbulent flow, reflected by spectral broadening on pulsed Doppler US. In addition to spectral broadening, a 3–4-fold increase in velocity documented on spectral Doppler US heralds PVS (see Fig. 9.10). CT or MRI confirm the diagnosis with the benefit of multiplanar reformatted images along the plane of the PV, in the case of CT, or with the benefit

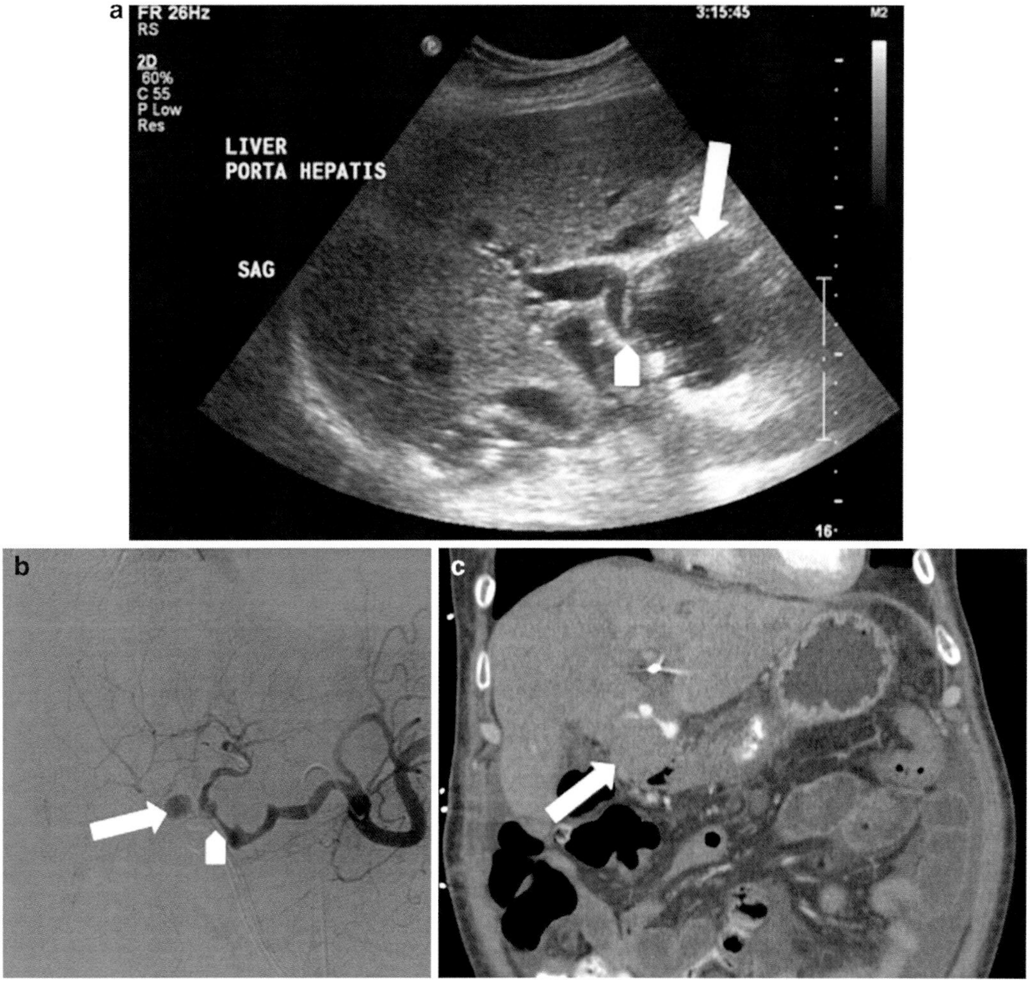

Fig. 9.8 Hepatic artery pseudoaneurysm. Sagittal gray-scale US image through a transplanted liver through the porta hepatis (**a**) shows an ovoid anechoic structure (*arrow*) adjacent to the hepatic artery (*arrowhead*). An image from a subsequent conventional catheter arteriogram (**b**) reveals a spherical collection of contrast (*arrow*) corresponding to the central nidus of a large hepatic arterial pseudoaneurysm at the anastomotic site resulting in arterial stenosis (*arrowhead*). Compression by the mostly thrombosed pseudoaneurysm (*arrow*) is better portrayed on the coronally-reformatted CT image (**c**)

of directly coronally (and/or sagittally) acquired images in the case of MRI (Fig. 9.10).

Posttransplantation complications of the IVC occur rarely – in approximately 1–4% of cases [29, 30]. IVC stenosis develops at either the proximal or distal anastomotic sites. Stenoses arise from a number of causes, including surgical technique and mass effect from hepatic regeneration or adjacent fluid collection. The US diagnosis of IVC stenosis reiterates the features of PVS – narrowing on gray-scale images with a 3–4-fold increase in velocity on spectral Doppler (see Fig. 9.11). Supporting findings include dampening of the upstream HV triphasic waveform and HV distention. CT and MRI reveal similar findings – diminution in the caliber of the retrohepatic IVC, intraluminal filling defect/thrombus and upstream distention of the IVC and/or HVs (Fig. 9.11). Clinical findings support the diagnostic imaging findings.

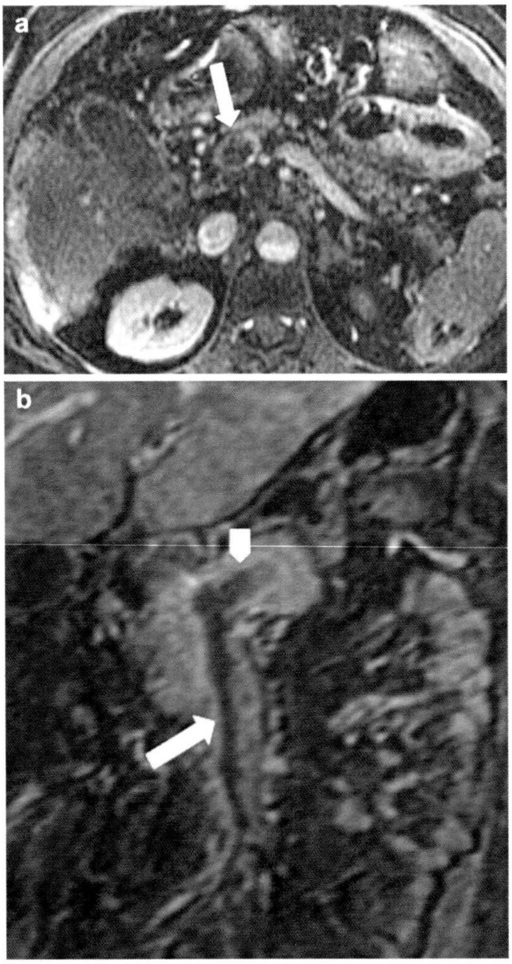

Fig. 9.9 Portal vein thrombosis. The axial contrast-enhanced MR image (**a**) shows hypointense filling defect within the main portal vein (*arrow*). The coronal contrast-enhanced MR image (**b**) shows the thrombus extending into the superior mesenteric (*arrow*) and splenic vein (*arrowhead*)

Lower extremity edema suggests IVC disease and ascites is prominent in HV pathology but is usually absent in PV pathology even though portal hypertension is present in both.

Portal Venous Disorders

The portal vein is susceptible to injury from disease infiltrating its destination – the liver – or arising from its source – the gastrointestinal tract. Portal venous thrombosis and portal hypertension constitute the main complications. Portal venous aneurysms are rare and virtually all other disorders arise postprocedurally, such as portal venous stenosis (after transplantation).

Portal Venous Thrombosis

PVT develops in the setting of diminished portal venous blood flow due to cirrhosis, abdominal septic conditions, hypercoagulable states, or tumoral invasion (Chaps. 8 and 12). With chronicity, collaterals develop in the porta hepatis to reconstitute portal venous flow, simulating the appearance of a sponge-like collection of serpiginous channels replacing the main portal vein (cavernomatous transformation).

All cross-sectional imaging modalities adeptly identify PVT. On US, variably echogenic material replaces the anechoic lumen of the PV, with absent color and spectral Doppler signal (Fig. 9.12) [31, 32]. Partial preservation of color/spectral Doppler signal indicates partially occlusive PVT. Insonation of the superior mesenteric and splenic veins – routinely included in surveillance studies for patients with chronic liver disease – potentially detects superior mesenteric venous (SMV) and/or splenic venous (SV) thrombus.

CT and MRI often corroborate US findings of PVT. After an appropriate delay (usually 45–60 s) following the intravenous administration of contrast, lack of enhancement, hypodense defects on CT or hypointense filling on MR signal the presence of PVT (see Fig. 9.9) [33, 34]. Compared to US, MR and CT scan allow for a more reliable detection of SMV and SV thrombus (see Fig. 9.9). MRI offers noncontrast techniques to supplement or obviate contrast-enhanced imaging (in the setting of severe renal insufficiency). Time-of-flight sequences – time-consuming and prone to motion artifact – have largely been replaced by steady-state techniques for unenhanced MR imaging. Steady-state images preserve high signal in fluid-filled objects regardless of flow or motion, which induces dephasing and signal loss on other types of pulse sequences. PVT findings on steady-state images simulate the appearance on contrast-enhanced images – a hypointense filling defect

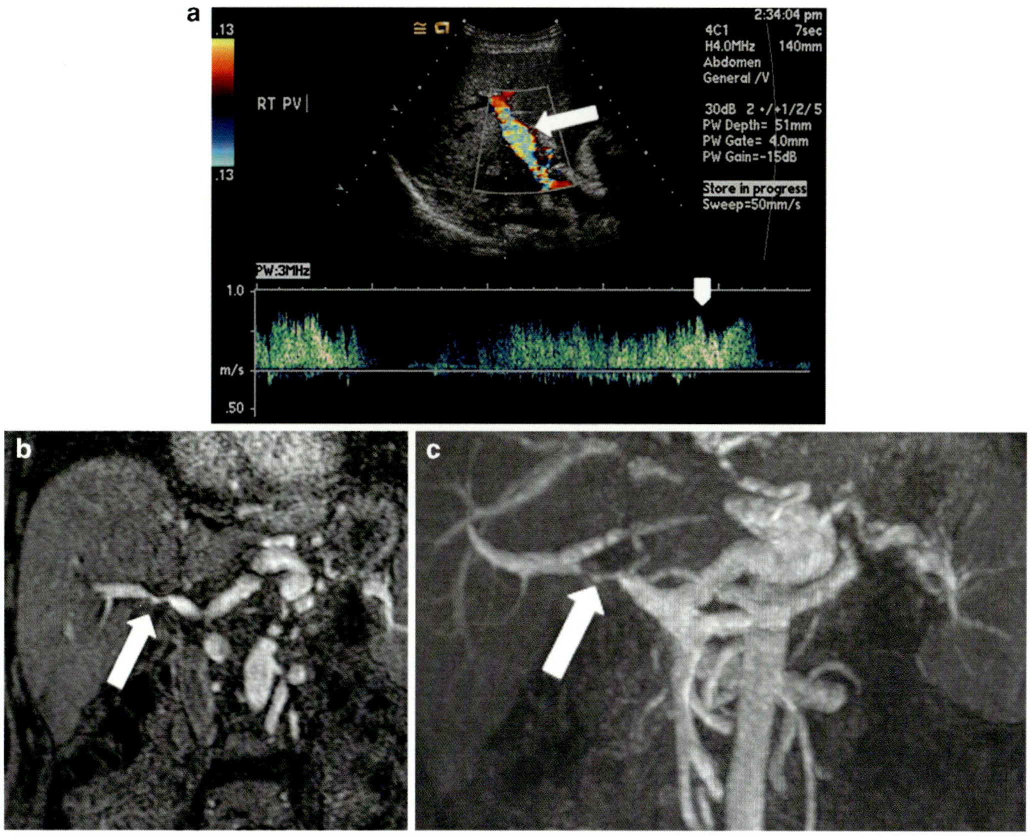

Fig. 9.10 Portal vein stenosis. The color Doppler US (**a**) shows heterogeneous color in the portal vein (*arrow*) in a transplanted liver indicating turbulent flow with elevated velocities recorded in the spectral waveform reaching up to 75 cm/s (*arrowhead*). Coronally-reformatted contrast-enhanced (**b**) and maximal intensity projectional (**c**) images depict a focal narrowing at the anastomotic site (*arrow*)

replacing the normally hyperintense background of the PV.

Especially in the context of known HCC or chronic liver disease, bland PVT must be differentiated from tumor thrombus. US excels in this capacity by harnessing the power of color Doppler. Color Doppler signal within PVT connotes blood flow, which implies viable, solid tissue compared to inert clot without a blood supply. Enhancement – or an increase in density or intensity on CT or MRI, respectively – between pre- and postcontrast images establishes the diagnosis of tumor thrombus on CT and MRI (Fig. 9.13). Conversely, absent enhancement confirms bland thrombus. Of course, identifying the underlying malignancy increases diagnostic confidence and helps plan subsequent treatment.

More commonly in the setting of benign disease, collateral channels develop to reconstitute portal venous flow – known as cavernous transformation of the portal vein. This pattern typically evolves over a time period of at least 12 months [35, 36], and conjures the appearance of convoluted, tubular, interconnected channels coursing within the porta hepatis, ramifying according to portal venous branching. US depicts clustered tubular anechoic structures in the porta hepatis with color Doppler flow and velocities of approximately 2–7 cm/s less than normal portal venous flow [37, 38]. CT and MRI reveal enhancing tubular structures in the porta hepatis smaller than the normal main portal vein (Fig. 9.14). With smaller caliber vessels, cavernous transformation appears more mass-like or infiltrative;

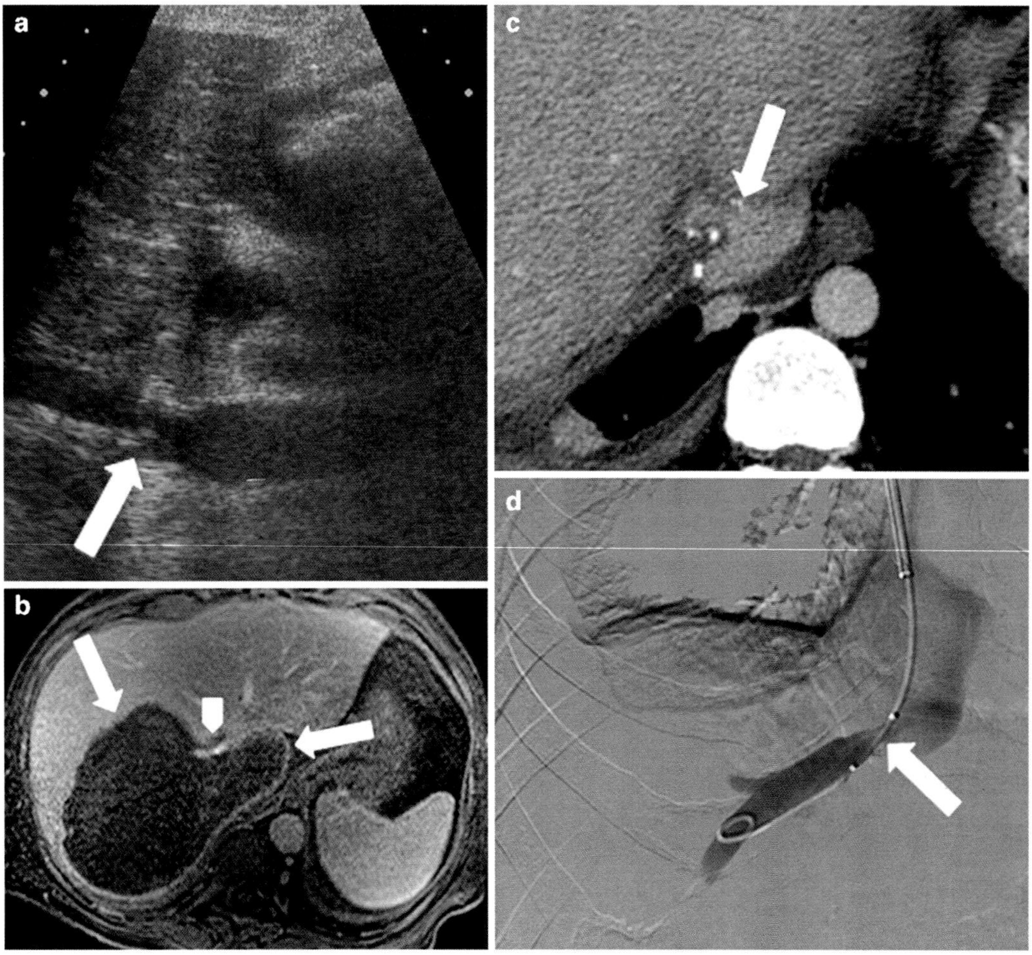

Fig. 9.11 IVC stenosis. Gray-scale sagittal US image (**a**) through a transplanted liver reveals an abrupt narrowing of the intrahepatic IVC (*arrow*). (**b**) An axial contrast-enhanced MR image shows a large perihepatic fluid collection (*arrows*) compressing and displacing the intrahepatic IVC (*arrowhead*). Axial enhanced CT image (**c**) through the distal IVC anastomosis in a different transplant patient reveals mild stenosis at the anastomotic site (*arrow*), shown not to be hemodynamically significant at catheter venography (**d**)

time-of-flight techniques specific for flow confirm the diagnosis and exclude malignancy and inflammatory etiologies.

Portal Venous Aneurysm

Portal venous aneurysms are rare and generally incidental – arising either as a congenital anomaly or as a complication of portal hypertension [39]. Aneurysms tend to occur at bifurcations – the SMV/SV or intrahepatic bifurcations. US depicts an anechoic fusiform or saccular structure continuous with the portal vein (see Fig. 9.15), usually with turbulent flow. Enhanced CT and MRI reveal a fusiform or saccular component of the portal vein, with enhancement intensity identical to portal enhancement (Fig. 9.15).

Portal Hypertension

Portal hypertension (HTN) is defined as portosystemic pressure gradient (wedged HV pressure vs. free HV pressure or direct PV pressure vs. IVC pressure) greater than 5 mmHg. The two major pathogenic factors responsible for portal

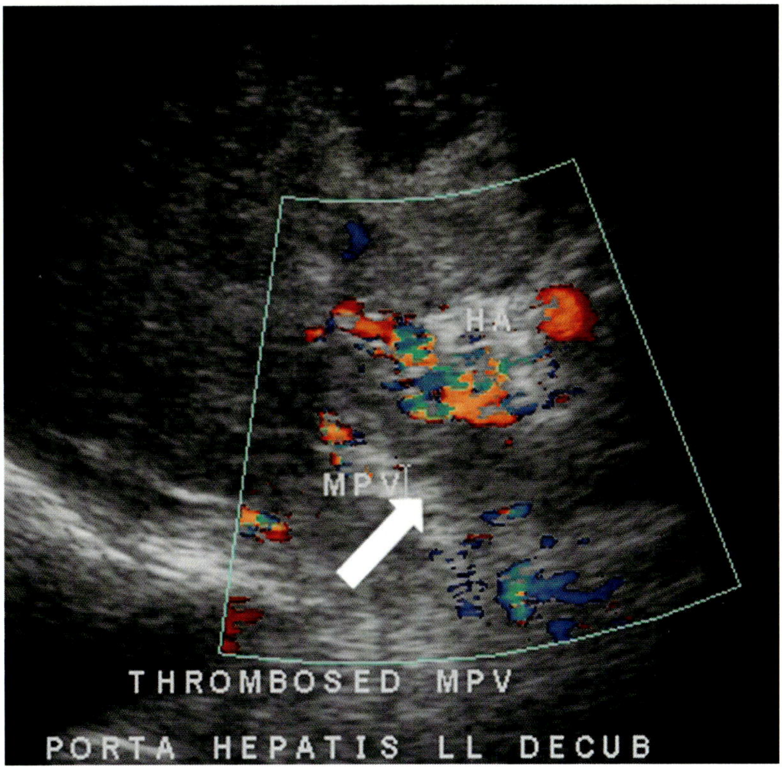

Fig. 9.12 Portal vein thrombosis on ultrasound. Color Doppler sagittal US image through the porta hepatis shows absence of color in the main portal vein (*arrow*) indicating absent flow and intraluminal thrombus

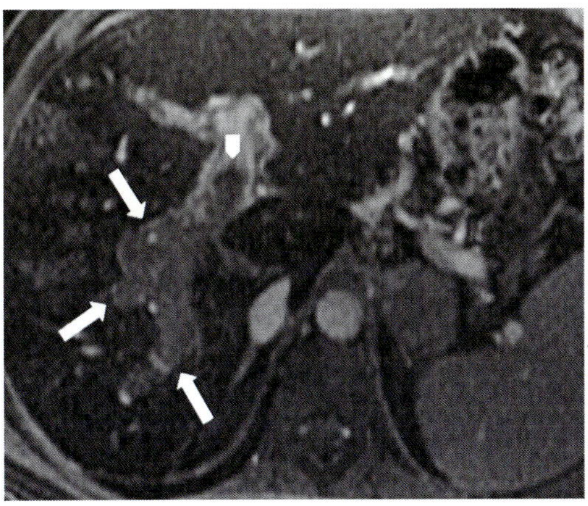

Fig. 9.13 Tumor thrombus on MRI. Axial enhanced image through the liver shows extensive intraluminal material corresponding to tumor thrombus within the right portal venous branches (*arrows*), which is relatively hyperintense to bland thrombus more centrally near the portal bifurcation (*arrowhead*) as a consequence of enhancement

venous hypertension are increased resistance and increased portal venous inflow (Chaps. 6 and 7).

While a vast array of diseases can lead to portal hypertension, cirrhosis is the main cause. While the imaging features of cirrhosis are independent of portal hypertension, they frequently coexist and alert the radiologist to the possibility of portal hypertension. Parenchymal nodularity and a characteristic segmental atrophy–hypertrophy pattern – right lobar and medial segmental atrophy and caudate lobar and lateral segmental hypertrophy – typify advanced cirrhosis. Textural heterogeneity and coarseness dominate the ultrasound appearance of cirrhosis; surface nodularity is best appreciated with surrounding ascites (Fig. 9.16a) [40]. Doppler interrogation of the hepatic vasculature confirms underlying liver disease with an increase in HA velocity and resistive index [(peak systolic velocity – end diastolic velocity)/peak systolic velocity], loss of the triphasic HV flow pattern, and loss of respiratory variation in the portal venous flow pattern (Fig. 9.16b) [41, 42]. Portal venous flow gradually diminishes until direction reverses and flow is hepatofugal [43]. CT and MRI display cirrhotic morphologic features more vividly (Fig. 9.17). Except in the case of PVT, flow derangements are not

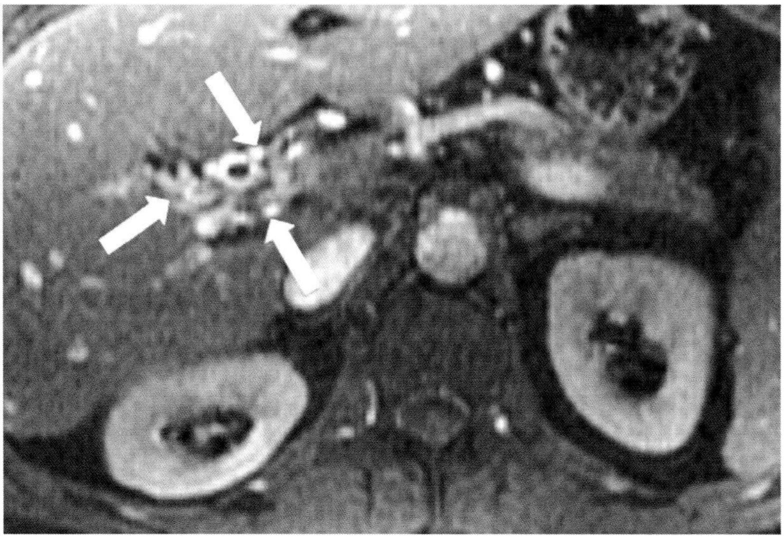

Fig. 9.14 Cavernous transformation of the portal vein. Axial enhanced MR image through the porta hepatis shows a cluster of small enhancing tubular structures (*arrows*) with no dominant vascular channel in a patient with long-standing portal venous occlusion and cavernous transformation

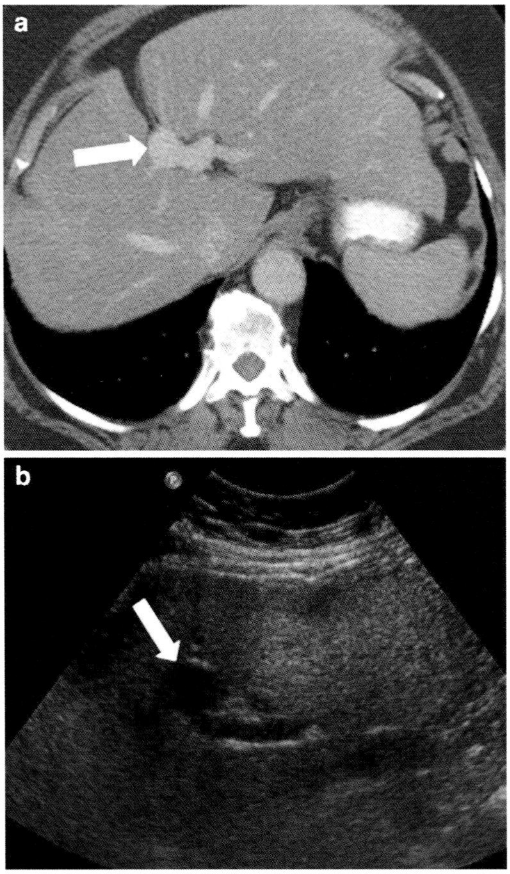

Fig. 9.15 Portal venous aneurysm. Axial enhanced CT image (**a**) and (**b**) sagittal gray-scale US image show a saccular protrusion from left portal bifurcation (*arrow*)

detectable on CT images. While technically feasible, MR flow characterization is not routinely performed.

CT and MRI portray the constellation of secondary findings in portal hypertension more comprehensively than US (Table 9.3) [44]. While visible on all modalities, ascitic fluid (see Fig. 9.17) is most conspicuous on MR images (because of extreme T2 hyperintensity and tissue contrast) and most comprehensively imaged on CT because of the potential to easily cover the entire abdomen and pelvis on a single examination. Portosystemic collaterals (Table 9.4) are most clearly depicted with CT and MRI (see Fig. 9.17). Varices blend in with adjacent soft tissue structures on unenhanced CT and most enhanced MR images and are generally better visualized with intravenous contrast. Steady-state MR images obtained without intravenous contrast are the exception. Accurately measuring splenic size to assess for splenomegaly benefits from the multiplanar capabilities of MRI and multiplanar reformatting potentially of multidetector CT. Enlargement of the cisterna chyli has been shown to be associated with portal hypertension and is most conspicuous on MR imaging [45]. The cisterna chyli courses through the right retrocrural space as a fluid-filled tubular

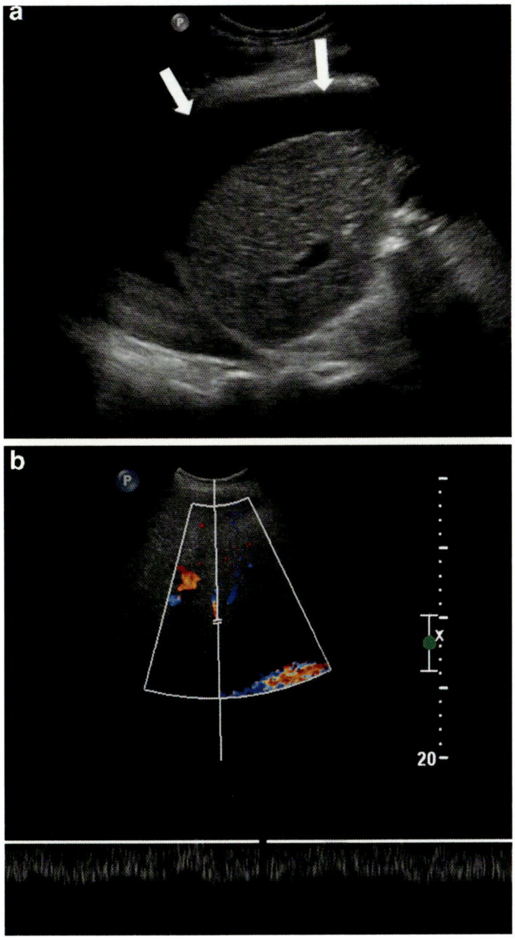

Fig. 9.16 Cirrhosis on ultrasound. Sagittal image transecting the margin of the liver (**a**) shows surrounding anechoic ascites (*arrows*) outlining the mildly nodular liver contour and providing a good acoustic window to visualize relatively coarse and heterogeneous echotexture. (**b**) Axial image though the liver with pulsed Doppler spectral waveform of the middle hepatic vein shows monotonous, continuous flow without the normal triphasic pattern (see Fig. 9.5)

structure, exhibiting enhancement only on delayed images (at least 5 min or more after contrast administration) [46].

Transhepatic Portosystemic Shunt (TIPS)

The TIPS procedure involves deployment of an expandable stent conduit between the portal and hepatic venous circulations in the setting of portal hypertension for the treatment of hemorrhage from gastroesophageal varices, intractable ascites, hepatorenal syndrome, and Budd-Chiari syndrome [47, 48]. The high incidence of TIPS failure (up to 50% within 6 months [49, 50]) warrants periodic surveillance. The next best option after transhepatic pressure gradient monitoring – which is not practically available – is US. US provides a surrogate measure of pressure gradient in the form of velocity, which is supplemented with gray-scale and color Doppler imaging. Following an immediate postprocedural baseline study, TIPS surveillance entails 3, 6-month, and biannual examinations.

The echogenic walls of the TIPS shunt surround the anechoic lumen on gray-scale images (Fig. 9.18). Variably echogenic material replacing the anechoic lumen indicates TIPS thrombosis, which is corroborated by absence of color Doppler flow. While absent flow is one of the criteria for TIPS failure, other findings require spectral Doppler imaging, and include: low peak shunt velocity (<50–90 cm/s), high peak shunt velocity (>190 cm/s), low mean PV velocity (<30 cm/s), antegrade flow in the intrahepatic PVs, and change in shunt velocity (>50 cm/s) compared with immediate postprocedural imaging or between studies [51, 52].

CT and MRI rely on contrast enhancement to document TIPS patency. The metallic wall appears dense on CT images and induces susceptibility artifact appearing dark on MR images (see Fig. 9.18). Lack of enhancement indicates occlusion.

Hepatic Arterial Disorders

Outside the setting of transplantation or percutaneous intervention, hepatic arterial disorders are rare. Except after transplantation, stenosis generally occurs only in the form of median arcuate ligament (MAL) syndrome. Interventions account for many cases of HA dissection and aneurysm; traumatic injury and underlying systemic diseases are also implicated. Inflammatory arteritides account for some instances of HA aneurysms – exemplified by polyarteritis nodosa (PAN).

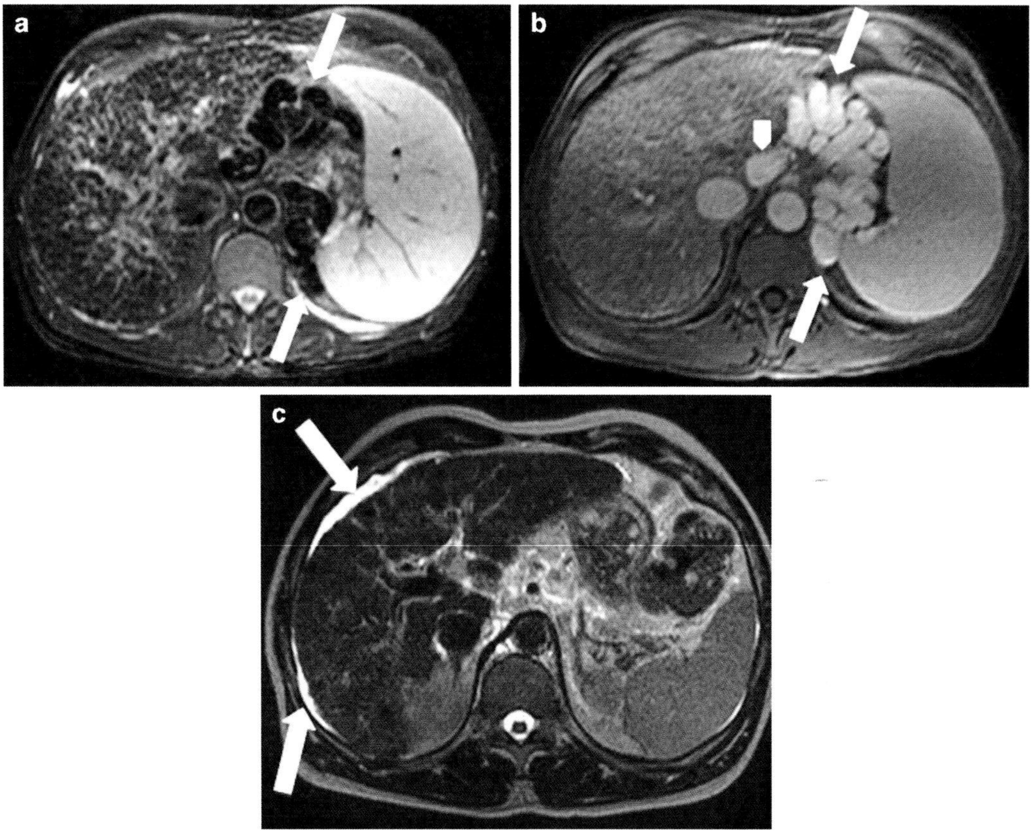

Fig. 9.17 Findings of cirrhosis and portal hypertension. Axial T2-weighted MR image (**a**) shows diffusely nodular, cirrhotic liver parenchyma and splenomegaly. The serpiginous hypointensities in the splenic hilum (*arrows*) achieve equal enhancement intensity on the postcontrast image (**b**) with the portal vein (*arrowhead*), indicating vascular etiology and corresponding to portosystemic splenorenal collaterals. (**c**) Axial T2-weighted MR image in a different cirrhotic patient reveals markedly hyperintense perihepatic ascitic fluid (*arrows*)

Table 9.3 Constellation of findings in portal hypertension

PV enlargement
PV flow reversal
Enlarged HA
Portosystemic collaterals
Ascites (or mesenteric edema)
Splenomegaly
Cisterna chyli enlargement

Table 9.4 Portosystemic collaterals

Paraumbilical
Splenorenal
Gastroesophageal
Paraesophageal
Submucosal esophageal
Mesenteric
Mesenteric-rectal
Retroperitoneal
Pancreaticoduodenal-paravertebral

Median Arcuate Ligament Syndrome

The MAL is a fibrous band interconnecting the diaphragmatic crura along the ventral aspect of the hiatus. While the MAL typically passes above the celiac axis, occasional proximity to the celiac axis (up to 25% of patients) results in arterial compression and potential MAL syndrome, manifest by epigastric pain and weight loss. While historically the diagnosis was established with conventional angiography (CA), CTA and MRA now constitute the mainstay in the diagnosis of MAL syndrome [53].

A characteristic extrinsic indentation along the ventral aspect of the proximal celiac axis

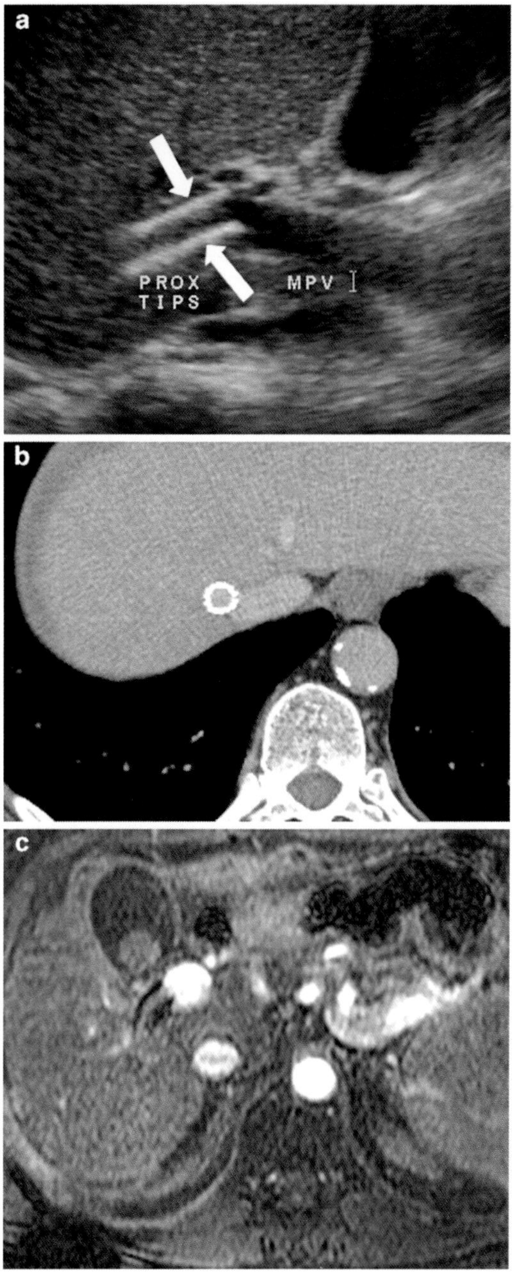

Fig. 9.18 The transjugular intrahepatic portosystemic shunt (TIPS). Sagittally-oriented gray-scale US image (**a**) depicts the portal-TIPS anastomosis and shows the parallel echogenic walls of the shunt (*arrows*). The metallic walls of the stent are dense – or bright – on the enhanced CT image (**b**), and hypointense – or dark – with blooming on the enhanced MR image (**c**)

describes the angiographic finding of MAL syndrome (Fig. 9.19). Expiration exaggerates this appearance and the ability to compare inspiratory with expiratory findings confers an advantage to CA in establishing this diagnosis. Poststenotic dilatation develops in severe compression/stenosis, which may also be associated with collateralization from the SMA.

CTA circumvents the need for direct arterial access and generates angiographic images with the use of multiplanar reformatting and volume-rendered images. The diagnosis hinges on the appearance of the celiac axis on sagittally-reformatted images. The MAL-induced celiac axis narrowing has a hooked configuration in the sagittal projection (see Fig. 9.19) [54]. Poststenotic dilatation and collateral vessels increase diagnostic confidence. MRA yields identical findings and also offers the opportunity for reformatting and multiplanar acquisition. Direct sagittal acquisition obviates the need for multiplanar reformatting.

Spectral analysis supplements the US diagnosis of MAL syndrome. An increase in elevated systolic velocity with expiration with superimposed turbulence suggests the diagnosis, which is established with reversion to normal velocities in the erect position [55].

Hepatic Artery Dissection

Visceral artery dissection usually represents extension of abdominal aortic dissection. Isolated visceral artery dissections are rare [56] and an underlying predisposing factor, such as hypertension, percutaneous intervention, surgery, and peritonitis, usually accompanies the disorder [57]. Although CTA and MRA represent the most straightforward imaging methods to establish this diagnosis, this can also be accomplished by US and CA.

The *sine qua non* of a dissection is the presence of an intimal flap, which appears as a linear hypointensity surrounded by avidly enhancing true and variably enhancing false lumens on contrast-enhanced CT and MR images (see Fig. 9.20). The same appearance is demonstrated on steady-state MR images without contrast. Unenhanced time-of-flight images potentially show the same finding, but are excessively degraded by breathing motion artifact. Among visceral arteries,

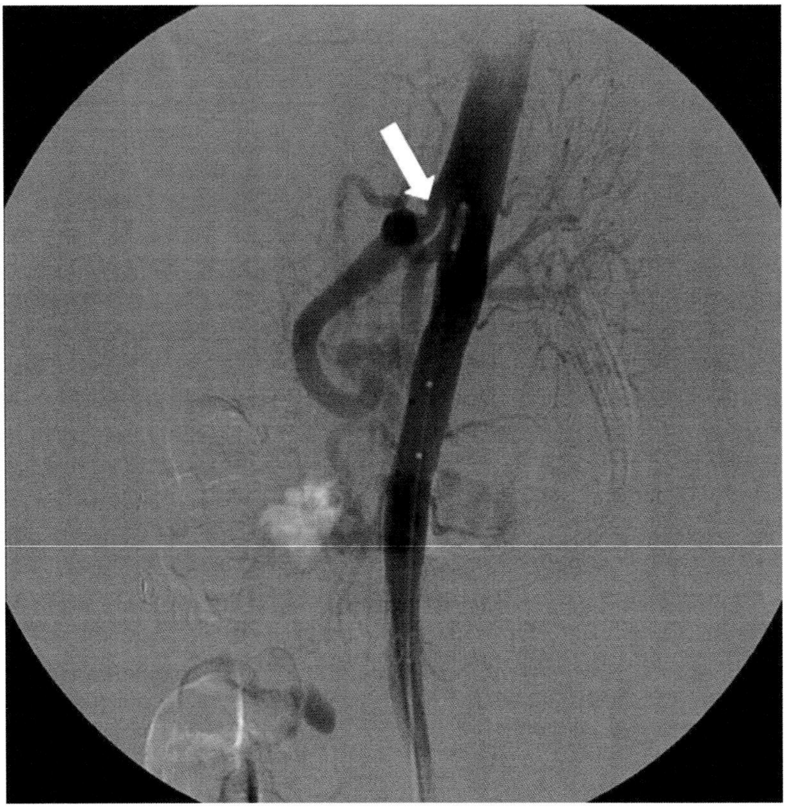

Fig. 9.19 Median arcuate ligament compression. Sagittal subtracted digital angiographic image shows a mild narrowing and extrinsic impression on the origin of the celiac axis (*arrow*), which is not hemodynamically significant

dissection occurs more commonly in the SMA, followed by the celiac axis and its branches. An echogenic intimal flap separates the true and false lumens on US images (Fig. 9.20).

Pertinent issues such as extent, relationship to branch vessels and patency can be assessed using noninvasive imaging. CA is usually reserved for symptomatic patients anticipating intervention. CA imaging findings depend on the unpredictable enhancement of the false lumen and eccentric compression on the true lumen by the false lumen. Stent placement is a percutaneous therapeutic option for symptomatic cases.

Hepatic Artery Aneurysm

Visceral aneurysms incur a high risk of rupture and life-threatening hemorrhage. Accordingly, treatment threshold is low and pretreatment imaging assists in planning. Among the splanchnic arterial aneurysms, the splenic artery is most commonly involved. Splenic artery aneurysms incur a risk of rupture of approximately 10% and generally involve the main extrasplenic trunk of the vessel. Treatment options include ligation and embolization.

After splenic artery, HA aneurysms are the most frequent [58]. True aneurysms are distinguished from the previously discussed pseudoaneurysms by the presence of an intact – albeit usually diseased and stressed – vessel wall. While pseudoaneurysms are usually the result of iatrogenic or blunt trauma, true aneurysms usually arise from arteriosclerosis, inflammatory arteritis or cystic medial necrosis. The appearance is similar, although the true aneurysm usually exhibits fusiform morphology compared with the saccular morphology of the pseudoaneurysm. Enhancement commensurate with neighboring arterial structures signifies arterial origin on enhanced CT and MR images. Continuity with the parent vessel on gray-scale US images with turbulent arterial flow on spectral waveforms typifies HA aneurysm.

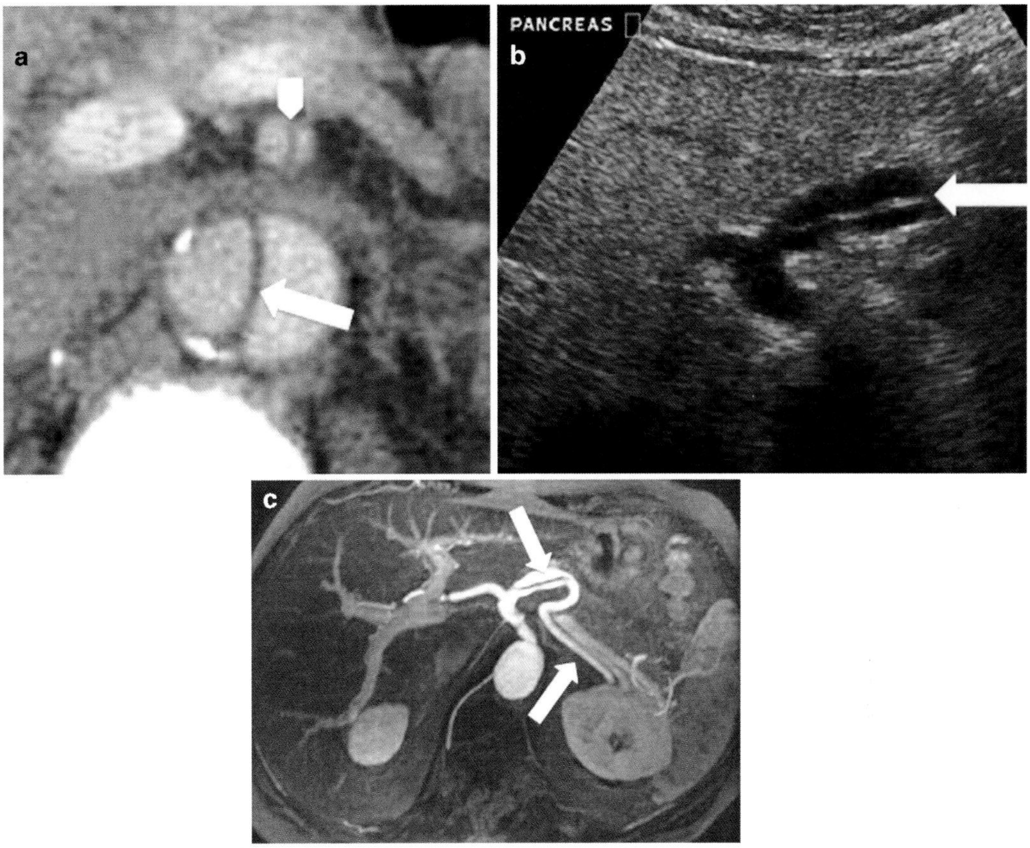

Fig. 9.20 Celiac dissection. Axial enhanced CT image (**a**) shows an intimal flap (*arrow*) of an aortic dissection extending into the celiac axis (*arrowhead*). Sagittal gray-scale US image (**b**) shows the echogenic intimal flap extending distally into the splenic artery (*arrow*) and the maximal intensity MR image (**c**) reveals the extent of the dissection throughout the course of the splenic artery (*arrows*)

Differentiation of extrahepatic from intrahepatic location potentially guides treatment. Extrahepatic aneurysms are generally ligated, while intrahepatic aneurysms may require partial hepatic resection. Nonetheless, surgical treatment incurs a high risk of death and percutaneous treatment is preferred. Selective injection of the celiac axis during CA enhances the common HA and clearly depicts the relationship of the aneurysm (or pseudoaneurysm) to the HA prior to embolization.

Hepatic Arteritis

Multiple hepatic arterial aneurysms raise the suspicion of an underlying disorder, such as mycotic infection, intravenous drug abuse, autoimmune disorders, fibromuscular dysplasia (FMD), or primary necrotizing vasculitis (such as PAN). Mycotic aneurysms typically manifest with febrile illness, a history of endocarditis or a history of intravenous drug abuse.

FMD most commonly affects the renal and carotid arteries, but other vessels are potentially involved [59]. Among the multiple histologic subtypes (Table 9.5), medial fibroplasia accounts for 85% of the cases and exhibits the classic "string-of-beads" appearance of stenoses alternating with fusiform or saccular aneurysms (Fig. 9.21). Given a high spatial resolution, CA remains the diagnostic gold standard. CTA or MRA have limited sensitivity in the setting of mild disease and lack the ability to assess the functional significance of stenoses.

Table 9.5 FMD distribution types

Type	Prevalence (%)	Imaging appearance
Intimal fibroplasia	1–2	Narrow annular bands with poststenotic dilatation
Medial fibroplasia	85	"String of beads" appearance
Medial hyperplasia	5–15	Long smooth stricture
Subadventitial fibroplasia	20	Long irregular narrowing
Medial dissection	5–10	Intimal flap with false lumen
Adventitial fibroplasia	<1	Long segmental stenosis

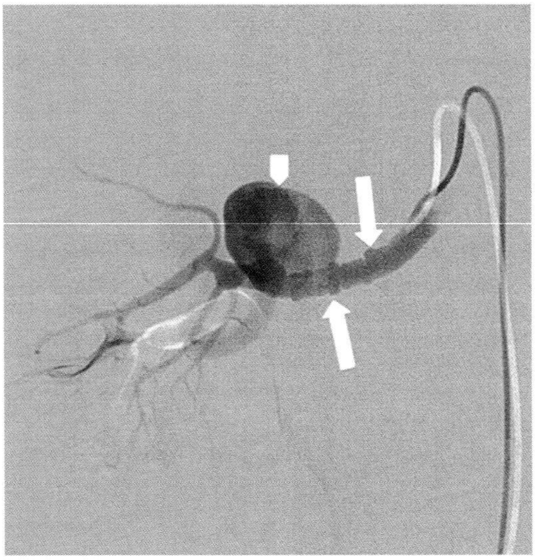

Fig. 9.21 Fibromuscular dysplasia with string-of-beads appearance. Selective injection of the right renal artery shows the classic string-of-beads appearance (*arrows*) complicated by a large aneurysm (*arrowhead*). Findings in the hepatic circulation are typically identical

Pressure measurements obtained during CA interrogate functional significance and direct access enables treatment, if necessary.

PAN is a systemic autoimmune inflammatory arteritis of small and medium-sized vessels that affects the liver approximately 50% of the time. Organs most commonly involved include the following, in descending order of frequency: the kidneys, the heart, the gastrointestinal tract, the liver, the spleen, and the pancreas.

Microaneurysms – usually measuring between 2 and 5 mm – are the most characteristic finding of PAN [60]. At least ten microaneurysms typically afflict involved visceral arterial beds and tend to occur at branching points. Other findings include segmental stenoses, dilatation, occlusions, and infarctions. CA is considered the gold standard for the diagnosis of PAN; other modalities have limited utility.

Multiple other rare vasculitides infrequently affect visceral and hepatic vasculature, including systemic lupus erythematosus, Wegener's granulomatosis, Churg–Strauss Disease and syndrome and leukocytoclastic vasculitis. Radiographic findings overlap and clinical findings direct the diagnostic work-up.

Hepatic Vein/Inferior Vena Cava Disorders

Budd-Chiari syndrome (BCS) is the umbrella term for this protean group of disorders. The common denominator is hepatic venous outflow obstruction, leading to portal venous flow impedance, portal hypertension, ascites, and hepatic morphologic derangements. While etiologic discussion of BCS often entails disease classification according to the level of vascular obstruction – either the IVC, the hepatic veins, or hepatic venules – temporal phase (acute vs. chronic) better classifies the radiographic appearance [61].

Acute BCS most commonly involves obstruction of the IVC and/or hepatic veins. The imaging findings include primary findings of vessel stenosis or occlusion and secondary findings involving the affected liver parenchyma. All imaging modalities demonstrate the primary vascular findings. Enhanced CT and MR images (and unenhanced steady-state MR images) generally show a relatively dark filling defect corresponding to thrombus against the bright backdrop of a normal, patent vessel lumen (Fig. 9.22). Given

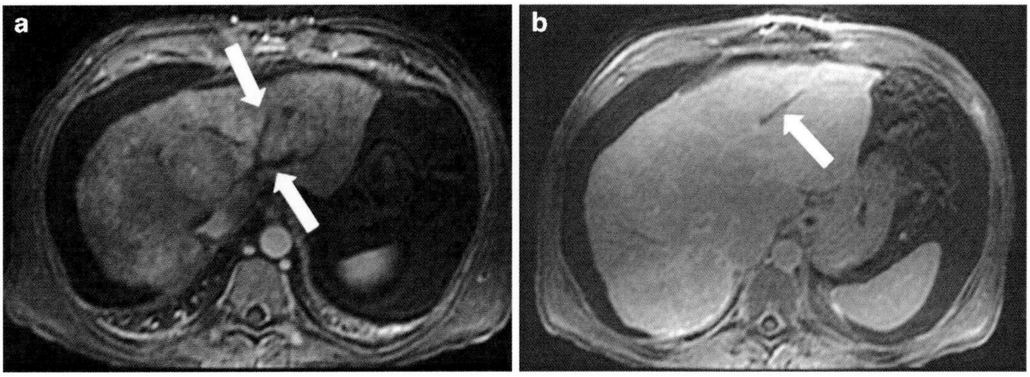

Fig. 9.22 Vascular thrombosis in Budd-Chiari syndrome. Axial portal phase (**a**) and delayed (**b**) enhanced MR images show extensive thrombus within the hepatic veins (*arrows*)

the long transit time from the peripheral injection site and the inevitable dispersion of contrast material, contrast enhancement in hepatic veins/IVC is diminished compared with arterial structures. The superior tissue contrast and contrast enhancement of MR compared with CT recommends MR for detecting venous thrombus and occlusion.

On US, a thrombus is seen as partial or complete echogenic filling defects within the anechoic lumen of the normal vessel. The absence of color Doppler from the occluded vessel confirms absence of flow. Other BCS findings on color and spectral Doppler US include: HV flow reversal; absent HV; PV flow derangement (including hepatofugal flow); and slow, reduced or balanced IVC flow.

By virtue of superior tissue contrast, MRI characterizes secondary acute parenchymal changes best, followed by CT and US. Congested, edematous peripheral hepatic parenchyma, without the benefit of the separate venous drainage outflow of the caudate lobe, appears hyperintense with diminished enhancement compared with the more adequately drained central liver, which more avidly enhances (Fig. 9.23). The enhancement pattern is demonstrated on CT and both modalities clearly depict the characteristic central hypertrophy–peripheral atrophy pattern that eventually develops. Parenchymal changes largely elude US detection.

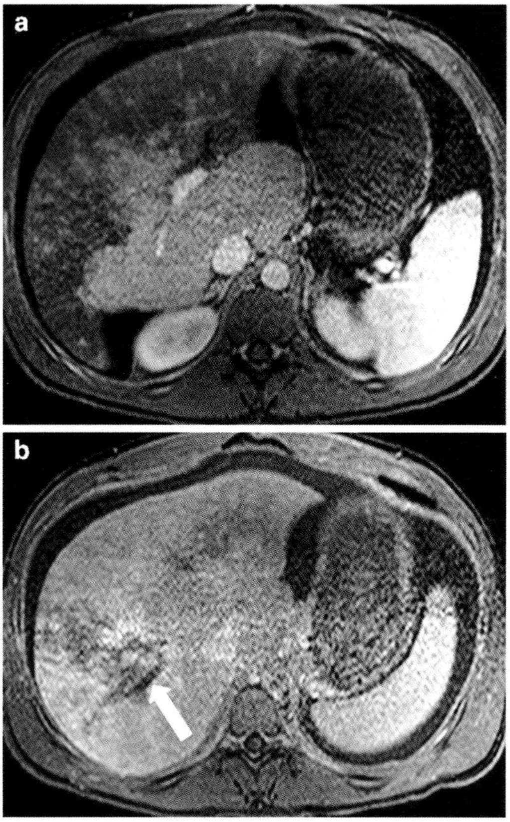

Fig. 9.23 Parenchymal changes in acute Budd–Chiari syndrome. Axial portal phase (**a**) and delayed (**b**) enhanced MR images show central hypertrophy and peripheral atrophy of the liver parenchyma. Peripheral congestion and better central drainage explains the more avid early enhancement of the central liver. The delayed image shows thrombosed right hepatic vein (*arrow*)

Over time, the characteristic enhancement pattern fades and the atrophy–hypertrophy pattern may be less striking as fibrosis ensues and regenerative nodules develop. These vary in size from 0.5 to 4 cm and are best detected and characterized on MR images. Regenerative nodules are typically mildly T1-hyperintense because of: (1) the increased water content and T1-hypointensity of surrounding, congested tissue and, (2) increased copper content. Mild hypointensity to isointensity typifies the appearance of RNs on T2-weighted images [62].

Intrahepatic collaterals occasionally have a pathognomonic appearance (most commonly detected on MR images), referred to as "comma-shaped" collaterals. Collateral vessels are sought when reversed flow is detected on color or spectral Doppler imaging and are most obvious when draining into inferior hepatic veins, unobstructed hepatic veins, or the IVC.

References

1. Michels NA. Blood supply and anatomy of the upper abdominal organs with a descriptive atlas. Philadelphia: Lippincott Williams and Wilkins; 1955.
2. Vandamme JPJ, Bonte J, Van der Scheueren G. A reevaluation of hepatic and cystic arteries: the importance of aberrant hepatic branches. Acta Anat. 1969;73:192–209.
3. Suzuki T, Nakayasu A, Kawabe K, et al. Surgical significance of anatomic variations of the hepatic artery. Am J Surg. 1971;122:505–12.
4. Dittman W. Hepatic angiography. Semin Liver Dis. 1982;2:41–8.
5. Ruzicka FF, Rossi P. Normal vascular anatomy of the abdominal viscera. Radiol Clin North Am. 1970;8: 3–29.
6. Blumgart L, Fong Y. Surgery of the liver and biliary tract. New York: Saunders; 2000. p. 1625–8.
7. Weinreb J, Kumari S, Phillips G, Pochaczevsky R. Portal vein measurements by real-time sonography. AJR Am J Roentgenol. 1982; 139(3):497–9. In: Siegel MJ. Pediatric sonography. New York: Raven Press; 1995. p. 175.
8. Gallego C, Velasco M, Marcuello P, Tejedor D, et al. Congenital and acquired anomalies of the portal venous system. Radiographics. 2002;22:141–59.
9. Covey AM, Brody LA, Getrajdman GI, Sofocleous CT, Brown KT. Incidence, patterns, and clinical relevance of variant portal vein anatomy. AJR Am J Roentgenol. 2004;183:1055–64.
10. Silva MA, Jambulingam PS, Gunson BK, Mayer D, Buckels JA, Mirza DF, et al. Hepatic artery thrombosis following orthotopic liver transplantation: a 10-year experience from a single centre in the United Kingdom. Liver Transpl. 2005;21(1):146–51.
11. Stange BI, Glanemann M, Nuessler NC, Settmacher U, Steinmuller T, Neuhaus P. Hepatic artery thrombosis after adult liver transplantation. Liver Transpl. 2003;6:612–20.
12. Vivarelli M, Cucchetti A, LaBarba G, et al. Ischemic arterial complications after liver transplantation in the adult. Arch Surg. 2004;139:1069–74.
13. Ito K, Siegelman ES, Stolpen AH, Mitchell DG. Pictorial essay: MR imaging of complications after liver transplantation. AJR Am J Roentgenol. 2000; 175:1145–9.
14. Caiado AHM, Blasbalg R, Marcelino ASZ, da Cunha Pinho M, Chammas MC, da Costa Leite C, et al. Complications of liver transplantation: multimodality imaging approach. RadioGraphics. 2007;27(5): 1401–17.
15. Pandharipande PV, Lee VS, Morgan GR, Teperman LW, Krinsky GA, Rofsky NM, et al. Vascular and extravascular complications of liver transplantation: comprehensive evaluation with three-dimensional contrast-enhanced volumetric MR imaging and MR cholangiopancreatography. AJR Am J Roentgenol. 2001;177:1101–7.
16. Quiroga S, Sebastia MC, Margarit C, Castells L, Boye R, Alvarez-Castells A. Complications of orthotopic liver transplantation: spectrum of findings with helical CT. RadioGraphics. 2001;21(5):1085–102.
17. Horrow MM, Blumenthal BM, Reich DJ, Manzarbeitia C. Sonographic diagnosis and outcome of hepatic artery thrombosis after orthotopic liver transplantation in adults. AJR Am J Roentgenol. 2007;189:346–51.
18. Kawamoto S, Soyer PA, Fishman EK, Bluemke DA. Nonneoplastic liver disease: evaluation with CT and MR imaging. Radiographics. 1998;18: 827–48.
19. Lipson JA, Qayyum A, Avrin DE, Westphalen A, Yeh BM, Coakley FV. Pictorial essay: CT and MRI of hepatic contour abnormalities. AJR Am J Roentgenol. 2005;184:75–81.
20. Balci NC, Semelka RC, Noone TC, Siegelman ES, de Beeck BO, Brown JJ, et al. Pyogenic hepatic abscesses: MRI findings on T1- and T2-weighted and serial gadolinium-enhanced gradient-echo images. J Magn Reson Imaging. 1999;9(2): 285–90.
21. Abbasoglu O, Levy MF, Vodapally MS, Goldstein RM, Husberg BS, Gonwa TA, et al. Hepatic artery stenosis after liver transplantation–incidence, presentation, treatment, and long term outcome. Transplantation. 1997;63(2):250–5.
22. Nghiem HV, Tran K, Winter III TC, et al. Imaging of complications in liver transplantation. Radiographics. 1996;16(4):825–40.

23. Marshall MM, Muiesan P, Srinivasan P, et al. Hepatic artery pseudoaneurysms following liver transplantation: incidence, presenting features and management. Clin Radiol. 2001;56:579–87.
24. Karatzas T, Lykaki-Karatzas E, Webb M. Vascular complications, treatment and outcome following orthotopic liver transplantation. Transpl Proc. 1997;29: 2853–5.
25. Glockner JF, Forauer AR. Vascular or ischemic complications after liver transplantation. AJR Am J Roentgenol. 1999;173:1055–9.
26. Quiroga S, Sebastia C, Margarit C, et al. Complications of orthotopic liver transplantation: spectrum of findings with helical CT. Radiographics. 2001;21: 1085–102.
27. Settmacher U, Nussler NC, Glanemann M, et al. Venous complications after orthotopic liver transplantation. Clin Transpl. 2000;14(3):235–41.
28. Nonami T, Yokoyama I, Iwatsuki S, Starzl TE. The incidence of portal vein thrombosis at liver transplantation. Hepatology. 2005;16(5):1195–8.
29. Glockner JF, Forauer AR, Solomon H, Varma CR, Perman WH. Three-dimensional gadolinium-enhanced MR angiography of vascular complications after liver transplantation. AJR Am J Roentgenol. 2000;174:1447–53.
30. Wozney P, Zajko AB, Bron KM, Point S, Starzl TE. Vascular complications after liver transplantation: a 5-year experience. AJR Am J Roentgenol. 1986;147: 657–63.
31. Tessler FN, Gehring BJ, Gomes AS, Perrella RR, Ragavendra N, Busuttil RW, et al. Diagnosis of portal vein thrombosis: value of color Doppler imaging. AJR Am J Roentgenol. 1991;157:293–6.
32. Rossi S, Rosa L, Ravetta V, Cascina A, Quaretti P, Azzaretti A, et al. Contrast-enhanced versus conventional and color Doppler sonography for the detection of thrombosis of the portal and hepatic venous systems. AJR Am J Roentgenol. 2006;186(3):763–73.
33. Novick SL, Fishman EK. Portal vein thrombosis: spectrum of helical CT and CT angiographic findings. Abdom Imaging. 1998;23(5):505–10.
34. Glockner JF, Forauer AR, Solomon H. Three-dimensional gadolinium-enhanced MR angiography of vascular complications after liver transplantation. AJR Am J Roentgenol. 2000;174(5):1447–53.
35. Kauzlaric D, Petrovic M, Barmeir E. Sonography of cavernous transformation of the portal vein. AJR Am J Roentgenol. 1984;142:383–4.
36. Aldrete JS, Slaughter RL, Han SY. Portal vein thrombosis resulting in portal hypertension in adults. Am J Gastroenterol. 1976;65:3–11.
37. Raby N, Meire HB. Duplex doppler ultrasound in the diagnosis of cavernous transformation of the portal vein. Br J Radiol. 1988;61:586–8.
38. Konno K, Ishida H, Uno A, et al. Cavernous transformation of the portal vein (CTPV): role of color Doppler sonography in the diagnosis. Eur J Ultrasound. 1996;3(3):231–40.
39. Vine HS, Sequira JC, Widrich WC, Sacks BA. Portal vein aneurysm. AJR. 1979;132:557–60.
40. Di Lelio A, Cestari C, Lomazzi A, Beretta L. Cirrhosis: diagnosis with sonographic study of the liver surface. Radiology. 1989;172:389–92.
41. Bolondi L, Bassi S, Gaiani S, et al. Liver cirrhosis: changes of doppler waveform of hepatic veins. Radiology. 1991;178:513–6.
42. Colli A, Cocciolo M, Riva C, et al. Abnormalities of doppler waveform of the hepatic veins in patients with chronic liver disease: correlation with histologic findings. AJR. 1994;162:833–7.
43. Nelson RC, Lovett KE, Chezmar JL, et al. Comparison of pulsed doppler sonography and angiography in patients with portal hypertension. AJR. 1987;149: 77–81.
44. Brancatelli G, Federle M, Ambrosini R, et al. Cirrhosis: CT and MRI imaging evaluation. Clin Imag. 2007;31(4):297–307.
45. Verma SK, Mitchell DG, Bergin D, et al. Dilated cisternae chyli: a sign of uncompensated cirrhosis at MR imaging. Abdom Imaging. 2009;34:211–6.
46. Verma SK, Mitchell DG, Bergin D, Mehta R, Chopra S, Choi D. The cisterna chyli: enhancement on delayed phase MR images after intravenous administration of gadolinium chelate. Radiology. 2007;244:791–6.
47. Ong JP, Sands M, Younossi ZM. Transjugular intrahepatic portosystemic shunts (TIPS): a decade later. J Clin Gastroenterol. 2000;30:14–28.
48. Jalan R, Lui HF, Redhead DN, et al. TIPSS 10 years on. Gut. 2000;46:578–81.
49. Otal P, Smayra T, Bureau C, et al. Preliminary results of a new expanded-polytetrafluouethylene-covered stent-graft for transjugular intrahepatic portosystemic shunt procedures. AJR. 2002;178:141–7.
50. Saxon RS, Ross PL, Mendel-Hartvig J, et al. Transjugular intrahepatic portosystemic shunt patency and the importance of stenosis location in the development of recurrent symptoms. Radiology. 1998;207:683–93.
51. Kanterman RY, Darcy MD, Middleton WD, et al. Doppler sonography findings associated with transjugular intrahepatic portosystemic shunt malfunction. AJR Am J Roentgenol. 1997;168:467–72.
52. Wachsberg RH. Doppler ultrasound evaluation of transjugular intrahepatic portosystemic shunt function. Ultrasound Q. 2003;19(3):139–48.
53. Shih M-C P, Angle JF, Leung DA, et al. CTA and MRA in mesenteric ischemia: part 2, normal findings and complications after surgical and endovascular treatment. AJR. 2007;188:462–71.
54. Horton KM, Talamini MA, Fishman KA. Median arcuate ligament syndrome: evaluation with CT angiography. Radiographics. 2005;25:1177–82.
55. Wolfman D, Bluth EI, Sossaman J. Median arcuate ligament syndrome. J Ultrasound Med. 2003;22:1377–80.
56. Takayama T, Miyata T, Shirakawwa M, et al. Isolated spontaneous dissection of the splanchnic arteries. J Vasc Surg. 2008;48(2):329–33.

57. Takeda H, Matsunaga N, Sakamoto I, et al. Spontaneous dissection of the celiac and hepatic arteries treated by transcatheter embolization. AJR. 1995;165: 1288–9.
58. Schick C, Ritter RG, Balzer JO, et al. Hepatic artery aneurysms: treatment options. Eur Radiol. 2004; 14(1):157–9.
59. Slovut DP, Olin JW. Fibromuscular dysplasia. N Engl J Med. 2004;350:1862–71.
60. Ha HK, Lee SH, Rha SE, et al. Radiologic features of vasculitis involving the gastrointestinal tract. Radiographics. 2000;20:779–94.
61. Brancatelli G, Vilgrain V, Federle MP, et al. Budd-Chiari syndrome: spectrum of imaging findings. AJR. 2007;188:168–76.
62. Vilgrain V, Lewin M, Vons C, et al. Hepatic nodules in Budd-Chiari syndrome: imaging features. Radiology. 1999;210:44.

10 Hepatic Vascular Pathology After Hematopoietic Cell Transplantation: Sinusoidal Obstruction Syndrome, Focal Nodular Hyperplasia, and Nodular Regenerative Hyperplasia

George B. McDonald

Abstract

Toxic injury to hepatic sinusoids may be caused by specific drugs and irradiation that are used to prepare patients for transplantation. The clinical disease resulting from sinusoidal injury is sinusoidal obstruction syndrome (SOS), which presents within 1–3 weeks of the completion of conditioning therapy. The frequency of SOS as a complication of transplant has declined markedly in recent years, following the recognition that only certain conditioning regimens (notably those containing cyclophosphamide or total body irradiation) caused SOS and that patients with underlying necroinflammatory and fibrotic liver diseases were at highest risk for fatal SOS. Avoiding the toxins that cause sinusoidal injury prevents SOS, a more promising approach than treatment of patients with severe liver dysfunction and multiorgan failure.

Other hepatic vascular pathology can be seen after transplant, including reversed portal venous flow, portal venous thrombosis, and rarely occlusion of hepatic veins. Nodular regenerative hyperplasia and focal nodular hyperplasia can be seen in long-term transplant survivors, usually as incidental findings.

Keywords

Toxic liver injury • Sinusoidal obstruction syndrome • Venocclusive disease • Nodular regenerative hyperplasia • Focal nodular hyperplasia

G.B. McDonald (✉)
Gastroenterology/Hepatology Section (D2-190), Fred Hutchinson Cancer Research Center and University of Washington School of Medicine, 1100 Fairview Avenue North, Seattle, WA 98109-1024, USA
e-mail: gmcdonal@fhcrc.org

Introduction

Toxic injury to hepatic sinusoids may be caused by specific drugs and irradiation that are used to prepare patients for transplant, the "conditioning therapy." The intent of conditioning therapy is twofold: to suppress the patient's immune system so that donor cells will not be rejected (in the

L.D. DeLeve and G. Garcia-Tsao (eds.), *Vascular Liver Disease: Mechanisms and Management*,
DOI 10.1007/978-1-4419-8327-5_10, © Springer Science+Business Media, LLC 2011

Table 10.1 Common hepatobiliary complications in the first 200 days after HCT

Complication	Current frequency	Timing
Sinusoidal obstruction syndrome (SOS)	0–20% (regimen dependent)	Onset before day 20
Cholestasis of sepsis (cholangitis lenta)	Common in neutropenic patients	Following sepsis or neutropenic fever (usually before day 30)
Acute GVHD involving the liver	~20% of allograft recipients Rare after autograft	Day 15–50
Acute viral hepatitis	Rare when prophylaxis is used against herpesviruses, hepatitis B	HSV, day 20–50 Adenovirus, day 30–80 VZV, day 80–250 HBV and HCV, during immune reconstitution
Fungal abscess	Rare when prophylaxis is used	Day 10–60
Drug-liver injury	Common but seldom severe	Day 0–100
Ischemic liver disease	Uncommon; confined to patients with SOS, shock or respiratory failure	Day 0–30
Biliary obstruction	Transient biliary sludge, uncommon Stones, chloromas rare	Day 15–60
Idiopathic hyperammonemia	Rare	Day 10–50
Iron overload	Very common	Present at baseline

GVHD Graft-versus-host disease; *HSV* herpe Simplex svirus; *VZV* varicella-zoster virus; *HBV* hepatitis B virus; *HCV* hepatitis C virus

case of allogeneic transplant) and to achieve tumor cell killing (in the case of malignant underlying disease). The clinical disease resulting from sinusoidal injury is sinusoidal obstruction syndrome (SOS), where signs and symptoms of liver injury can be seen within 1–3 weeks of the completion of conditioning therapy. The frequency of SOS as a complication of transplant has declined markedly in recent years, following the recognition that only certain conditioning regimens caused SOS and that patients with underlying necroinflammatory and fibrotic liver diseases were at highest risk for fatal SOS. Many centers now avoid the most liver-toxic conditioning regimens altogether and, when liver-toxic regimens are prescribed, they triage patients at risk to nonliver-toxic regimens, resulting in the near disappearance of SOS as a fatal complication of transplant in many centers. The portal and hepatic veins are also sites of injury in the aftermath of transplantation and two consequences of vascular liver injury can be seen in long-term transplant survivors (nodular regenerative hyperplasia (NRH) and focal nodular hyperplasia (FNH)).

However, it is unusual for a patient to have vascular liver injury as the sole explanation for liver dysfunction, as patients undergoing hematopoietic cell transplantation (HCT) are at risk of developing other forms of liver injury from complications of the medications used, infection related to immune deficiency, and in allogeneic graft recipients, graft-versus-host disease (GVHD) involving the liver [1] (Table 10.1). In clinical practice, the question is often not what liver disorder is present, but what combination of liver disorders.

Sinusoidal Obstruction Syndrome After Myeloablative Conditioning Regimens

Terminology and Historical Context

SOS is the clinical name for toxic liver injury that follows myeloablative conditioning therapy, characterized clinically by the development of hepatomegaly, ascites, and jaundice and histologically by diffuse damage in the centrilobular zone of the liver. Because the cardinal features of this injury involve sinusoidal pathology (disappearance of sinusoidal endothelial cells, loss of containment of blood cells within sinusoids, stellate cell activation, matrix deposition in sinusoids) and obstruction to sinusoidal blood flow that leads to circulatory compromise of centrilobular hepatocytes, the older name for this condition, veno-occlusive disease (VOD), was abandoned in 2002 [2]. The first reports of toxic sinusoidal injury in the transplant setting [3, 4] had called the disorder VOD because the end-stage histology resembled that of central vein fibrosis after chronic toxin ingestion [5]. However, in the setting of myeloablative conditioning therapy, involvement of hepatic venules is not essential to the development of signs and symptoms. Venular fibrosis and occlusion of central veins may develop later in the course of SOS.

Incidence of SOS

The reported incidence of SOS varies with the composition and intensity of the conditioning regimen, from as low as 0 after most reduced intensity regimens [6] to as high as 50% after cyclophosphamide (CY) 120 mg/kg plus total body irradiation (TBI) >14 Gy [7]. Other important contributors to variability in the incidence of SOS are: (1) large variations in the metabolism of CY from patient to patient in CY/TBI regimens [8–10]; (2) underlying fibro-inflammatory liver diseases such as hepatitis C [7, 11]; and (3) concomitant use of drugs during and after conditioning therapy that either affect the metabolism of myeloablative drugs (e.g., itraconazole) or cause concomitant liver injury (e.g., methotrexate, sirolimus, norethisterone) [12–14]. During the 1990s, the overall incidence of SOS among patients at our center was 38% (7% severe) following CY/TBI and 12% (2% severe) following targeted oral busulfan plus CY [8, 15]. However, the frequency and severity of SOS have fallen dramatically over the last few years, for several reasons: (1) doses of TBI >14 Gy are seldom used; (2) fludarabine is replacing CY in many centers; (3) patients at risk for SOS are being given conditioning regimens that do not contain either CY or TBI >12 Gy; (4) the incidence of chronic hepatitis C in transplant candidates is now very low; and (5) therapeutic drug monitoring allows personalized dosing of chemotherapy drugs that have extremely variable metabolism. An exception to the pattern of falling incidence rates for SOS may be in pediatric patients, particularly those receiving busulfan/melphalan conditioning regimens [16, 17]. A meta analysis suggests that prophylaxis with ursodeoxycholic acid (UDCA) prevents SOS [18], but the largest randomized trial of UDCA that specifically tracked SOS as an endpoint found no evidence of protection [19]. As the effect of UDCA is primarily on cholestatic liver disease, it seems likely that many patients diagnosed as having SOS on the basis of jaundice mostly had cholestatic and not sinusoidal liver injury.

Histology

Early Histologic Abnormalities

Initial histologic changes of SOS are dilation of sinusoids, extravasation of red cells through the space of Disse (often described as "hemorrhage" in zones 2 and 3 of the liver acinus), necrosis of perivenular hepatocytes, and widening of the subendothelial zone between the basement membrane and the adventitia of central veins and sublobular veins [2, 20]. Destruction of sinusoidal endothelium – the initiating injury in SOS – is what leads to "hemorrhage." Sinusoidal obstruction, ischemia, elevated sinusoidal pressures, and fragmentation of hepatocyte cords may result in dislodgement of hepatocytes into portal veins or into lumina of damaged central veins. Immunohistological studies demonstrate diffuse deposition of fibrinogen and Factor VIII/vWF, but not platelet antigens, in zone 3 of the liver acinus, in the midst of necrotic cells [21]. Similar changes have been seen by electron microscopy in the liver damaged by pyrrolizidine alkaloids [22].

Later Histologic Findings: Stellate Cell Proliferation and Collagenization

Within 2 weeks of the onset of clinical signs of SOS, curvilinear deposits of extracellular matrix can be seen in subendothelial spaces and in sinusoids. Immunostaining for activated stellate cells with α-smooth actin antibodies demonstrates a marked increase in the number of stellate cells lining sinusoids [23, 24] in which types I, III, and IV collagen are deposited [21]. Advanced, fatal SOS is characterized by extensive collagenization of sinusoids and venules. In some cases, a pattern of "reverse cirrhosis" develops, with coalescence of extinguished perivenular zones with fibrous bridging between central veins, simulating cardiac cirrhosis. The intensity of collagenization of sinusoids and central veins correlates with outcome [20].

Correlation of Histologic Findings with Clinical Signs

In retrospective autopsy studies of bone marrow transplant recipients, 20–30% of cases showing occluded venules had no clinical evidence of SOS [25, 26]. Furthermore, several perivenular lesions correlated with clinical signs of SOS in the absence of venular occlusion [25]. A coded review of the histological features in a cohort of 76 consecutive necropsy patients who had clinical evidence of SOS found that the strongest histological associations with clinically severe SOS were zone 3 (perivenular) hepatocyte necrosis and sinusoidal fibrosis, occluded hepatic venules and eccentric luminal narrowing/phlebosclerosis of venules [20]. Moreover, the number of these histologic changes was proportional to the clinical severity of SOS. Not surprisingly, the presence of ascites correlated with occluded venules, zone 3 sinusoidal fibrosis, and zone 3 hepatocyte necrosis [20]. Of patients with clinical evidence of severe SOS, 25% had no venular fibrosis at autopsy [20].

Clinical Presentation and Diagnosis

The first clinical signs of SOS are increase in liver size, right upper quadrant tenderness, renal sodium retention, and weight gain, occurring 10–20 days after the start of cyclophosphamide-based cytoreductive therapy [7] and later after other myeloablative regimens [27–29]. Patients then develop hyperbilirubinemia some 4–10 days later, usually before day 20 [7]. While the triad of hepatomegaly, weight gain, and jaundice has been useful for defining SOS for research purposes, there are usually additional clues to the clinical diagnosis (Table 10.2).

Table 10.2 Clinical, laboratory, and imaging manifestations of SOS

Usually present	May be present
Hepatomegaly (change from baseline)	Low urine sodium concentration or fractional excretion of sodium
Weight gain (usually abrupt)	
Jaundice	Peripheral edema, ascites, anasarca
	Elevation of serum Alanine aminotrasferase (ALT)
	Gallbladder wall edema on ultrasound, pain over gallbladder fossa
	Isolated weight gain
	Isolated jaundice
	Thrombocytopenia
	Appearance of esophageal varices
	Pleural effusions, pulmonary vascular congestion, hypoxemia
	Acute renal failure

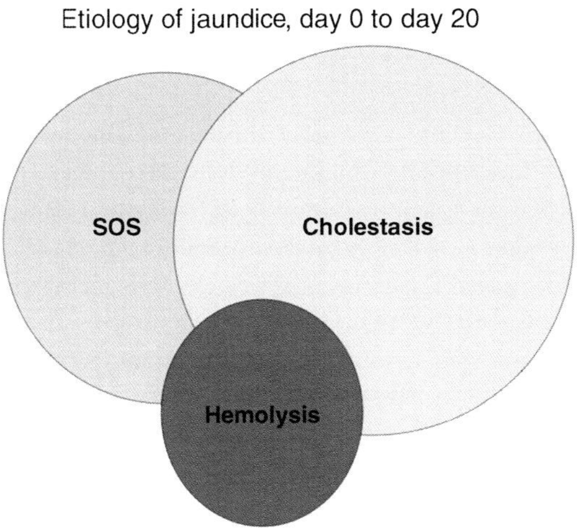

Fig. 10.1 Venn diagram illustrating the overlap of causes of jaundice in the weeks following myeloablative conditioning therapy and hematopoietic cell transplantation (HCT)

Ascites, renal and lung dysfunctions, and refractory thrombocytopenia strongly suggest SOS. However, cholestatic liver injury can be confused with SOS, particularly in the aftermath of sepsis syndrome and vigorous fluid resuscitation. Cholestasis often co-exists with SOS – a point that is often neglected in the studies of disease incidence and outcome (Fig. 10.1). After HCT, treatment of relapsed acute myeloid leukemia with gemtuzumab ozogamicin may also result in SOS [30, 31].

Laboratory Studies

Measurement of serum total serum bilirubin is a sensitive but nonspecific test for SOS, as jaundice may result from sepsis, acute GVHD, drug-liver injury, and cyclosporine therapy [1]. The most difficult diagnoses are in patients with several simultaneous causes of jaundice (see Fig. 10.1). Elevations of serum aspartate aminotransferase (AST) and alanine aminotransferase (ALT) can occur in the course of SOS from day 15 to 25, reflecting ischemic hepatocyte necrosis as a result of obstruction to sinusoidal blood flow [25, 32]. Extreme elevation of serum ALT is one marker of a poor prognosis [32]. Several plasma proteins have been reported to be abnormally high in patients with SOS, including endothelial cell markers (hyaluronic acid, von Willebrand factor, plasminogen activator inhibitor-1, tissue plasminogen activator), thrombopoietin, cytokines (tumor necrosis factor-α (TNFα), transforming growth factor-β (TGFβ), interleukins-1, -2, -6, and -8, soluble IL-2 receptor) and procollagen peptides. Some laboratory tests are abnormally low in patients with SOS, including the anticoagulant proteins – protein C and antithrombin III – and platelet count. It is not clear whether any of these tests have diagnostic or prognostic utility beyond the clinical criteria of weight gain, jaundice, and hepatomegaly, although levels of PAI-1 less than 120 ng/mL have been proposed as clinically useful in excluding a diagnosis of SOS [33]. Serum levels of collagen peptides, however, appear to reflect the extent of sinusoidal fibrosis, probably the most important prognostic variable [20]. None of these putative biomarkers is in wide clinical use.

Ultrasound, Computerized Tomography, and MR Imaging

Imaging studies of the liver are useful not only to demonstrate hepatomegaly, ascites, periportal edema, attenuated hepatic venous flow, and gall bladder wall edema consistent with SOS [34–36], but also to exclude other causes of hepatomegaly and jaundice. Abnormal findings later in the course of SOS may include an enlarged portal vein, slow or reversed flow in the portal vein or its segmental branches [37], high congestion index, portal vein thrombosis, and increased resistive index to hepatic artery flow [38]. Unfortunately, ultrasound findings very early in the course of SOS – when there is the greatest diagnostic uncertainty – do not appear to add to the information provided by clinical criteria [38]. There may be value in following flow parameters (portal flow, resistive indices to hepatic artery flow) as indices of improvement in sinusoidal blood flow.

Liver Biopsy and Hepatic Venous Pressure Gradient

A transvenous approach that allows both biopsy and hepatic venous pressure measurements is the most accurate test when there is uncertainty about the diagnosis of SOS [39, 40]. A transjugular liver biopsy can be done safely with platelet counts above 30,000/mm^3. Unlike cirrhosis, in SOS the interventional radiologist will find little resistance to the passage of a transvenous needle. Major complications include intrahepatic hematomas and perforation of the liver capsule resulting in hemoperitoneum. Laparoscopic needle biopsy is an alternative method of obtaining liver tissue [41]. In HCT patients, a hepatic venous pressure gradient using an occlusive balloon technique [42] above 10 mmHg is highly specific for SOS [39, 40].

Differential Diagnosis

Other causes of posttransplant jaundice seldom lead to renal sodium avidity, rapid weight gain, and hepatomegaly before the onset of jaundice. There are patients who present with jaundice and weight gain that can be confused with SOS [43, 44] but the most problematic are those in patients where both portal hypertension and cholestasis are present. The most common combinations of illnesses that mimic SOS are: (1) sepsis syndrome requiring large volumes of crystalloid, followed by renal insufficiency and sepsis-related cholestasis; (2) cholestatic liver disease, hemolysis, and congestive heart failure; and (3) hyperacute GVHD and sepsis syndrome. SOS may also co-exist with these disease processes. The triad of jaundice, renal insufficiency, and respiratory failure is common in severe SOS [45, 46] but can also be seen as a result of sepsis syndrome and multiorgan failure.

Clinical Course and Prognosis

Recovery from SOS occurs in more than 70% of patients with SOS that results from myeloablative conditioning regimens [7, 27]. Patients with severe SOS seldom die of liver failure, but rather from renal and cardiopulmonary failure [7, 45–47]. For research purposes, retrospective scoring of the severity of SOS categorizes the liver disease as mild (SOS that is clinically obvious, requires no treatment, and resolves completely), moderate (SOS that causes signs and symptoms requiring treatment such as diuretics or pain medications, but that resolves completely), or severe (SOS that requires treatment but that does not resolve before death or day 100), with the proviso that patients with liver disease of uncertain etiology are excluded from the analysis [7]. There is a range of clinical and laboratory findings that correspond to these operational definitions of disease severity (Table 10.3).

In real time, predicting the outcome early in the course of the disease is more difficult. A clinically useful model has been developed that predicts the outcome of SOS after cyclophosphamide-based regimens, derived from rates of increase of both bilirubin and weight in the first 2 weeks following transplant [48]. In some patients, there is a bimodal presentation of SOS, i.e., clinical signs of SOS appear in the first 2 weeks posttransplant, then wane, then reappear later; this pattern is associated with a worse prognosis [27]. In some cases, signs of SOS resolve, but ascites later recurs following development of inflammatory liver disease (e.g., GVHD). Development of respiratory and

Table 10.3 Clinical features of patients with SOS following cyclophosphamide-based myeloablative regimens for HCT

	Mild	Moderate	Severe
Weight gain (% increase)	7.0 ± 3.5	10.1 ± 5.3	15.5 ± 9.2
Maximum bilirubin (mg/dL)	4.7 ± 2.9	7.9 ± 6.6	26.0 ± 15.2
Percent with peripheral edema (%)	23	70	85
Percent with ascites (%)	5	16	48
Day 100 mortality (all causes) (%)	3	20	98

The data are observations through day 20 posttransplant, according to a retrospective assessment of the severity of disease, expressed as the mean and standard deviation [7]

renal failure, higher serum ALT, higher wedged hepatic venous pressure gradient, and development of portal vein thrombosis predict a poor prognosis [32, 39, 40, 46, 47, 49, 50].

Pathogenesis of SOS

There is no mystery as to the cause of SOS in the HCT setting – it is the components of myeloablative conditioning regimens that damage sinusoidal endothelial cells, setting off a cascade of events that result in sinusoidal obstruction to blood flow. The in vitro and animal models of toxic sinusoidal injury are discussed in detail in Chap. 2; this body of work has had an important impact on the incidence of severe SOS and mortality in patients undergoing HCT, particularly in the identification of cyclophosphamide as a sinusoidal endothelial cell toxin [51].

Chemotherapy Drugs in Conditioning Regimens

CY is common to the conditioning regimens with the highest incidence of fatal SOS – CY/TBI, BU/CY, and BCV (BCNU, CY and VP 16). The metabolism of CY is highly variable and unpredictable; patients who generate a greater quantity of toxic CY metabolites are more likely to develop severe SOS [7]. The liver toxin generated by CY metabolism is acrolein (a metabolite formed simultaneously along with the desired metabolite, phosphoramide mustard). Accurate methods to target the dose of CY to a metabolic endpoint, using the reporter molecule carboxyethyl phosphoramide mustard, can eliminate variable exposure to liver toxins, allow personalized CY dosing, and significantly reduce liver and kidney injury from the CY/TBI conditioning regimen [7, 10, 52].

Busulfan BU is another component of regimens with a high frequency of SOS, but BU itself does not appear to be hepatotoxic [53, 54]. In adults with chronic myeloid leukemia in chronic phase and children with acute leukemia, there is no correlation between BU exposure and SOS [55, 56]. BU may contribute to liver injury by inducing oxidative stress, reducing glutathione levels in hepatocytes and sinusoidal endothelial cells [53], and altering CY metabolism [15]. Co-administration of the BU/CY regimen with sirolimus increases the frequency of SOS [14].

Gemtuzumab ozogamicin may cause sinusoidal liver injury when used to treat patients with acute myeloid leukemia [31, 57]. The risk of SOS is 15–40% when high-dose gemtuzumab ozogamicin is given in proximity to a CY-based myeloablative regimen, but lower doses of gemtuzumab ozogamicin appear to eliminate this risk [31, 57]. Gemtuzumab may also cause SOS when given for relapsed acute myeloid leukemia after HCT [30, 31].

Total Body Irradiation

Doses of TBI 10–16 Gy (in the absence of chemotherapy) are less than the dose that causes radiation-induced liver disease. In combination with CY dosed at 120 mg/kg, however, there is a clear relationship between the total dose of TBI and the frequency of severe SOS. The frequency of severe SOS is approximately 1% after CY/TBI 10 Gy [58], 4–7% after CY/TBI 12–14 Gy [8], and 20% after CY/TBI >14 Gy [7, 8].

Intrahepatic Coagulation

Based on plasma studies in patients with SOS and an immunohistological study [21], some see SOS as a disease of disordered coagulation, in which damage to endothelium in the sinusoids and central veins leads to thrombosis. However, sinusoidal endothelial cells embolize downstream in SOS; heparin and antithrombin III infusions are ineffective in preventing fatal SOS; and thrombolytic therapy effects improvement in few patients. Genetic disorders predisposing to coagulation have no associations with SOS. Current evidence suggests that disordered coagulation in SOS is an epiphenomenon secondary to widespread centrilobular damage, not a cause of sinusoidal damage. However, thrombosis in the portal vein may result from a hypercoaguable state in patients with severe SOS [50].

Stellate Cells and Sinusoidal Fibrosis

Procollagen peptides appear in the serum of patients who develop more severe SOS [59], along with inhibitors of fibrolysis, consistent with the intense fibrosis in sinusoids and venular walls that is common in fatal SOS [20]. Immunohistology for α-smooth muscle actin in liver specimens from patients with SOS shows intense staining in sinusoids [23, 24].

Genetic Factors

Genetically determined differences in drug metabolism or susceptibility to toxic injury might explain some of the variability in the frequency of SOS. Small case-control studies using single nucleotide polymorphisms have reported associations between SOS and the carbamyl phosphate synthetase 1 c.4340C>A (*CPS1*), Factor 5 c.1691G>A (FV Leiden), *HFE* C282Y, and glutathione *S*-transferase (*GSTM1* and *GSTT1*) genes [60–62]. These associations could not be confirmed in a cohort of 147 Seattle patients receiving a uniform conditioning regimen (CY/TBI) (McDonald, unpublished observations). Detection of genetic polymorphisms that lead to SOS will require more highly powered studies.

Prevention of SOS in Patients Undergoing HCT

The only certain way to prevent fatal SOS is to avoid giving anyone conditioning therapy that damages hepatic sinusoidal endothelial cells. Prescribing a conditioning therapy that contains sinusoidal toxins to patients with underlying liver disease greatly increases the risk of fatal SOS. The two most common sinusoidal toxins are CY and TBI, but other chemotherapy drugs and radiolabeled antibodies have the potential for sinusoidal injury [8, 63, 64]. The challenge for transplant oncologists is to remove liver-toxic drugs from conditioning regimens without sacrificing engraftment or malignancy relapse rates. For a given myeloablative conditioning regimen, prevention of severe sinusoidal liver injury begins with an assessment of the risk in patients with underlying liver disease. Underlying liver disorders that increase the risk of severe sinusoidal liver injury following CY-based myeloablative conditioning regimens include chronic hepatitis C [11, 16] and by inference and clinical experience, other fibroinflammatory disorders (nonalcoholic steatohepatitis, alcoholic hepatitis, cirrhosis, lobular fibrosis, extramedullary hematopoiesis with sinusoidal fibrosis, prior liver irradiation, and recent gemtuzumab ozogamicin therapy) [7, 27, 57]. Patients who have experienced SOS following conventional chemotherapy, or who have undergone a previous myeloablative HCT, are also at risk.

Patients at risk for fatal SOS have several options (Fig. 10.2): (1) conventional therapy that does not involve HCT; (2) a reduced-intensity conditioning regimen [6]; (3) a myeloablative regimen that does not contain CY, e.g., targeted busulfan-fludarabine for allogeneic [65, 66] or BEAM (high-dose carmustine, etoposide, cytarabine, and melphalan) [67] for autologous HCT; (4) modification of CY-based regimens, i.e., personalized CY dosing or reduction in CY total dose and/or reduction of TBI doses [10, 52] ; and (5) use of pharmacologic approaches to prevent sinusoidal liver injury.

If a CY/TBI regimen must be used for a patient at risk for fatal SOS, modifications should be considered for both CY and TBI dosing. The total dose of CY should be 90–110 mg/kg range [9, 10] and TBI doses should not exceed 12 Gy unless there is an oncologic imperative for higher doses. Shielding the liver during TBI will lessen liver injury but leads to relapse of underlying hematological disease [68]. Accurate methods are available to target CY doses to a metabolic endpoint, based on exposure to the CY metabolites 4-hydroxy CY and carboxyethyl phosphoramide mustard [9, 10, 52].

If a BU/CY regimen must be used for a patient at risk for fatal SOS, liver toxicity may be less frequent if CY is given before targeted BU [69] or if dosing of CY is delayed for 1–2 days after completion of BU [70]. BU and phenytoin to prevent BU-related seizures result in increased exposure to toxic CY metabolites when CY is given second in order, compared to giving CY first [15]. A lower incidence of SOS has been reported following intravenous BU/CY, compared to oral BU/CY, when neither BU formulation was adjusted for metabolism [71]. The metabolism of

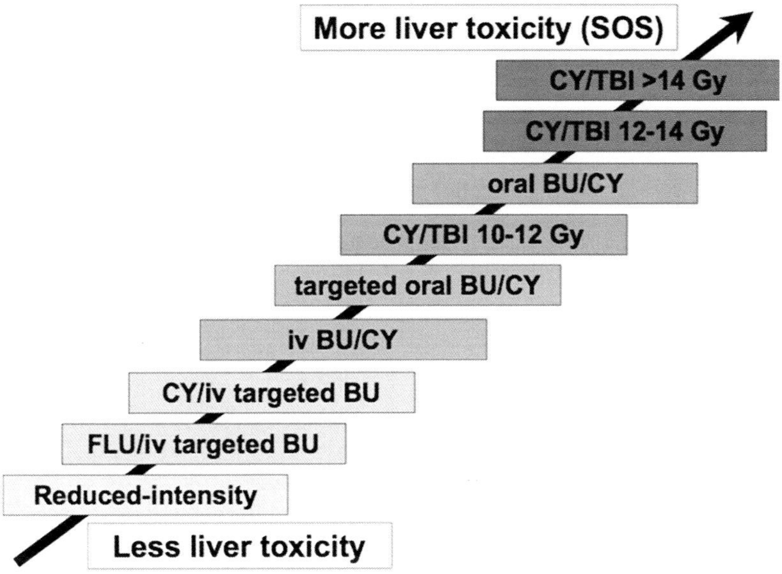

Fig. 10.2 Schematic ladder illustrating the potential for sinusoidal liver injury among conditioning regimens, from lowest to highest risk. CY = cyclophosphamide; TBI = total body irradiation; BU = busulfan; FLU = fludarabine

intravenous BU is variable, with a several-fold range in AUC_{BU}, a problem that can be addressed only with therapeutic drug monitoring [72]. Liver toxicity has remained a complication of conditioning with both targeted oral BU/CY [15, 73, 74] and weight-based dosing of iv BU/CY [71, 75, 76].

Pharmaceutical prevention of SOS has been achieved in animal models of liver injury but these strategies, particularly repletion of intracellular GSH [77] or inhibition of matrix metalloproteinase enzymes [78] have not been studied in the clinical setting. Infusion of defibrotide has been reported to be effective as prophylaxis [79, 80]; preliminary results from a large randomized trial in children reported less liver disease and better outcomes in those receiving defibrotide [81]. Prospective studies have shown no benefit from use of prophylactic heparin [82, 83] or antithrombin III [84] in preventing fatal SOS. A meta analysis suggested that UDCA may prevent SOS [18], but a large randomized trial showed no effect of UDCA on the frequency of SOS [19].

Treatment of Patients with SOS Following Myeloablative Therapy

Over 70% of patients diagnosed with SOS on clinical grounds will recover spontaneously with supportive care (management of sodium and water balance, preservation of renal blood flow, and repeated paracenteses for ascites that is associated with discomfort or pulmonary compromise). Patient with a poor prognosis can be recognized soon after disease onset by steep rises in total serum bilirubin and body weight, serum ALT values >750 U/L, portal pressures over 20 mmHg, development of portal vein thrombosis, and especially by multiorgan failure requiring dialysis, hemofiltration, or mechanical ventilation [32, 45–48, 50, 85]. There are no satisfactory therapies for severe SOS and multiorgan failure; the best current results are with intravenous defibrotide (25 mg/kg/day) therapy, i.e., a 46% complete response rate, defined as resolution of both jaundice and multiorgan failure [86, 87]. Defibrotide, a mixture of porcine oligodeoxyribonucleotides, has antithrombotic and profibrinolytic effects in vitro and in vivo. However, its mechanism of action in the treatment of SOS is not known, and clinical responses often take weeks to occur [88, 89]. The complete recovery of some patients with severe SOS and multi-organ failure suggests that the drug has biologic effects in man [86, 87, 90]. AASLD Practice Guidelines are neutral on the use of defibrotide for treatment of SOS [64]. Because cholestasis commonly co-exists with SOS and because it is impossible to know which clinical signs of liver injury are caused by cholestasis and which by sinusoidal injury, randomized trials will be needed to define the role of defibrotide in SOS treatment.

Numerous other approaches to treat severe SOS have been reported (tissue plasminogen activator, intravenous *N*-acetylcysteine, human antithrombin III concentrate, activated protein C, prostaglandin E_1, prednisone, topical nitrate, vitamin E plus glutamine, and use of a liver assist device), but none can be currently recommended [64]. Transjugular intrahepatic portosystemic shunts (TIPS) have been placed in patients with SOS to reduce portal pressure and mobilize ascites, but neither serum bilirubin levels nor patient outcomes were improved [91] and TIPS placement has resulted in death [92]. Patients with persistent ascites and normal serum bilirubin have undergone successful portosystemic shunts but in these cases, jaundice had resolved completely. Peritoneovenous shunts for intractable ascites have been unsuccessful. Successful liver transplants for severe SOS have been reported [93–95] but in most centers, patients with severe SOS are low-priority candidates for liver transplant because of the hazards that they will develop GVHD and that their underlying malignancy (the indication for HCT) will recur. When severe SOS develops in a patient with a benign condition (a rare event) or in a patient with a favorable outcome post-HCT (e.g., chronic myeloid leukemia in chronic phase), liver transplantation should be considered. Prevention of sinusoidal injury carries more promise for improving HCT outcomes than treatment of patients with severe liver dysfunction and multiorgan failure.

Other Hepatic Vascular Problems Before Day 200 Posttransplant

Portal Vein Abnormalities

Except for portal vein pathology at baseline (usually seen in patients with underlying cirrhosis, previous abdominal sepsis, or hematologic disorders such as polycythemia vera), almost all portal vein pathologies that develop in the 200-day period after HCT is related to SOS. In severe SOS, Doppler ultrasound may show slack or reversed flow [37]. Portal vein thrombosis in patients with severe SOS appears to result from the combination of flow abnormalities plus a procoagulant state, related to low circulating levels of antithrombin III and protein C [50].

Hepatic Vein Abnormalities

Except for patients who come to transplant with a history of Budd–Chiari syndrome (related to hematologic or clotting disorders), almost all hepatic vein abnormalities before day 200 are related to either SOS or mold infection. In severe SOS, Doppler ultrasound may show attenuation of hepatic vein flow along with a decrease in the caliber of the hepatic veins as a result of hepatomegaly [34–36]. Rarely, in patients who are deeply immune suppressed (usually because of drugs used to treat GVHD), intravascular infection caused by organisms from *Mucor* or *Rhizopus* genera may involve the hepatic veins, causing Budd–Chiari Syndrome. The diagnosis of hepatic vein obstruction is made by ultrasound. Mold infections in general and intravascular mold infections especially are now rare, owing to the broader spectrum of prophylactic fungal agents and preemptive therapy with systemic antifungal drugs [96].

Liver Lesions Related to Vascular Injury in Long-Term Survivors of Hematopoietic Cell Transplant

Nodular Regenerative Hyperplasia

Some patients who receive high-dose chemotherapy in oncology and immunology practices will develop hepatic nodularity without fibrosis or liver dysfunction because of exposure to chemotherapy drugs with vascular toxicity [63]. The most common causes are chronic dosing of 6-thioguanine or azathioprine. This process is usually clinically silent unless signs of portal hypertension, particularly ascites, develop. It is surprising that NRH has been described more frequently as a histological entity after HCT than as a clinical problem, given the frequency of SOS in past years [20, 97].

Focal Nodular Hyperplasia

Incidental FNH lesions were discovered during MRI liver imaging in 12% of transplant survivors [98]. These lesions have characteristic central scars that differentiate them from hepatocellular carcinoma and fungal lesions, and can be multiple throughout the liver. The likely cause is sinusoidal injury caused by myeloablative conditioning regimens. The natural history of FNH lesions in this population is not known.

Acknowledgments Dr. McDonald's research in the area of liver injury after hematopoietic cell transplantation has been supported by the National Institutes of Health, National Cancer Institute, CA 15704 and CA 18029.

References

1. McDonald GB. Hepatobiliary complications of hematopoieic cell transplant, 40 years on. Hepatology. 2010;51:1450–60.
2. Deleve LD, Shulman HM, McDonald GB. Toxic injury to hepatic sinusoids: sinusoidal obstruction syndrome (venocclusive disease). Semin Liver Dis. 2002;22:27–41.
3. Berk PD, Popper H, Krueger GRF, Decter J, Herzig J, Graw RGJ. Veno-occlusive disease of the liver after allogeneic bone marrow transplantation. Ann Intern Med. 1979;90:158–64.
4. Jacobs P, Miller JL, Uys CJ, Dietrich BE. Fatal veno-occlusive disease of the liver after chemotherapy, whole-body irradiation and bone marrow transplantation for refractory acute leukaemia. S Afr Med J. 1979;55:5–10.
5. Bras G, Jeliffe DB, Stuart KL. Veno-occlusive disease of the liver wit non-portal type of cirrhosis occurring in Jamaica. Arch Pathol. 1954;57:285–300.
6. Hogan WJ, Maris M, Storer B, Sandmaier BM, Maloney DG, Schoch G, et al. Hepatic injury after nonmyeloablative conditioning followed by allogeneic hematopoietic cell transplantation: a study of 193 patients. Blood. 2004;103:76–82.
7. McDonald GB, Hinds MS, Fisher LB, Schoch HG, Wolford JL, Banaji M, et al. Venocclusive disease of the liver and multiorgan failure after bone marrow transplantation: a cohort study of 355 patients. Ann Intern Med. 1993;118:255–67.
8. McDonald GB, Slattery JT, Bouvier ME, Ren S, Batchelder AL, Kalhorn TF, et al. Cyclophosphamide metabolism, liver toxicity, and mortality following hematopoietic stem cell transplantation. Blood. 2003;101:2043–8.
9. McDonald GB, McCune JS, Batchelder A, Cole S, Phillips B, Ren AG, et al. Metabolism-based cyclophosphamide dosing for hematopoietic cell transplant. Clin Pharmacol Ther. 2005;78:298–308.
10. McCune JS, Batchelder AL, Guthrie KA, Witherspoon R, Appelbaum FR, Phillips B, et al. Personalized dosing of cyclophosphamide in the total body irradiation – cyclophosphamide conditioning regimen: a phase II trial in patients with hematologic malignancy. Clin Pharmacol Ther. 2009;85:615–22.
11. Strasser SI, Myerson D, Spurgeon CL, Sullivan KM, Storer B, Schoch HG, et al. Hepatitis C virus infection after bone marrow transplantation: a cohort study with 10 year follow-up. Hepatology. 1999;29:1893–9.
12. Marr KA, Leisenring W, Crippa F, Slattery JT, Corey L, Boeckh M, et al. Cyclophosphamide metabolism is affected by azole antifungals. Blood. 2004;103:1557–9.
13. Hagglund H, Remberger M, Klaesson S, Lonnqvist B, Ljungman P, Ringden O. Norethisterone treatment, a major risk-factor for veno-occlusive disease in the liver after allogeneic bone marrow transplantation. Blood. 1998;92:4568–72.
14. Cutler C, Stevenson K, Haesook TK, Richardson PG, Vincent TH, Linden E, et al. Sirolimus is associated with veno-occlusive disease of the liver after myeloblative allogeneic stem cell transplantation. Blood. 2008;112:4425–31.
15. McCune JS, Batchelder A, Deeg HJ, Gooley TA, Cole SL, Phillips B, et al. Cyclophosphamide following

targeted oral busufan as conditioning for hematopoietic cell transplantation: pharmacokinetics, liver toxicity, and mortality. Biol Blood Marrow Transplant. 2007;13:853–62.
16. Corbacioglu S, Honig M, Lahr G, Stohr S, Berry G, Friedrich W, et al. Stem cell transplantation in children with infantile osteopetrosis is associated with a high incidence of VOD, which could be prevented with defibrotide. Bone Marrow Transplant. 2006;38:547–53.
17. Cheuk DK, Wang P, Lee TL, Chiang AK, Ha SY, Lau YL, et al. Risk factors and mortality predictors of hepatic veno-occlusive disease after pediatric hematopoietic stem cell transplantation. Bone Marrow Transplant. 2007;40:935–44.
18. Tay J, Tinmouth A, Fergusson D, Huebsch L, Allan DS. Systematic review of controlled clinical trials on the use of ursodeoxycholic acid for the prevention of hepatic veno-occlusive disease in hematopoietic stem cell transplantation. Biol Blood Marrow Transplant. 2007;13:206–17.
19. Ruutu T, Eriksson B, Remes K, Juvonen E, Volin L, Remberger M, et al. Ursodeoxycholic acid for the prevention of hepatic complications in allogeneic stem cell transplantation. Blood. 2002;100:1977–83.
20. Shulman HM, Fisher LB, Schoch HG, Henne KW, McDonald GB. Venocclusive disease of the liver after marrow transplantation: histologic correlates of clinical signs and symptoms. Hepatology. 1994;19:1171–80.
21. Shulman HM, Gown AM, Nugent DJ. Hepatic veno-occlusive disease after bone marrow transplantation. Immunohistochemical identification of the material within occluded central venules. Am J Pathol. 1987;127:549–58.
22. Vonnahme F-J. Die leber des Menschen. Rasterelektronen-mikroskopischer Atlas. 1st ed. Freiburg: S. Karger; 1993.
23. Watanabe K, Iwaki H, Satoh M, Ikeda T, Ichimiya S, Suzuki N, et al. Veno-occlusive disease of the liver following bone marrow transplantation: a clinical-pathological study of autopsy cases. Artif Organs. 1996;20:1145–50.
24. Sato Y, Asada Y, Hara S, Marutsuka K, Tamura K, Hayashi T, et al. Hepatic stellate cells (Ito cells) in veno-occlusive disease of the liver after allogeneic bone marrow transplantation. Histopathology. 1999;34:66–70.
25. Shulman HM, McDonald GB, Matthews D, Doney KC, Kopecky KJ, Gauvreau JM, et al. An analysis of hepatic venocclusive disease and centrilobular hepatic degeneration following bone marrow transplantation. Gastroenterology. 1980;79:1178–91.
26. Jones RJ, Lee KS, Beschorner WE, Vogel VG, Grochow LB, Braine HG, et al. Veno-occlusive disease of the liver following bone marrow transplantation. Transplantation. 1987;44:778–83.
27. Lee JL, Gooley T, Bensinger W, Schiffman K, McDonald GB. Venocclusive disease of the liver after busulfan, melphalan, and thioTEPA conditioning therapy: incidence, risk factors, and outcome. Biol Blood Marrow Transplant. 1999;5:306–15.
28. Toh HC, McAfee SL, Sackstein R, Cox BF, Colby C, Spitzer TR. Late onset veno-occlusive disease following high-dose chemotherapy and stem cell transplantation. Bone Marrow Transplant. 1999;24:891–5.
29. Hasegawa S, Horibe K, Kawabe T, Kato K, Kojima S, Matsuyama T, et al. Veno-occlusive disease of the liver after allogeneic bone marrow transplantation in children with hematologic malignancies: incidence, onset time and risk factors. Bone Marrow Transplant. 1998;22:1191–7.
30. Rajvanshi P, Shulman HM, Sievers EL, McDonald GB. Hepatic sinusoidal obstruction following gemtuzumab ozogamicin (Mylotarg) therapy. Blood. 2002;99:4245–6.
31. McKoy JM, Angelotta C, Bennett CL, Tallman MS, Wadleigh M, Evens AM, et al. Gemtuzumab ozogamicin-associated sinusoidal obstructive syndrome (SOS): an overview from the research on adverse drug events and reports (RADAR) project. Leuk Res. 2007;31:599–604.
32. Sakai M, Strasser SI, Shulman HM, McDonald SJ, Schoch HG, McDonald GB. Severe hepatocellular necrosis after hematopoietic cell transplant: incidence, etiology, and outcome. Bone Marrow Transplant. 2009;44:441–447.
33. Pihusch M, Wegner H, Goehring P, Salat C, Pihusch V, Hiller E, et al. Diagnosis of hepatic veno-occlusive disease by plasminogen activator inhibitor-1 plasma antigen levels: a prospective analysis in 350 allogeneic hematopoietic stem cell recipients. Transplantation. 2005;80:1376–82.
34. Lassau N, Auperin A, Leclere J, Bennaceur A, Valteau-Couanet D, Hartmann O. Prognostic value of Doppler-ultrasonography in hepatic veno-occlusive disease. Transplantation. 2002;74:60–6.
35. Erturk SM, Mortele KJ, Binkert CA, Glickman JN, Oliva M-R, Ros PR, et al. CT features of hepatic venoocclusive disease and hepatic graft-versus-host disease in patients after hematopoietic stem cell transplantation. AJR Am J Roentgenol. 2006;186:1497–501.
36. Coy DL, Ormazabal A, Godwin JD, Lalani T. Imaging evaluation of pulmonary and abdominal complications following hematopoietic stem cell transplantation. Radiographics. 2005;25:305–17.
37. Hashiguchi M, Okamura T, Yoshimoto K, Ono N, Imamura R, Yakushiji K, et al. Demonstration of reversed flow in segmental branches of the portal vein with hand-held color Doppler ultrasonography after hematopoietic stem cell transplantation. Bone Marrow Transplant. 2005;36:1071–5.
38. McCarville MB, Hoffer FA, Howard SC, Goloubeva O, Kauffman WM. Hepatic veno-occlusive disease in children undergoing bone-marrow transplantation: usefulness of sonographic findings. Pediatr Radiol. 2001;31:102–5.
39. Carreras E, Granena A, Navasa M, Bruguera M, Marco V, Sierra J, et al. Transjugular liver biopsy in bone marrow transplantation. Bone Marrow Transplant. 1993;11:21–6.

40. Shulman HM, Gooley T, Dudley MD, Kofler T, Feldman R, Dwyer D, et al. Utility of transvenous liver biopsies and wedged hepatic venous pressure measurements in sixty marrow transplant recipients. Transplantation. 1995;59:1015–22.
41. Choi SW, Islam S, Greenson JK, Levine J, Hutchinson R, Yanik G, et al. The use of laparoscopic liver biopsies in pediatric patients with hepatic dysfunction following allogeneic hematopoietic stem cell transplantation. Bone Marrow Transplant. 2005;36:891–6.
42. Groszmann RJ, Wongcharatrawee S. The hepatic venous pressure gradient: anything worth doing should be done right. Hepatology. 2004;39:280–2.
43. Vukelja SJ, Baker WJ, Jeffreys P, Reeb BA, Pick T. Nonbacterial thrombotic endocarditis clinically mimicking veno-occlusive disease of the liver complicating autologous bone marrow transplantation. Am J Clin Oncol. 1992;15:500–2.
44. Costa F, Choy CG, Seiter K, Hann L, Thung SN, Michaeli J. Hepatic outflow obstruction and liver failure due to leukemic cell infiltration in chronic lymphocytic leukemia. Leuk Lymphoma. 1998;30:403–10.
45. Rubenfeld GD, Crawford SW. Withdrawing life support from mechanically ventilated recipients of bone marrow transplants: a case for evidence-based guidelines. Ann Intern Med. 1996;125:625–33.
46. Coppell JA, Richardson PG, Soiffer RJ, Martin PL, Kernan NA, Chen A, et al. Hepatic veno-occlusive disease following stem cell transplantation: incidence, clinical course and outcome. Biol Blood Marrow Transplant. 2010;16:157–68.
47. Hingorani SR, Guthrie K, Batchelder A, Schoch G, Aboulhosn N, Manchion J, et al. Acute renal failure after myeloablative hematopoietic cell transplant: incidence and risk factors. Kidney Int. 2005;67:272–7.
48. Bearman SI, Anderson GL, Mori M, Hinds MS, Shulman HM, McDonald GB. Venocclusive disease of the liver: development of a model for predicting fatal outcome after marrow transplantation. J Clin Oncol. 1993;11:1729–36.
49. Bearman SI, Lee JL, Baron AE, McDonald GB. Treatment of hepatic venocclusive disease with recombinant human tissue plasminogen activator and heparin in 42 marrow transplant patients. Blood. 1997;89:1501–6.
50. Kikuchi K, Rudolph R, Murakami C, Kowdley KV, McDonald GB. Portal vein thrombosis after hematopoietic cell transplantation: frequency, treatment, and outcome. Bone Marrow Transplant. 2002;29:329–33.
51. DeLeve LD, Wang XD, Huybrechts MM. Cellular target of cyclophosphamide toxicity in the murine liver-role of glutathione and site of metabolic activation. Hepatology. 1996;24:830–7.
52. Salinger DH, McCune JS, Ren AG, Shen DD, Slattery JT, Phillips B, et al. Real-time dose adjustment of cyclophosphamide in a preparative regimen for hematopoietic cell transplant: a Bayesian pharmacokinetic approach. Clin Cancer Res. 2006;12:4888–98.
53. DeLeve LD, Wang X. Role of oxidative stress and glutathione in busulfan toxicity in cultured murine hepatocytes. Pharmacology. 2000;60:143–54.
54. Jenke A, Freiberg-Richter J, Wilhelm S, Freund M, Renner UD, Bornhauser M, et al. Accidental busulfan overdose during conditioning for stem cell transplantation. Bone Marrow Transplant. 2005;35:125–8.
55. Slattery JT, Clift RA, Buckner CD, Radich J, Storer B, Bensinger WI, et al. Marrow transplantation for chronic myeloid leukemia – the influence of plasma busulfan levels on the outcome of transplantation. Blood. 1997;89:3055–60.
56. Shaw PJ, Scharping CE, Brian RJ, Earl JW. Busulfan pharmacokinetics using a single daily high-dose regimen in children with acute leukemia. Blood. 1994;84:2357–62.
57. Wadleigh M, Richardson PG, Zahrieh D, Lee SJ, Cutler C, Ho V, et al. Prior gemtuzumab ozogamicin exposure significantly increases the risk of veno-occlusive disease in patients who undergo myeloablative allogeneic stem cell transplantation. Blood. 2003;102:1578–82.
58. Ringden O, Ruutu T, Remberger M, Nikoskelainen J, Volin L, Vindelov L, et al. A randomized trial comparing busulfan with total body irradiation as conditioning in allogeneic marrow transplant recipients with leukemia: a report from the Nordic Bone Marrow Transplantation Group. Blood. 1994;83:2723–30.
59. Pihusch M, Wegner H, Goehring P, Salat C, Pihusch V, Andreesen R, et al. Protein C and procollagen III peptide levels in patients with hepatic dysfunction after allogeneic hematopoietic stem cell transplantation. Bone Marrow Transplant. 2005;36:631–7.
60. Kallianpur AR, Hall LD, Yadav M, Byrne DW, Speroff T, Dittus RS, et al. The hemochromatosis C282Y allele: a risk factor for hepatic veno-occlusive disease after hematopoietic stem cell transplantation. Bone Marrow Transplant. 2005;35:1155–64.
61. Kallianpur AR. Genomic screening and complications of hematopoietic stem cell transplantation: has the time come? Bone Marrow Transplant. 2005;35:1–16.
62. Srivastava A, Poonkuzhali B, Shaji RV, George B, Mathews V, Chandy M, et al. Glutathione S-transferase M1 polymorphism: a risk factor for hepatic venoocclusive disease in bone marrow transplantation. Blood. 2004;104:1574–7.
63. McDonald GB, Frieze D. A problem-oriented approach to liver disease in oncology patients. Gut. 2008;57:987–1003.
64. DeLeve LD, Valla DC, Garcia-Tsao G, American Association for the Study Liver D. Vascular disorders of the liver. Hepatology. 2009;49:1729–64.
65. Bornhauser M, Storer B, Slattery J, Appelbaum F, Deeg H, Hansen J, et al. Conditioning with fludarabine and targeted busulfan for transplantation of allogeneic hematopoietic stem cells. Blood. 2003;102:820–6.
66. de Lima M, Couriel D, Thall PF, Wang X, Madden T, Jones R, et al. Once-daily intravenous busulfan and

fludarabine: clinical and pharmacokinetic results of a myeloablative, reduced-toxicity conditioning regimen for allogeneic stem cell transplantation in AML and MDS. Blood. 2004;104:857–64.
67. Puig N, de la Rubia J, Remigia MJ, Jarque I, Martin G, Cupelli L, et al. Morbidity and transplant-related mortality of CBV and BEAM preparative regimens for patients with lymphoid malignancies undergoing autologous stem-cell transplantation. Leuk Lymphoma. 2006;47:1488–94.
68. Anderson JE, Appelbaum FR, Schoch G, Barnett T, Chauncey TR, Flowers ME, et al. Relapse after allogeneic bone marrow transplantation for refractory anemia is increased by shielding lungs and liver during total body irradiation. Biol Blood Marrow Transplant. 2001;7:163–70.
69. Meresse V, Hartmann O, Vassal G, Benhamou E, Vatteau-Couenet D, Brugieres L, et al. Risk factors of hepatic venocclusive disease after high-dose busulfan-containing regimens followed by autologous bone marrow transplantation: a study in 136 children. Bone Marrow Transplant. 1992;10:135–41.
70. Hassan M, Ljungman P, Ringden O, Hassan Z, Oberg G, Nilsson C, et al. The effect of busulphan on the pharmacokinetics of cyclophosphamide and its 4-hydroxy metabolite: time interval influence on therapeutic efficacy and therapy-related toxicity. Bone Marrow Transplant. 2000;25:915–24.
71. Lee J-H, Choi S-J, Lee J-H, Kim S-E, Park C-J, Chi H-S, et al. Decreased incidence of hepatic veno-occlusive disease and fewer hemostatic derangements associated with intravenous busulfan vs oral busulfan in adults conditioned with busulfan + cyclophosphamide for allogeneic bone marrow transplantation. Ann Hematol. 2005;84:321–30.
72. Geddes M, Kangarloo SB, Naveed F, Quinlan D, Chauhry MA, Stewart D, et al. High busulfan exposure is associated with worse outcomes in a daily IV busulfan and fludarabine allogeneic transplant regimen. Biol Blood Marrow Transplant. 2008;14:220–8.
73. Radich JP, Gooley T, Bensinger W, Chauncey T, Clift R, Flowers M, et al. HLA-matched related hematopoietic cell transplantation for chronic-phase CML using a targeted busulfan and cyclophosphamide preparative regimen. Blood. 2003;102:31–5.
74. Deeg HJ, Storer BE, Boeckh M, Martin PJ, McCune JS, Myerson D, et al. Reduced incidence of acute and chronic graft-versus-host disease with the addition of thymoglobulin to a targeted busulfan/cyclophosphamide regimen. Biol Blood Marrow Transplant. 2006;12:573–84.
75. Kashyap A, Wingard J, Cagnoni P, Roy J, Tarantolo S, Hu W, et al. Intravenous versus oral busulfan as part of a busulfan/cyclophosphamide preparative regimen for allogeneic hematopoietic stem cell transplantation: decreased incidence of hepatic venoocclusive disease (HVOD), HVOD-related mortality, and overall 100-day mortality. Biol Blood Marrow Transplant. 2002;8:493–500.
76. Williams CB, Day SD, Reed MD, Copelan EA, Bechtel T, Leather HL, et al. Dose modification protocol using intravenous busulfan (Busulfex) and cyclophosphamide followed by autologous or allogeneic peripheral blood stem cell transplantation in patients with hematologic malignancies. Biol Blood Marrow Transplant. 2004;10:614–23.
77. Wang X, Kanel GC, DeLeve LD. Support of sinusoidal endothelial cell glutathione prevents hepatic veno-occlusive disease in the rat. Hepatology. 2000;31:428–34.
78. Deleve LD, Wang X, Tsai J, Kanel G, Strasberg S, Tokes ZA. Sinusoidal obstruction syndrome (veno-occlusive disease) in the rat is prevented by matrix metalloproteinase inhibition. Gastroenterology. 2003;125:882–90.
79. Chalandon Y, Roosnek E, Mermillod B, Newton A, Ozsahin H, Wacker P, et al. Prevention of veno-occlusive disease with defibrotide after allogeneic stem cell transplantation. Biol Blood Marrow Transplant. 2004;10:347–54.
80. Versluys B, Bhattacharaya R, Steward C, Cornish J, Oakhill A, Goulden N. Prophylaxis with defibrotide prevents veno-occlusive disease in stem cell transplantation after gemtuzumab ozogamicin exposure. Blood. 2004;103:1968.
81. Corbacioglu S. Cesaro S, Faraci M, Valteau-Couanet D, Gruhu B, Boeleus JJ, et al., Detibrotide prevents hepatic VOD and reduces significantly VOD-associated Complications in Childrens at high risk: final results of a prospective phase 11/111 multicentre study. Bone Marrow Transplant. 2010;45:51.
82. Imran H, Tleyjeh IM, Zirakzadeh A, Rodriguez V, Khan SP. Use of prophylactic anticoagulation and the risk of hepatic veno-occlusive disease in patients undergoing hematopoietic stem cell transplantation: a systematic review and meta-analysis. Bone Marrow Transplant. 2006;37:677–86.
83. Bearman SI, Hinds MS, Wolford JL, Petersen FB, Nugent DL, Slichter SJ, et al. A pilot study of continuous infusion heparin for the prevention of hepatic venocclusive disease after bone marrow transplantation. Bone Marrow Transplant. 1990;5:407–11.
84. Budinger MD, Bouvier M, Shah A, McDonald GB. Results of a phase I trial of antithrombin III as prophylaxis in bone marrow transplant patients at risk for venocclusive disease. Blood. 1996;88:172a.
85. Gooley TA, Rajvanshi P, Schoch HG, McDonald GB. Serum bilirubin levels and mortality after myeloablative allogeneic hematopoietic cell transplantation. Hepatology. 2005;41:345–52.
86. Richardson PG, Soiffer RJ, Antin JH, Uno H, Jin Z, Kurtzberg J, et al. Defibrotide for the treatment of severe hepatic veno-occlusive disease and multi-organ failure post stem cell transplantation: a multi-center, randomized, dose-finding trial. Biol Blood Marrow Transplant. 2010;16:1005–17.
87. Corbacioglu S, Greil J, Peters C, Wulffraat N, Laws HJ, Dilloo D, et al. Defibrotide in the treatment of children with veno-occlusive disease (VOD): a retrospective multicentre study demonstrates therapeutic efficacy upon early intervention [erratum in Bone Marrow Transplant. 2004;33:673]. Bone Marrow Transplant. 2004;33:189–95.

88. Kornblum N, Ayyanar K, Benimetskaya L, Richardson P, Iacobelli M, Stein CA. Defibrotide, a polydisperse mixture of single-stranded phosphodiester oligonucleotides with lifesaving activity in severe hepatic veno-occlusive disease: clinical outcomes and potential mechanisms of action. Oligonucleotides. 2006;16:105–14.
89. Benimetskaya L, Wu S, Voskresenskiy AM, Echart C, Zhou JF, Shin J, et al. Angiogenesis alteration by defibrotide: implications for its mechanism of action in severe hepatic veno-occlusive disease. Blood. 2008;112:4343–52.
90. Lazarus HM, McCrae KR. SOS! Defibrotide to the rescue. Blood. 2008;112:3924–5.
91. Azoulay D, Castaing D, Lemoine A, Hargreaves GM, Bismuth H. Transjugular intrahepatic portosystemic shunts (TIPS) for severe veno-occlusive disease of the liver following bone marrow transplantation. Bone Marrow Transplant. 2000;25:987–92.
92. Meacher R, Venkatesh B, Lipman J. Acute respiratory distress syndrome precipitated by transjugular intrahepatic porto-systemic shunting for severe hepatic veno-occlusive disease. Is it due to pulmonary leucostasis? Intensive Care Med. 1999;25:1332–3.
93. Koenecke C, Kleine M, Schrem H, Krug U, Nashan B, Neipp M, et al. Sinusoidal obstruction syndrome of the liver after hematopoietic stem cell transplantation: decision making for orthotopic liver transplantation. Int J Hematol. 2006;83:271–4.
94. Mellgren K, Fasth A, Saalman R, Olausson M, Abrahamsson J. Liver transplantation after stem cell transplantation with the same living donor in a monozygotic twin with acute myeloid leukemia. Ann Hematol. 2005;84:755–7.
95. Kim ID, Egawa H, Marui Y, Kaihara S, Haga H, Lin YW, et al. A successful liver transplantation for refractory hepatic veno-occlusive disease originating from cord blood transplantation. Am J Transplant. 2002;2:796–800.
96. Ullmann AJ, Lipton JH, Vesole DH, Chandrasekar P, Langston A, Tarantolo SR, et al. Posaconazole or fluconazole for prophylaxis in severe graft-versus-host disease. N Engl J Med. 2007;356:335–47.
97. Snover DC, Weisdorf S, Bloomer J, McGlave P, Weisdorf D. Nodular regenerative hyperplasia of the liver following bone marrow transplantation. Hepatology. 1989;9:443–8.
98. Sudour H, Mainard L, Baumann C, Clement L, Salmon A, Bordigoni P. Focal hepatic hyperplasia following hematopoietic stem cell transplantation. Bone Marrow Transplant. 2009;43:127–32.

Management: Cirrhotic Portal Hypertension

11

Joseph K. Lim and Guadalupe Garcia-Tsao

Abstract

Gastroesophageal varices are a direct consequence of portal hypertension, the main complication of cirrhosis. An understanding of the pathophysiology of portal hypertension has led to significant improvements in the prevention and treatment of variceal hemorrhage. However, variceal hemorrhage continues to carry a significant mortality. By screening all patients with cirrhosis for varices, applying prophylaxis appropriately, actively managing acute variceal hemorrhage, and aggressively preventing recurrence, survival can be improved. Future directions include better risk stratification for a more individualized care, determining the role of noninvasive markers of varices and portal pressure and the development of novel pharmacotherapeutic agents.

Keywords

Variceal hemorrhage • Esophagogastric varices • Cirrhosis • Portal hypertension

Portal hypertension is the main complication of cirrhosis and is responsible for the development of most of the complications that mark the transition from the compensated to the decompensated stage [1]. These complications are ascites, encephalopathy and variceal hemorrhage, with the latter being the one associated with the highest morbidity and mortality.

Gastroesophageal varices are portosystemic collaterals that result directly from a high pressure in the portal venous system, either by dilatation of preexisting vascular channels or by formation of new vessels (neoangiogenesis) [2]. Although portal hypertension may result from many conditions that impede blood flow at several points within the portal venous system (Table 11.1), cirrhosis is the main cause of portal hypertension in the Western world, representing approximately 90% of all cases.

This chapter reviews the management of varices and variceal hemorrhage in patients with cirrhosis and is based on practice guidelines [3, 4] that in turn are based on evidence in the literature that has been summarized and prioritized at consensus conferences [5, 6]. Although the

G. Garcia-Tsao (✉)
Section of Digestive Diseases, Yale University School of Medicine, 333 Cedar Street, LMP 1080, New Haven, CT 06520, USA
and
Section of Digestive Diseases, VA Connecticut Health Care System, West Haven, CT, USA
e-mail: guadalupe.garcia-tsao@yale.edu

L.D. DeLeve and G. Garcia-Tsao (eds.), *Vascular Liver Disease: Mechanisms and Management*, DOI 10.1007/978-1-4419-8327-5_11,

recommendations apply to patients with cirrhosis, they may be extended to patients with other causes of portal hypertension.

Natural History

Gastroesophageal varices are present in approximately 50% of patients with cirrhosis, and correlate with the stage of liver disease. Presence and size of varices depend on the severity of liver disease as assessed by the Child–Turcotte–Pugh (Child) classification (Table 11.2). Data from a U.S. endoscopic database comprising 881 patients with cirrhosis, found varices in 52% of the cases, more frequently in Child B/C (72%) than in Child A (42%) patients. Of those with varices, Child B/C were more likely to have large varices than patients with Child class A ($p=0.02$) [7]. Although varices are typically present only in the cirrhotic stage of any chronic liver disease, their presence has been described in noncirrhotic stages of primary biliary cirrhosis (by virtue of its initial presinusoidal involvement) [8] and in individuals with chronic hepatitis C infection and bridging fibrosis [9], although this may be the result of fibrosis underestimation due to biopsy sampling error [10].

Varices develop at a rate of 7–8% per year [11]. Among those with small varices, the rate of growth to large varices is approximately 7–8% per year, and is more common among those with Child B or C cirrhosis and red wale markings on varices [12]. Among individuals with varices, only one-third will experience hemorrhage, and this is estimated to occur at a rate of 5–15% per year depending on the presence of risk factors, with variceal size, red wale marks on varices, and advanced liver disease (Child B or C) identifying patients at a high risk of variceal hemorrhage [13] (Table 11.3).

Although epidemiologic data are limited, available studies suggest that variceal bleeding accounts for 6–14% of all cases of upper gastrointestinal bleeding, and approximately 50–60% of these occur in patients with cirrhosis. The largest cohort was reported in a French study describing 2,133 patients, 468 with cirrhosis. Variceal hemorrhage was the cause of bleeding in 59% of the patients with cirrhosis [14].

Six-week mortality with each episode of variceal hemorrhage is still around 15–25% and also depends on the severity of liver disease [15, 16]. While mortality in Child A patients is essentially

Table 11.1 Causes of portal hypertension

Prehepatic portal hypertension [normal wedged hepatic venous pressure (WHVP), free hepatic venous pressure (FHVP), and hepatic venous pressure gradient (HVPG)]:
• Portal vein thrombosis
• Splenic vein thrombosis
Intrahepatic portal hypertension (increased WHVP, normal FHVP, increased HVPG):
• Presinusoidal: schistosomiasis, early primary biliary cirrhosis, nodular regenerative hyperplasia
• Sinusoidal: cirrhosis
• Postsinusoidal: sinusoidal obstruction syndrome
Posthepatic portal hypertension (increased WHVP and FHVP with normal HVG):
• Budd–Chiari syndrome
• Congestive heart failure
• Constrictive pericarditis

Table 11.2 Child–Turcotte–Pugh (CTP) classification of the severity of cirrhosis

	Points[a]		
	1	2	3
Encephalopathy	None	Grade 1–2 (or precipitant-induced)	Grade 3–4 (or chronic)
Ascites	None	Mild/moderate (diuretic-responsive)	Severe (diuretic-refractory)
Bilirubin (mg/dL)	<2	2–3	>3
Albumin (g/dL)	>3.5	2.8–3.5	<2.8
PT (seconds prolonged)	<4	4–6	>6
INR	<1.7	1.7–2.3	>2.3

PT Prothrombin time; *INR* international normalized ratio
[a]5–6 points=CTP class A; 7–9 points=CTP class B; 10–15 points=CTP class C

Table 11.3 One-year probability (%) of developing variceal hemorrhage according to risk factors

	Child class A			Child class B			Child class C		
Red wale markings	Small varices	Medium varices	Large varices	Small varices	Medium varices	Large varices	Small varices	Medium varices	Large varices
Absent	6	10	15	10	16	26	20	30	42
Mild	8	12	19	15	23	33	28	38	54
Moderate	12	16	24	20	30	42	36	48	64
Severe	16	23	34	28	40	52	44	60	76

Modified from North Italian Endoscopic Club for the Study and Treatment of Esophageal Varices [13]

nil, mortality in Child C patients is ~30% [15–18]. Late rebleeding occurs in approximately 60–70% of untreated patients, usually within 1–2 years of the initial hemorrhage [19, 20].

Evaluation of Portal Hypertension

Since portal hypertension is the driving force behind the development of varices and variceal hemorrhage, it is reasonable to assume that measurements of portal pressure will be predictive of outcome. Portal pressure can be assessed through several approaches. Direct measurements require catheterization of the portal vein, which is feasible but technically difficult and impractical for routine clinical use. The preferred approach is indirect measurement of portal venous pressure through catheterization of the hepatic vein using a balloon-tipped catheter, which is introduced from either the internal jugular vein or the femoral vein under fluoroscopic guidance [21]. It is a simple, safe and reproducible method and, like measurement of wedged capillary pulmonary pressure, is performed by inflating a balloon in a large branch of the hepatic vein, thereby obtaining the wedged hepatic venous pressure (WHVP). The balloon is then deflated and the free hepatic venous pressure (FHVP) is obtained [2]. These measurements are performed in triplicate and recorded on a multichannel recorder [22, 23]. The hepatic venous pressure gradient (HVPG) is calculated by subtracting the FHVP from the WHVP. Normal HVPG ranges between 3 and 5 mmHg. Because it represents a measure of sinusoidal pressure, it will only be elevated in sinusoidal and postsinusoidal causes of portal hypertension (see Table 11.1).

As expected, HVPG measurements have been important in the prediction of outcomes in patients with varices and variceal hemorrhage.

In a prospective longitudinal study that included 212 patients with compensated cirrhosis without varices, an HVPG >10 mmHg was the strongest predictor of the development of varices [11]; while 26% of patients with HVPG <10 developed varices in a median follow-up of 55 months, this occurred in 44% of those with an HVPG >10 mmHg ($p=0.004$). Variceal development was slower in patients who achieved a reduction in HVPG after the first year of follow-up. The best cutoff was a reduction of >10%. This same cutoff was recently identified as predictive of a lower rate of first variceal hemorrhage in patients with large varices undergoing primary prophylactic therapy [24].

In a cross-sectional study comparing patients with and without varices, all patients with varices had an HVPG of at least 12 mmHg, while a percentage of patients without varices had pressures below 12 mmHg [25]. More importantly, prospective studies have shown that if the HVPG is reduced (either pharmacologically or spontaneously) to levels below 12 mmHg, the risk of bleeding from varices is essentially eliminated [20, 26]. Moreover, a reduction in HVPG in this setting is also predictive of lower recurrent hemorrhage. In patients in whom the HVPG decreases by >20% from baseline, the risk of recurrent variceal hemorrhage is significantly lower (7–13%) than in patients in whom such reduction does not occur (46–65%) [20, 27, 28].

In a cross-sectional study of patients admitted with variceal hemorrhage, an HVPG >20 mmHg was found to be the best predictor of a poor outcome; patients with an HVPG (measured within 24 h from admission) >20 mmHg had higher rates of treatment failure or early rebleeding (83% vs. 29%) and higher 1-year mortality (64% vs. 20%) compared to patients with an HVPG <20 mmHg [29]. This was confirmed in two subsequent studies [15, 30], one of which was a recent study that used current standards of care in the management of variceal hemorrhage [15].

Of note, data regarding prognostic value of HVPG applies to patients with alcoholic and viral cirrhosis, which comprise the majority of patients included in these studies, and in whom the HVPG correlates well with direct measurements of portal pressure [31].

Although evidence shows that HVPG is an ideal method to stratify patients with these types of cirrhosis and portal hypertension, it is invasive and its use is not widespread in the United States. Standardization of the technique is needed to help bring the HVPG into wider clinical use [6].

Diagnosis of Varices

Esophagogastroduodenoscopy (EGD) is the diagnostic test of choice to identify gastroesophageal varices. Traditional endoscopic assessment incorporates classification of size in three groups: F1 (small, minimal enlargement of veins beyond mucosal surface with flattening upon full insufflation), F2 (medium, tortuous veins occupying less than one-third of the esophageal lumen without flattening upon full air insufflation), and F3 (large >5 mm, occupying greater than one-third of the esophageal lumen). Simpler two-classification systems (small <5 mm vs. large >5 mm) may be preferred as treatment recommendations for medium-sized varices are identical to those for large varices [13, 32].

EGD should be performed at the time of diagnosis of cirrhosis, and repeated in 3 years if no varices are identified, and in 2 years if small varices are identified and β-blocker prophylaxis is not initiated [3, 4].

Because only 15–25% of patients with cirrhosis will have medium to large varices at the time of initial screening [7], simple noninvasive screening methods based on a few laboratory and/or ultrasonographic variables have been evaluated in the hope of selecting high-risk patients for EGD, thereby reducing the number of unnecessary procedures in patients without varices. Perhaps the most solid of these methods is the platelet/spleen size ratio. This ratio is calculated by dividing the platelet count (in mm^3) by the maximum spleen bipolar diameter (in mm) as determined by ultrasonography. A ratio above 909 has a high negative predictive value (i.e., patients with this ratio are unlikely to have varices) [33]. However, this method has not been entirely validated and is not recommended for use in clinical practice [34, 35].

On the other hand, newer, relatively less invasive approaches have been examined that could be used as substitutes for EGD in determining the presence and size of varices. Such methods include capsule endoscopy [36], transient elastography [37], and multidetector computed tomographic esophagography [38]. The most investigated method is capsule endoscopy, with the two largest studies (288 and 120 patients, respectively) showing sensitivities of 84 and 77%, respectively, for the presence of varices and of 78 and 84%, respectively, for the presence of varices that would require primary prophylaxis [36, 39]. This indicates that 16–22% of the patients who required prophylactic therapy, would have not received it, an unacceptably high rate. In fact, recent recommendations from the European Society of Gastrointestinal Endoscopy conclude that the usefulness of capsule endoscopy must be weighed against the wide availability of EGD, its good tolerability and relatively low cost. Moreover, EGD allows a complete examination of the stomach and duodenum during the same procedure and biopsy sampling [40]. As such, EGD remains the gold-standard diagnostic tool for all patients with cirrhosis.

Management Principles

Rationale for the Management of Varices and Variceal Hemorrhage

Several approaches have been developed in the management of gastroesophageal varices and variceal hemorrhage, including pharmacological,

Table 11.4 Therapeutic effects on portal flow, resistance, and pressure of different therapies for portal hypertension

Treatment	Portal flow	Portal resistance	Portal pressure
Vasoconstrictors (β-blockers)	↓↓	↑	↓
Venodilators			
Nitrates	↓	–	↓
Simvastatin	–	↓	
Endoscopic therapy (band ligation/sclerotherapy)	–	–	–
Transjugular intrahepatic portosystemic shunt (TIPS)/shunt therapy	↑	↓↓↓	↓↓↓

Modified from Garcia-Tsao et al. [3]

endoscopic, radiologic, and surgical therapies. Pharmacological therapies are based on ameliorating the intrahepatic (Chap. 6) and extrahepatic mechanisms (Chap. 7) that lead to and maintain portal hypertension.

Vasoconstrictors, such as nonselective β-blockers (NSBB), vasopressin (and analogs) and somatostatin (and analogs), produce splanchnic vasoconstriction and thereby reduce portal venous inflow. Importantly, the reduction in portal inflow induced by NSBB (propranolol, nadolol) is mostly due to β-2 adrenergic blockade (which leads to unopposed adrenergic splanchnic vasoconstriction). Therefore, selective β-1 blockers (atenolol, metoprolol), that reduce flow by reducing cardiac output, are not as effective and their use is not recommended.

Venodilators would theoretically act by producing intrahepatic vasodilatation. However, available vasodilators appear to decrease portal pressure through hypotension and a consequent decrease in flow [41]. It has been observed with vasodilators such as angiotensin-receptor antagonists that hypotension is a potentially deleterious effect in patients with cirrhosis, as it can lead to sodium retention and deterioration in renal function [42, 43]. An exception may be simvastatin, which increases intrahepatic nitric oxide and has recently been shown to cause a modest decrease in portal pressure without changes in hepatic blood flow or systemic blood pressure [44].

Combining a vasoconstrictor and a vasodilator leads to a synergistic reduction in HVPG [45, 46] and this may be the mechanism of action of carvedilol. In large doses (~30 mg/day) carvedilol was shown to lead to a greater reduction in HVPG than propranolol although, as occurs with other vasodilators, it decreased mean arterial pressure and worsened sodium retention [47].

Endoscopic therapies, such as variceal ligation (using rubber bands), sclerotherapy (injection of a sclerosing agent) or variceal obturation (using tissue adhesives), act locally and do not have a direct effect on portal flow or resistance. They can cause varices to disappear ("eradication"), however since portal pressure is not resolved, varices will eventually recur. Other shorter-term temporizing local measures include balloon tamponade and placement of expandable esophageal stents.

The transjugular intrahepatic portosystemic shunt (TIPS) or surgical shunt normalizes portal pressure by bypassing the site of increased resistance.

The mechanisms by which current therapies affect portal venous inflow, portal resistance, and portal pressure are summarized in Table 11.4.

Management Recommendations

An EGD should be performed at the time of initial diagnosis of cirrhosis and management will depend on findings at this screening endoscopy, specifically presence and size of varices, as outlined below and as summarized in Table 11.5.

Prevention of Varices in Patients with Cirrhosis but Without Varices (Pre-Primary Prophylaxis)

Decreasing portal pressure at earlier stages of cirrhosis could theoretically prevent the development of varices. In fact, in an animal model of portal hypertension, propranolol reduced the

Table 11.5 Management of varices following screening EGD in patients without prior variceal hemorrhage

No varices	Repeat endoscopy in 3 years (or in 1 year if Child B/C)		
Small varices	• High-risk for hemorrhage (Child B/C or red wale signs on EGD)	Nonselective β-blocker (NSBB)	Propranolol (10–20 mg BID) or nadolol (20–40 mg QD) Titrate to maximal tolerable dose or HR 55–60 bpm No need for repeat EGD
	• Low-risk for hemorrhage (Child A, no red wale signs)	NSBB optional Repeat endoscopy in 2 years if the choice is not to start NSBB	
Medium/large varices	• NSBB	Propranolol (10–20 mg BID) or nadolol (20–40 mg QD) Titrate to maximal tolerated dose or HR 55–60 bpm No need for repeat EGD	
	OR • Endoscopic variceal ligation (EVL)	Repeat band ligation every 1–2 wks until variceal obliteration Surveillance EGD 1–3 months after obliteration, then every 6–12 months	

BID twice a day; *QD* once daily; *EGD* esophagogastroduodenoscopy
Modified from Garcia-Tsao and Lim [4]

development of portosystemic collaterals [48]. However, a large multicenter, placebo-controlled, randomized controlled trial of timolol (an NSBB) performed in 213 patients with cirrhosis, portal hypertension (HVPG >5 mmHg) but without varices showed no differences between study groups in the development of gastroesophageal varices or variceal hemorrhage (39% vs. 40%, $p=0.89$) after a mean follow-up of 54.9 months [11]. Severe adverse events were more prevalent in the timolol group vs. the placebo group (18% vs. 6%, $p=0.006$) [11]. Interestingly, patients who achieved a reduction (≥10% from baseline) in HVPG after the first year of follow-up had a lower rate of variceal development and the proportion of portal pressure "responders" was greater in the timolol than in the placebo group (53% vs. 38%, $p=0.04$). However, given the overall results of the trial, NSBB cannot be recommended for primary prevention of variceal development.

B. Prevention of Variceal Bleeding in Patients with Cirrhosis and Varices (Primary Prophylaxis)

Many therapies have been examined to prevent first variceal hemorrhage [49]. The first approach was prophylactic portacaval surgical shunts. Although very useful in preventing hemorrhage, shunting was associated with severe encephalopathy and, more importantly, with a decrease in survival [49]. Therefore, the use of prophylactic shunt therapy and, by extension, the use of TIPS in this setting should be proscribed [3, 32].

The second approach in the prevention of first variceal hemorrhage was endoscopic sclerotherapy. However, uncertain results from a meta-analysis (with significant heterogeneity among trials) [49], a high rate of complications, and the emergence of more effective therapies, led to its abandonment.

The two currently effective therapies for prevention of first variceal hemorrhage are NSBB and endoscopic variceal ligation (EVL), each of which can be considered first-line therapies.

Evidence for Nonselective β-Blockers

A meta-analysis of 11 randomized controlled trials involving 1,189 patients demonstrated that patients with all-size varices randomized to NSBBs had a significantly lower risk for first hemorrhage compared to no therapy/placebo (15% vs. 25%) during a mean follow-up period of 24 months, consistent with a relative risk reduction of 40% [50]. These results were particularly significant in patients with medium/large varices in whom first variceal hemorrhage was 14% compared to 30% in control groups. Notably, NSBB also reduce bleeding from portal hypertensive gastropathy [51]. Importantly, patients on primary prophylactic therapy in whom HVPG is reduced by >10% have been shown to have not only a lower probability of developing hemorrhage [24], but also a lower probability of developing ascites, spontaneous bacterial peritonitis and hepatorenal syndrome [52, 53]. Therefore, unlike local therapies, NSBB not only decreases variceal hemorrhage but may also change the natural history of cirrhosis by ameliorating portal hypertension.

NSBB should be initiated at a dose of 20–40 mg (twice a day for propranolol, once a day for nadolol). Because the β-2 effect is more important in reducing portal pressure than the β-1 effect, there is no correlation between the decrease in HVPG and a decrease in heart rate (a β-1 effect) [54]. Therefore, the dose of NSBBs should be titrated to the maximal tolerated dose or to a heart rate of 55–60 beats/min (bpm) and should be maintained indefinitely [55]. Once on NSBB, there is no need to repeat EGD.

The major limitations to the use of NSBB are that approximately 15% of patients may have absolute or relative contraindications to therapy (e.g., asthma, insulin-dependent diabetes mellitus, peripheral vascular disease) and that another 15% require dose-reduction or discontinuation due to its common side-effects (e.g., fatigue, weakness, lightheadedness, shortness of breath) that resolve upon discontinuation but that deter patients from using them [56]. Although nadolol appears to have fewer side-effects than propranolol as reported in clinical trials, and may have superior adherence due to once-daily dosing, no direct comparisons are available to confirm these observations.

More recently, carvedilol, an NSBB with intrinsic anti-α-1 adrenergic activity, was compared to EVL in a randomized clinical trial [57]. This NSBB, by having a vasodilatory activity, mimics the combination of propranolol and prazosin, which has a large portal pressure-reducing effect. Patients randomized to carvedilol (at a dose of 12.5 mg/day, a dose lower than that associated with hypotension) had a significantly lower rate of first variceal hemorrhage compared to EVL (10% vs. 23%, $p=0.04$). The results are promising but certain methodological problems limit its conclusions and the results should be confirmed in future studies, comparing carvedilol to NSBB, before its use can be widely recommended [58].

Evidence for Endoscopic Variceal Ligation

For many years, NSBB were the only prophylactic therapy recommended for patients with medium/large varices. This changed when EVL emerged as a new local therapy that, compared to sclerotherapy, was safer and more effective [59].

A number of trials have been performed comparing NSBB vs. EVL and have been summarized in meta-analyses. Two earlier analyses, one including 8 trials (596 subjects) and a second including 12 trials (839 subjects) showed a lower rate of first variceal hemorrhage with EVL compared to NSBB, without differences in mortality [60, 61]. Notably, first hemorrhage rate in patients randomized to NSBB (21%) in the latter meta-analysis is higher than rates observed in primary prophylactic trials of no therapy vs. NSBB (14%). More recent meta-analyses show that when trials with an appropriate treatment allocation and a longer follow-up are analyzed, the benefit of EVL disappears [62] and it also disappears when only trials that include 100 patients or more are analyzed [58].

EVL should be performed at the time of initial endoscopy and repeated every 1–2 weeks until variceal obliteration has been achieved, followed by surveillance EGD in 1–3 months, and then every 6–12 months (indefinitely) to confirm absence of variceal growth requiring repeat ligation.

The major limitation of EVL is the small but important risk for severe complications such as ligation-induced ulcers and/or bleeding, with three fatal cases reported in clinical trials. Therefore, although the number of side-effects is greater with NSBB than with EVL [60, 61], no lethal side-effects have been reported with the use of NSBB. Other side-effects of EVL such as transient dysphagia and chest discomfort occur in approximately 10–15% of individuals. Due to the frequency of shallow ulcers, which form after varices have sloughed off following ligation, proton pump inhibitors may be used to promote healing, although clinical trials have been inconclusive [63].

Recommendations for Primary Prophylaxis

For patients with medium/large varices, both EVL and NSBBs are effective for primary prevention of first variceal hemorrhage, and the decision for either approach is best made by clinicians in the context of local expertise and individual patient characteristics. There are centers that perform predominantly EVL while others prefer the approach of starting with NSBB and switching to EVL if there is intolerance to NSBB.

Small varices with red wale marks or that are present in Child B/C patients have the same risk of first hemorrhage as patients with large varices (see Table 11.3), and therefore it is recommended that these patients be started on NSBB (since small varices are not always easy to ligate) [6].

In patients with small low-risk varices, the role of NSBBs is less clear. A study performed in a homogeneous population of patients with low-risk small varices demonstrated that nadolol resulted in a slower progression to large varices compared to placebo (11% vs. 37% over a 3-year follow-up period) [64]. Expert panels have concluded that NSBBs are optional in these patients and those who do not undergo β-blockade should have surveillance endoscopies every 2 years (or annually, if decompensated) [6].

Treatment of Acute Variceal Hemorrhage

Variceal hemorrhage is the most common etiology for acute gastrointestinal bleeding in patients with cirrhosis, and should be suspected at the time of initial presentation. The diagnosis is confirmed on the basis of active bleeding from a varix, a white nipple or clot adherent to or overlying a varix, or the presence of varices without other potential sources for bleeding. Variceal bleeding is associated with significant morbidity and mortality, although recent studies have confirmed that the mortality has decreased significantly over the last 20 years from approximately 40 to 15–20%, which is believed to be attributable to improvements in critical care management and increased efficacy of pharmacologic and endoscopic therapies, specifically prophylactic antibiotics and EVL, respectively [65–67]. Management recommendations for acute variceal hemorrhage are summarized in Table 11.6.

General Management

The primary goals of management in patients with suspected acute variceal bleeding are prompt resuscitation, confirmation of diagnosis, endoscopic hemostasis, and prevention of associated complications. The first steps include basic life support through an assessment of airway (A), breathing (B), and circulation (C) to optimize oxygen support to tissues, which includes securing an adequate airway and venous access, and admission to an intensive care unit for critical care monitoring. In individuals with impaired mental status due to alcohol, substance withdrawal, or encephalopathy, elective or emergent intubation with mechanical ventilation should be considered. Volume resuscitation should be initiated cautiously with colloids and blood transfusions to achieve hemodynamic stability (systolic blood pressure of 90–100 mmHg and a heart rate <100 bpm) while keeping a hemoglobin of 7–8 g/dL. Evidence for this recommendation is supported by a recent trial in which patients were randomized to liberal transfusion vs. a restrictive strategy (aiming to maintain the hemoglobin at 7–8 g/dL) and showed that therapeutic failure was lower (16% vs. 28%) and 6-week survival probability was higher (82% vs. 69%) in the restrictive strategy group [68]. Fresh frozen plasma and platelet transfusions are not recommended in the setting of severe coagulopathy and thrombocytopenia because they are often inadequate in correcting the coagulopathy and may induce volume overload and rebound increases in portal pressure. Recombinant factor VIIa (rFVIIa) was thought to have a potential role based on a multicenter placebo-controlled trial which demonstrated

Table 11.6 Management of acute variceal hemorrhage

Diagnosis	Any of the following findings on EGD: Active bleeding from varix Stigmata of variceal hemorrhage (white nipple sign) Presence of gastroesophageal varices without alternative source of hemorrhage
General management	Cautious transfusion of fluids and blood products, aiming to maintain a hemoglobin of 7–8 g/dL Antibiotic prophylaxis (3–7 days) with: Norfloxacin 400 mg BID or ciprofloxacin 500 mg BID (PO) or 400 mg BID (IV) Ceftriaxone 1 g/day (IV) particularly in centers with known quinolone-resistance and in patients with two or more of the following : malnutrition, ascites, encephalopathy, serum bilirubin >3 mg/dL
Specific initial management	Pharmacological therapy initiated as soon as diagnosis is suspected Octreotide 50 μg IV bolus followed by continuous infusion 50 μg/h (3–5 days) Terlipressin 2 mg IV every 4–6 h followed by 1 mg IV every 4 h (5 days) (not available in the United States) EGD within 12 h of initial hemorrhage with definite endoscopic therapy with EVL Consider preemptive TIPS (first 24–48 hours) in Child C patients
Rescue management	Considered in patients who have failed pharmacological and endoscopic therapy TIPS Low threshold to do TIPS in patients with bleeding gastric varices Balloon tamponade as bridge to TIPS

EGD esophagogastroduodenoscopy; *BID* twice a day; *PO* orally; *IV* intravenously; *EVL* endoscopic variceal ligation; *TIPS* transjugular intrahepatic portosystemic shunt
Modified from Garcia-Tsao and Lim [4]

improvement in hemostasis in a subgroup of patients with Child B/C cirrhosis. However, a subsequent multicenter trial performed specifically in this subgroup of patients could not find any differences in control of acute hemorrhage, acute rebleeding, and 5-day mortality between study groups [18]. Therefore, rFVIIa cannot be recommended in the management of acute variceal hemorrhage.

Bacterial infections remain one of the most common complications in cirrhotic patients who experience upper GI hemorrhage, and represent a strong negative prognostic factor for survival. A short-term course of antibiotics decreases not only rates of bacterial infection, but also rates of variceal rebleeding and mortality [69, 70]. As such, the use of short-term prophylactic antibiotics is considered standard-of-care for all patients with cirrhosis and GI bleeding with or without ascites. The antibiotic regimen supported by consensus consists of oral norfloxacin 400 mg twice daily for 7 days [71], which aims to achieve selective eradication of gram-negative bacteria in the gut, the theoretical source for bacteria. However, norfloxacin is not always available and has been substituted by oral or intravenous ciprofloxacin. Intravenous ceftriaxone appears to be superior to oral norfloxacin in high-risk patients based on a recent trial performed in Child B/C cirrhotic patients in which patients with two or more risk factors (malnutrition, ascites, encephalopathy, serum bilirubin >3 mg/dL) had lower rates of bacterial infection in the IV ceftriaxone group [72]. However, six of the seven patients with bacterial infections in the oral norfloxacin group demonstrated infection with quinolone-resistant organisms, and therefore the prevalence of quinolone resistance in various practice settings may be relevant to the selection of antibiotic coverage.

Specific Therapies to Control Bleeding

Control of acute variceal bleeding should consist of a combination of pharmacologic and endoscopic therapy. A diagnostic and therapeutic EGD should be performed as soon as possible after hemodynamic stability is achieved, and at minimum within a 12 h time as per standard practice guidelines [3, 4]. Rescue therapies should be used if these initial hemostatic methods fail to control bleeding.

Pharmacologic Therapies

Pharmacological therapy is considered first-line therapy for acute variceal bleeding, and should be initiated at the time of initial diagnosis of upper GI bleeding in a patient with cirrhosis, prior to diagnostic EGD. A meta-analysis of 15 controlled trials revealed similar efficacy between emergency sclerotherapy and pharmacologic therapy (vasopressin, terlipressin, somatostatin, or octreotide) in the initial control of acute variceal bleeding, with fewer side-effects observed with pharmacologic therapy, supporting its role in initial management [73]. The choice of vasoactive agent is determined primarily on local availability and cost.

Vasopressin and Related Analogs

Vasopressin acts on V1 receptors in arterial smooth muscle and is the most potent splanchnic vasoconstrictor. Its use is limited primarily due to adverse effects related to its powerful vasoconstrictive properties, including hypertension, myocardial and peripheral ischemia, arrhythmias, bowel ischemia, and limb gangrene. As such, vasopressin can only be administered for a period of 24 h at its highest effective dose of 0.2–0.4 units/min continuous infusion, which may be increased up to a maximum of 0.8 units/min. The addition of nitroglycerin further improves control of bleeding and reduces ischemic complications of vasopressin [45]. Therefore, vasopressin should only be administered in combination with nitroglycerin, which is administered at 40 μg/min, which may be increased up to a maximum of 400 μg/min. The use of vasopressin plus nitroglycerin has essentially been abandoned in favor of safer therapies, such as terlipressin, a synthetic triglycyl lysine analog with a longer half-life and significantly fewer side-effects than vasopressin plus nitroglycerin. It is effective in controlling acute variceal hemorrhage and represents the only pharmacologic agent to demonstrate an improvement in survival [74]. It may be administered at the time of initial diagnosis of GI bleeding prior to EGD, initially at a dose of 2 mg every 4–6 h up to 48 or 24 h post hemostasis, and then maintained for up to 5 days at a dose of 1 mg every 4 h [75]. However, it is not presently approved for use in the United States.

Somatostatin and Related Analogs

Somatostatin reduces portal pressure through splanchnic vasoconstriction mediated through a combination of inhibition of vasodilatory peptide release (e.g., glucagon) and a local vasoconstrictive effect. It has a short half-life of 1–3 min, and is dosed with an initial bolus of 250 μg followed by a continuous intravenous infusion of 250–500 μg/h for up to 5 days. Although minor side-effects such as nausea, vomiting, and hyperglycemia may be seen in up to 30% of patients, major side-effects are quite rare. Randomized controlled trials have demonstrated significant improvement in control of acute variceal bleeding when compared to controls, although it does not improve mortality. Octreotide, a long-acting somatostatin analog with a half-life of 80–120 min, is dosed with an initial bolus of 50 μg followed by a continuous intravenous infusion of 50 μg/h for up to 5 days. Due primarily to the rapid development of tachyphylaxis, its portal pressure-reducing effect is transient [76], and its efficacy as a single agent in acute variceal bleeding remains controversial. However, it appears to be useful as an adjunct to endoscopic therapy [77], and is presently used in combination with EVL as first-line treatment of acute variceal bleeding in the United States. Vapreotide, a cyclic long-acting somatostatin analog, also appears to improve control of acute variceal hemorrhage [78], but is not available in the United States.

Endoscopic Therapies

A meta-analysis of 10 randomized controlled trials involving 404 patients demonstrated an almost statistically significant benefit of EVL compared to sclerotherapy in the initial control of acute variceal hemorrhage, with a pooled relative risk of 0.53 (CI 0.28–1.01) [61]. This meta-analysis did not include a more recent trial that showed that EVL was associated with significantly lower treatment failure, fewer side-effects and improved survival, compared to sclerotherapy [17]. Therefore, EVL should be the endoscopic therapy of choice with sclerotherapy reserved for cases in which EVL is not technically feasible.

Placing greater than six bands at the time of initial endoscopic hemostasis does not appear to improve rates of variceal rebleeding, variceal recurrence, or 6 week or 1 year mortality, and increases procedural time and rate of misfired bands and is therefore not recommended [79].

Rescue Therapies

Although acute hemostasis is achieved in 80–90% of patients with standard therapies, the remaining 10–20% fail to achieve initial control of bleeding or experience early rebleeding. While repeat endoscopic intervention can be pursued in the case of rebleeding beyond 48 h from admission or when endoscopic therapy was thought to be insufficient, rescue or salvage therapies should be considered in other types of failure, particularly in patients with advanced liver disease.

Transjugular Intrahepatic Portosystemic Shunt

TIPS is effective in achieving hemostasis from acute variceal hemorrhage in 90–95% of cases. However, mortality after salvage TIPS is 20–30% higher than reported in elective conditions. As mentioned in Chap. 15, early (within the first 48 h) TIPS placement in high-risk patients (HVPG >20 mmHg or Child C) with variceal hemorrhage has been associated with better outcomes and an improvement in survival [30, 80]. Therefore, it can be considered in this small subset of patients with acute variceal hemorrhage.

Balloon Tamponade and Local Therapies

In addition to shunt therapies, balloon tamponade with a Sengstaken–Blakemore, Linton, or Minnesota tube is effective in achieving temporary control of active variceal hemorrhage in 60–90% of patients, and may represent a life-saving salvage therapy in patients who have failed standard therapies. However, rebleeding in occurs in up to 50% of cases after balloon deflation, and its use is associated with severe, potentially fatal complications such as aspiration pneumonia, airway obstruction, and esophageal necrosis and perforation. Therefore, it should only be used by clinicians experienced in its use, accompanied in most cases by elective endotracheal intubation for airway protection, and restricted to individuals with uncontrolled bleeding as a bridge to definitive therapy such as TIPS [5]. Lastly, endoscopic placement of self-expanding metallic stents demonstrated efficacy in achieving hemostasis in two pilot studies performed in patients with uncontrolled bleeding with low associated complication rate, and may represent a future alternative salvage therapy [81, 82].

Prevention of Recurrent Variceal Hemorrhage in Patients with Cirrhosis Who Have Recovered From an Episode of Variceal Hemorrhage (Secondary Prophylaxis)

While the risk of first variceal hemorrhage is only about 12% per year in untreated patients with varices, the risk of recurrent variceal hemorrhage in untreated patients (within 1–2 years from the index bleed) is around 60–70% and is greatest in those with advanced liver disease [20]. This indicates that: (a) combination therapies that will likely be associated with a higher probability of side-effects are warranted in this setting (not so in primary prophylaxis) and (b) prophylaxis of recurrent hemorrhage should be initiated as soon as the episode of acute variceal hemorrhage is controlled and patients have remained bleed-free for minimum 24 h. Individuals who have undergone TIPS for control of acute hemorrhage require no further intervention. Additionally, patients who are eligible for transplant (MELD score >15) should be referred for transplant evaluation.

Management recommendations for secondary prevention of variceal bleeding are summarized in Table 11.7.

Table 11.7 Prevention of recurrent variceal hemorrhage

First-line combination therapy	NSBB	Propranolol (20 mg BID) or nadolol (40 mg QD) Titrate to maximum tolerated dosage or HR 55–60 bpm No need for repeat EGD
	EVL	Repeat band ligation every 1–2 weeks until variceal obliteration Surveillance EGD 1–3 months after obliteration, then every 6–12 months
Second-line therapy (if pharmacologic + endoscopic treatment has failed)	TIPS or Shunt surgery (CTP class A patients, where available)	

NSBB non-selective beta-blockers; *HR* heart rate; *EGD* esophagogastroduodenoscopy; *BID* twice a day; *QD* once daily; *EVL* endoscopic variceal ligation; *TIPS* transjugular intrahepatic portosystemic shunt; *CTP* Child–Turcotte–Pugh
Modified from Garcia-Tsao and Lim [4]

Table 11.8 Comparison of different current therapies to prevent recurrent variceal hemorrhage

Therapy	Number of studies (references)	Median follow-up (months)	Recurrent variceal hemorrhage	Recurrent gastrointestinal hemorrhage	Death
EVL alone	7 [86–91, 93]	15 (12–25)	32% (23–46)	47% (18–58)	25% (3–42)
NSBB + isosorbide mononitrate (ISMN)	5 [88–92]	14 (8–24)	32% (24–46)	37% (35–47)	19% (13–33)
EVL + drugs[a]	4 [87, 90, 92, 93]	16 (15–22)	12% (12–18)	20% (14–28)	14% (2–20)

[a] Either NSBB alone or NSBB + ISMN

Pharmacological and Endoscopic Therapy

EVL is the most effective endoscopic therapy [59] and the combination of NSBB plus isosorbide mononitrate (ISMN) is the most effective pharmacological therapy, although it is associated with a higher rate of side-effects [50, 83].

Meta-analysis of trials comparing EVL vs. combination pharmacological therapy (NSBB plus ISMN) have demonstrated that both therapies are equivalent, although the long-term (82-month) follow-up of one of these studies showed that combination pharmacological therapy (NSBB plus ISMN) was associated with a better long (82-month)-term survival compared to EVL [84]. However, this trial did not explore combination EVL + NSBB. A recent meta-analysis of 4 studies including 404 patients showed a benefit of combination EVL + drugs compared to EVL alone [85]. A review of data obtained from published randomized trials comparing EVL alone vs. EVL + NSBB [86, 87], EVL alone vs. NSBB + ISMN [88–91], EVL + BB/ISMN vs. BB/ISMN alone [92] or EVL alone [93], shows that, at equivalent follow-up times, the combination EVL plus drugs is associated with the lowest rates of recurrent variceal hemorrhage (12%), overall gastrointestinal hemorrhage (20%) and death (17%) (Table 11.8).

Therefore, the current standard-of-care for secondary prevention is a combination of EVL and NSBB. In patients who are not candidates or refuse EVL, the combination of NSBB plus ISMN should be attempted, although in our experience, this combination is poorly tolerated.

Shunt Therapy

Shunt therapies, either surgical shunt or TIPS, are very effective in preventing rebleeding; however, they increase the risk of hepatic encephalopathy, without an impact on survival [94, 95]. Therefore, shunt therapy should not be used as a first-line treatment, but as a rescue therapy for patients who have failed pharmacologic plus endoscopic treatment. The choice of shunt therapy depends on local expertise and patient characteristics, as detailed in Chap. 16.

Role of HVPG

The lowest rates of recurrent variceal hemorrhage (approximately 10%) are observed in individuals who have a hemodynamic response to pharmacologic therapy, defined as a decrease in HVPG to <12 mmHg or a decrease of >20% from baseline levels [20, 28]. As such, the more rational approach would be to monitor HVPG in order to assess the hemodynamic effects of pharmacotherapy, and guide the use of pharmacotherapy vs. EVL based on hemodynamic response. A recent controlled trial randomized patients to HVPG-guided pharmacotherapy (nadolol plus ISMN or prazosin) vs. combined pharmacotherapy and endoscopic therapy (nadolol plus EVL) with baseline hemodynamic studies performed at baseline and within 1 month [96]. Individuals in the HVPG-guided pharmacotherapy arm (who required 2–3 HVPG measurements) demonstrated higher rates of hemodynamic response (74% vs. 32%, p <0.01), and HVPG responders (in both groups) experienced less frequent variceal rebleeding compared to nonresponders (15% vs. 57%, p <0.01) [96]. Overall however, the rates of recurrent hemorrhage were similar between groups: 23% (5/22) in the nadolol plus EVL group and 26% (7/27) in the HVPG-guided pharmacotherapy group.

The need for separate HVPG procedures to assess response to therapy can be obviated by assessing acute hemodynamic response to intravenous propranolol (0.15 mg/kg) during the same procedure. This was found to be predictive of variceal bleeding in a retrospective cohort of 166 cirrhotic patients on pharmacotherapy for primary or secondary prophylaxis. HVPG acute responders to propranolol were found to have significantly decreased risk of variceal rebleeding at 2 years following initial hemorrhage compared to nonresponders (23% vs. 46%, $p = 0.032$) with improved survival (95% vs. 65%, $p = 0.003$) [97]. This was confirmed in another study performed in patients on nadolol for primary prophylaxis, which also showed a good correlation ($r = 0.62$) between the acute and chronic HVPG response [24].

Recognizing the limitations of reliable and reproducible HVPG measurement in clinical practice and the lack of evidence, additional data are needed to more clearly define the role of HVPG in secondary prophylaxis of variceal hemorrhage.

Conclusions

In summary, gastroesophageal varices remain a significant source of morbidity and mortality in patients with cirrhosis and portal hypertension. Advances in our understanding of the pathophysiology of portal hypertension, the hemodynamic changes produced by pharmacologic agents, and short-term and long-term effects of endoscopic therapies have led to significant improvements in our ability to prevent and control variceal hemorrhage in at-risk individuals. Despite an abundance of evidence to support the current role of pharmacotherapy, endoscopic therapy, and shunt therapy, many questions remain unanswered regarding the role of noninvasive markers, HVPG, novel pharmacotherapeutic agents, and new endoscopic, radiologic, and surgical techniques in the future management of gastroesophageal variceal bleeding. Our current evidence supports the following recommendations:

1. Screening EGD should be performed in all individuals with cirrhosis to evaluate for the presence and size of gastroesophageal varices.
2. Patients without varices on screening EGD do not require prophylaxis with NSBB but should undergo surveillance EGD in 2–3 years depending on the stage of liver disease.
3. Patients with small nonbleeding varices and high-risk for hemorrhage (Child B/C or red wale markings on endoscopy) should initiate NSBB for primary prophylaxis; low-risk individuals may continue surveillance EGD in 1–2 years depending on disease stage.
4. Patients with medium/large nonbleeding varices can receive prophylaxis with either NSBB or EVL, although a rational approach would be to start NSBB and switch to EVL in case of intolerance to NSBB.
5. Patients with bleeding esophageal varices should undergo cautious resuscitation in an intensive care unit with volume support and blood products to achieve a hemoglobin goal of 7–8 g/dL.
6. A short course of prophylactic antibiotics with oral norfloxacin or intravenous ciprofloxacin or ceftriaxone should be administered in all cirrhotic patients admitted with upper GI hemorrhage.

7. Pharmacologic therapy with terlipressin, somatostatin or a somatostatin analog should be initiated at the time of initial presentation once variceal hemorrhage is suspected, prior to EGD.
8. EGD should be performed as soon as possible, or within 12 h, to establish the diagnosis and perform therapeutic hemostasis with EVL if indicated.
9. EVL plus NSBB represents the preferred strategy for prevention of recurrent variceal hemorrhage, with NSBB plus ISMN reserved for patients who are unwilling or unable to undergo EVL.
10. Patients with bleeding gastroesophageal varices should be considered for transplant evaluation.

References

1. D'Amico G, Garcia-Tsao G, Pagliaro L. Natural history and prognostic indicators of survival in cirrhosis. A systematic review of 118 studies. J Hepatol 2006; 44:217–231.
2. Garcia-Tsao G, Bosch J. Management of varices and variceal hemorrhage in cirrhosis. N Engl J Med 2010; 362(9):823–832.
3. Garcia-Tsao G, Sanyal AJ, Grace ND, Carey W. Prevention and management of gastroesophageal varices and variceal hemorrhage in cirrhosis. Hepatology 2007; 46(3):922–938.
4. Garcia-Tsao G, Lim JK. Management and treatment of patients with cirrhosis and portal hypertension: recommendations from the Department of Veterans Affairs Hepatitis C Resource Center Program and the National Hepatitis C Program. Am J Gastroenterol 2009; 104(7):1802–1829.
5. de Franchis R. Evolving Consensus in Portal Hypertension Report of the Baveno IV Consensus Workshop on methodology of diagnosis and therapy in portal hypertension. J Hepatol 2005; 43(1): 167–176.
6. Garcia-Tsao G, Bosch J, Groszmann RJ. Portal hypertension and variceal bleeding – unresolved issues. Summary of an American Association for the Study of Liver Diseases and European Association for the Study of the Liver Single-Topic Conference. Hepatology 2008; 47(5):1764–1772.
7. Kovalak M, Lake J, Mattek N, Eisen G, Lieberman D, Zaman A. Endoscopic screening for varices in cirrhotic patients: data from a national endoscopic database. Gastrointest Endosc 2007; 65(1):82–88.
8. Navasa M, Pares A, Bruguera M, Caballeria J, Bosch J, Rodes J. Portal hypertension in primary biliary cirrhosis. Relationship with histological features. J Hepatol 1987; 5(3):292–298.
9. Sanyal AJ, Fontana RJ, DiBisceglie AM, Everhart JE, Doherty MC, Everson GT et al. The prevalence and risk factors associated with esophageal varices in subjects with hepatitis C and advanced fibrosis. Gastrointest Endosc 2006; 64:855–864.
10. Blasco A, Forns X, Carrion JA, Garcia-Pagan JC, Gilabert R, Rimola A et al. Hepatic venous pressure gradient identifies patients at risk of severe hepatitis C recurrence after liver transplantation. Hepatology 2006; 43(3):492–499.
11. Groszmann RJ, Garcia-Tsao G, Bosch J, Grace ND, Burroughs AK, Planas R et al. Beta-blockers to prevent gastroesophageal varices in patients with cirrhosis. N Engl J Med 2005; 353:2254–2261.
12. Merli M, Nicolini G, Angeloni S, Rinaldi V, De Santis A, Merkel C et al. Incidence and natural history of small esophageal varices in cirrhotic patients. J Hepatol 2003; 38(3):266–272.
13. North Italian Endoscopic Club for the Study and Treatment of Esophageal Varices. Prediction of the first variceal hemorrhage in patients with cirrhosis of the liver and esophageal varices. A prospective multicenter study. N Engl J Med 1988; 319:983–989.
14. Lecleire S, Di Fiore F, Merle V, Herve S, Duhamel C, Rudelli A et al. Acute upper gastrointestinal bleeding in patients with liver cirrhosis and in noncirrhotic patients: epidemiology and predictive factors of mortality in a prospective multicenter population-based study. J Clin Gastroenterol 2005; 39(4):321–327.
15. Abraldes JG, Villanueva C, Banares R, Aracil C, Catalina MV, Garci A-P et al. Hepatic venous pressure gradient and prognosis in patients with acute variceal bleeding treated with pharmacologic and endoscopic therapy. J Hepatol 2008; 48(2):229–236.
16. Augustin S, Muntaner L, Altamirano JT, Gonzalez A, Saperas E, Dot J et al. Predicting early mortality after acute variceal hemorrhage based on classification and regression tree analysis. Clin Gastroenterol Hepatol 2009; 7(12):1347–1354.
17. Villanueva C, Piqueras M, Aracil C, Gomez C, Lopez-Balaguer JM, Gonzalez B et al. A randomized controlled trial comparing ligation and sclerotherapy as emergency endoscopic treatment added to somatostatin in acute variceal bleeding. J Hepatol 2006; 45(4):560–567.
18. Bosch J, Thabut D, Albillos A, Carbonell N, Spicak J, Massard J et al. Recombinant factor VIIa for variceal bleeding in patients with advanced cirrhosis: A randomized, controlled trial. Hepatology 2008;47(5): 1604–1614.
19. El-Serag HB, Everhart JE. Improved survival after variceal hemorrhage over an 11-year period in the Department of Veterans Affairs. Am J Gastroenterol 2000; 95:3566–3573.
20. Bosch J, Garcia-Pagan JC. Prevention of variceal rebleeding. Lancet 2003; 361(9361):952–954.
21. Groszmann RJ, Glickmann MM, Blei A, Storer EH, Conn HO. Wedged and free hepatic venous pressure

measured with a balloon catheter. Gastroenterology 1979; 76(2):253–258.
22. Groszmann RJ, Wongcharatrawee S. The hepatic venous pressure gradient: Anything worth doing should be done right. Hepatology 2004; 39(2):280–283.
23. Bosch J, Garcia-Pagan JC, Berzigotti A, Abraldes JG. Measurement of portal pressure and its role in the management of chronic liver disease. Semin Liver Dis 2006; 26(4):348–362.
24. Villanueva C, Aracil C, Colomo A, Hernandez-Gea V, Lopez-Balaguer JM, Alvarez-Urturi C et al. Acute hemodynamic response to beta-blockers and prediction of long-term outcome in primary prophylaxis of variceal bleeding. Gastroenterology 2009; 137(1): 119–128.
25. Garcia-Tsao G, Groszmann RJ, Fisher RL, Conn HO, Atterbury CE, Glickman M. Portal pressure, presence of gastroesophageal varices and variceal bleeding. Hepatology 1985; 5(3):419–424.
26. Groszmann RJ, Bosch J, Grace N, Conn HO, Garcia-Tsao G, Navasa M et al. Hemodynamic events in a prospective randomized trial of propranolol vs placebo in the prevention of the first variceal hemorrhage. Gastroenterology 1990; 99(5):1401–1407.
27. Feu F, Garcia-Pagan JC, Bosch J, Luca A, Teres J, Escorsell A et al. Relation between portal pressure response to pharmacotherapy and risk of recurrent variceal haemorrhage in patients with cirrhosis. Lancet 1995; 346:1056–1059.
28. D'Amico G, Garcia-Pagan JC, Luca A, Bosch J. HVPG reduction and prevention of variceal bleeding in cirrhosis. A systematic review. Gastroenterology 2006; 131:1611–1624.
29. Moitinho E, Escorsell A, Bandi JC, Salmeron JM, Garcia-Pagan JC, Rodes J et al. Prognostic value of early measurements of portal pressure in acute variceal bleeding. Gastroenterology 1999; 117:626–631.
30. Monescillo A, Martinez-Lagares F, Ruiz-del-Arbol L, Sierra A, Guevara C, Jimenez E et al. Influence of portal hypertension and its early decompression by TIPS placement on the outcome of variceal bleeding. Hepatology 2004; 40(4):793–801.
31. Perello A, Escorsell A, Bru C, Gilabert R, Moitinho E, Garcia-Pagan JC et al. Wedged hepatic venous pressure adequately reflects portal pressure in hepatitis C virus-related cirrhosis. Hepatology 1999; 30: 1393–1397.
32. de Franchis R, Pascal JP, Burroughs AK, Henderson JM, Fleig W, Groszmann RJ et al. Definitions, methodology and therapeutic strategies in portal hypertension. A Consensus Development Workshop. J Hepatol 1992; 15:256–261.
33. Giannini E, Botta F, Borro P, Risso D, Romagnoli P, Fasoli A et al. Platelet count/spleen diameter ratio: proposal and validation of a non-invasive parameter to predict the presence of oesophageal varices in patients with liver cirrhosis. Gut 2003; 52(8):1200–1205.
34. D'Amico G, Morabito A. Noninvasive markers of esophageal varices: another round, not the last. Hepatology 2004; 39(1):30–34.
35. de Franchis R. Non-invasive (and minimally invasive) diagnosis of oesophageal varices. J Hepatol 2008; 49(4):520–527.
36. de Franchis R, Eisen GM, Laine L, Fernandez-Urien I, Herrerias JM, Brown RD et al. Esophageal capsule endoscopy for screening and surveillance of esophageal varices in patients with portal hypertension. Hepatology 2008; 47(5):1595–1603.
37. Castera L, Le Bail B, Roudot-Thoraval F, Bernard PH, Foucher J, Merrouche W et al. Early detection in routine clinical practice of cirrhosis and oesophageal varices in chronic hepatitis C: comparison of transient elastography (FibroScan) with standard laboratory tests and non-invasive scores. J Hepatol 2009; 50(1):59–68.
38. Kim SH, Kim YJ, Lee JM, Choi KD, Chung YJ, Han JK et al. Esophageal varices in patients with cirrhosis: multidetector CT esophagography – comparison with endoscopy. Radiology 2007; 242(3):759–768.
39. Lapalus MG, Ben Soussan E, Gaudric M, Saurin JC, D'Halluin PN, Favre O et al. Esophageal capsule endoscopy vs. EGD for the evaluation of portal hypertension: a French prospective multicenter comparative study. Am J Gastroenterol 2009; 104(5): 1112–1118.
40. Ladas SD, Triantafyllou K, Spada C, Riccioni ME, Rey JF, Niv Y et al. European Society of Gastrointestinal Endoscopy (ESGE): recommendations (2009) on clinical use of video capsule endoscopy to investigate small-bowel, esophageal and colonic diseases. Endoscopy 2010; 42(3):220–227.
41. Blei AT, Garcia-Tsao G, Groszmann RJ, Kahrilas P, Ganger D, Fung HL. Hemodynamic evaluation of isosorbide dinitrate in alcoholic cirrhosis: Pharmacokinetic-hemodynamic interactions. Gastroenterology 1987; 93:576–583.
42. Gonzalez-Abraldes J, Albillos A, Banares R, Ruiz del Arbol L, Moitinho E, Rodriguez C et al. Randomized comparison of long-term losartan versus propranolol in lowering portal pressure in cirrhosis. Gastroenterology 2001; 121:382–388.
43. Schepke M, Werner E, Biecker E, Schiedermaier P, Heller J, Neef M et al. Hemodynamic effects of the angiotensin II receptor antagonist irbesartan in patients with cirrhosis and portal hypertension. Gastroenterology 2001; 121:389–395.
44. Abraldes JG, Albillos A, Banares R, Turnes J, Gonzalez R, Garcia-Pagan JC et al. Simvastatin lowers portal pressure in patients with cirrhosis and portal hypertension: a randomized controlled trial. Gastroenterology 2009; 136(5):1651–1658.
45. Groszmann RJ, Kravetz D, Bosch J, Glickman M, Bruix J, Bredfeldt JE et al. Nitroglycerin improves the hemodynamic response to vasopressin in portal hypertension. Hepatology 1982; 2:757–762.
46. Garcia-Pagan JC, Feu F, Bosch J, Rodes J. Propranolol compared with propranolol plus isosorbide-5-mononitrate for portal hypertension in cirrhosis. A randomized controlled study. Ann Intern Med 1991; 114:869–873.

47. Banares R, Moitinho E, Matilla A, Garcia-Pagan JC, Lampreave JL, Piera C et al. Randomized comparison of long-term carvedilol and propranolol administration in the treatment of portal hypertension in cirrhosis. Hepatology 2002; 36(6):1367–1373.
48. Sarin SK, Groszmann RJ, Mosca PG, Rojkind M, Stadecker MJ, Reuben A et al. Propranolol ameliorates the development of portal-systemic shunting in a chronic murine schistosomiasis model of portal hypertension. J Clin Invest 1991; 87:1032–1036.
49. D'Amico G, Pagliaro L, Bosch J. The treatment of portal hypertension: A meta-analytic review. Hepatology 1995; 22(1):332–354.
50. D'Amico G, Pagliaro L, Bosch J. Pharmacological treatment of portal hypertension: an evidence-based approach. Sem Liv Dis 1999; 19:475–505.
51. Perez-Ayuso RM, Pique JP, Bosch J, Panes J, Gonzalez A, Perez R et al. Propranolol in prevention of recurrent bleeding from severe portal hypertensive gastropathy in cirrhosis. Lancet 1991; 337:1431–1434.
52. Turnes J, Garcia-Pagan JC, Abraldes JG, Hernandez-Guerra M, Dell'era A, Bosch J. Pharmacological reduction of portal pressure and long-term risk of first variceal bleeding in patients with cirrhosis. Am J Gastroenterol 2006; 101(3):506–512.
53. Hernandez-Gea V, Colomo A, Aracil C, Concepcion M, Poca MC, Torras X et al. Relationship between changes in portal pressure and development of ascites in cirrhotic patients with severe portal hypertension. Hepatology 50[4 (Suppl)], 313A. 2009.Ref Type: Abstract
54. Garcia-Tsao G, Grace N, Groszmann RJ, Conn HO, Bermann MM, Patrick MJ et al. Short term effects of propranolol on portal venous pressure. Hepatology 1986; 6:101–106.
55. Abraczinkas DR, Ookubo R, Grace ND, Groszmann RJ, Bosch J, Garcia-Tsao G et al. Propranolol for the prevention of first variceal hemorrhage: A lifetime commitment? Hepatology 2001; 34:1096–1102.
56. Longacre AV, Imaeda A, Garcia-Tsao G, Fraenkel L. A pilot project examining the predicted preferences of patients and physicians in the primary prophylaxis of variceal hemorrhage. Hepatology 2008; 47: 169–176.
57. Tripathi D, Ferguson JW, Kochar N, Leithead JA, Therapondos G, McAvoy NC et al. Randomized controlled trial of carvedilol versus variceal band ligation for the prevention of the first variceal bleed. Hepatology 2009; 50(3):825–833.
58. Bosch J, Garcia-Tsao G. Pharmacological versus endoscopic therapy in the prevention of variceal hemorrhage: and the winner is.. Hepatology 2009; 50(3):674–677.
59. Laine L, Cook D. Endoscopic ligation compared with sclerotherapy for treatment of esophageal variceal bleeding. A meta-analysis. Ann Intern Med 1995; 123:280–287.
60. Khuroo MS, Khuroo NS, Farahat KL, Khuroo YS, Sofi AA, Dahab ST. Meta-analysis: endoscopic variceal ligation for primary prophylaxis of oesophageal variceal bleeding. Aliment Pharmacol Ther 2005; 21(4):347–361.
61. Garcia-Pagan JC, Bosch J. Endoscopic band ligation in the treatment of portal hypertension. Nat Clin Pract Gastroenterol Hepatol 2005; 2(11):526–535.
62. Gluud LL, Klingenberg S, Nikolova D, Gluud C. Banding ligation versus beta-blockers as primary prophylaxis in esophageal varices: systematic review of randomized trials. Am J Gastroenterol 2007; 102(12):2842–2848.
63. Shaheen NJ, Stuart E, Schmitz SM, Mitchell KL, Fried MW, Zacks S et al. Pantoprazole reduces the size of postbanding ulcers after variceal band ligation: a randomized, controlled trial. Hepatology 2005; 41(3):588–594.
64. Merkel C, Marin R, Angeli P, Zanella P, Felder M, Bernardinello E et al. A placebo-controlled clinical trial of nadolol in the prophylaxis of growth of small esophageal varices in cirrhosis. Gastroenterology 2004; 127(2):476–484.
65. Chalasani N, Kahi C, Francois F, Pinto A, Marathe A, Bini EJ et al. Improved patient survival after acute variceal bleeding: a multicenter, cohort study. Am J Gastroenterol 2003; 98(3):653–659.
66. Carbonell N, Pauwels A, Serfaty L, Fourdan O, Levy VG, Poupon R. Improved survival after variceal bleeding in patients with cirrhosis over the past two decades. Hepatology 2004; 40(3):652–659.
67. Stokkeland K, Brandt L, Ekbom A, Hultcrantz R. Improved prognosis for patients hospitalized with esophageal varices in Sweden 1969-2002. Hepatology 2006; 43(3):500–505.
68. Colomo A, Hernandez-Gea V, Muniz-Diaz E, Madoz P, Aracil C, Alvarez-Urturi C et al. Transfusion strategies in patients with cirrhosis and acute gastrointestinal bleeding. Hepatology 48[4 (Suppl)], 413A. 2008. Ref Type: Abstract
69. Bernard B, Grange JD, Khac EN, Amiot X, Opolon P, Poynard T. Antibiotic prophylaxis for the prevention of bacterial infections in cirrhotic patients with gastrointestinal bleeding: a meta-analysis. Hepatology 1999; 29:1655–1661.
70. Hou MC, Lin HC, Liu TT, Kuo BI, Lee FY, Chang FY et al. Antibiotic prophylaxis after endoscopic therapy prevents rebleeding in acute variceal hemorrhage: a randomized trial. Hepatology 2004; 39(3): 746–753.
71. Rimola A, Garcia-Tsao G, Navasa M, Piddock LJV, Planas R, Bernard B et al. Diagnosis, treatment and prophylaxis of spontaneous bacterial peritonitis: a consensus document. J Hepatol 2000; 32:142–153.
72. Fernandez J, Ruiz dA, Gomez C, Durandez R, Serradilla R, Guarner C et al. Norfloxacin vs ceftriaxone in the prophylaxis of infections in patients with advanced cirrhosis and hemorrhage. Gastroenterology 2006; 131(4):1049–1056.
73. D'Amico G, Pietrosi G, Tarantino I, Pagliaro L. Emergency sclerotherapy versus vasoactive drugs for variceal bleeding in cirrhosis: a Cochrane meta-analysis. Gastroenterology 2003; 124(5):1277–1291.

74. Ioannou GN, Doust J, Rockey DC. Systematic review: terlipressin in acute oesophageal variceal haemorrhage. Aliment Pharmacol Ther 2003; 17(1):53–64.
75. Escorsell A, Ruiz del Arbol L, Planas R, Albillos A, Banares R, Cales P et al. Multicenter randomized controlled trial of terlipressin versus sclerotherapy in the treatment of acute variceal bleeding: the TEST study. Hepatology 2000; 32:471–476.
76. Escorsell A, Bandi JC, Andreu V, Moitinho E, Garcia-Pagan JC, Bosch J et al. Desensitization to the effects of intravenous octreotide in cirrhotic patients with portal hypertension. Gastroenterology 2001; 120: 161–169.
77. Banares R, Albillos A, Rincon D, Alonso S, Gonzalez M, Ruiz-del-Arbol L et al. Endoscopic treatment versus endoscopic plus pharmacologic treatment for acute variceal bleeding: a meta-analysis. Hepatology 2002; 35:609–615.
78. Cales P, Masliah C, Bernard B, Garnier PP, Silvain C, Szostak-Talbodec N et al. Early administration of vapreotide for variceal bleeding in patients with cirrhosis. N Engl J Med 2001; 344:23–28.
79. Ramirez FC, Colon VJ, Landan D, Grade AJ, Evanich E. The effects of the number of rubber bands placed at each endoscopic session upon variceal outcomes: a prospective, randomized study. Am J Gastroenterol 2007; 102(7):1372–1376.
80. Garcia-Pagan JC, Caca K, Bureau C, Laleman W, Appenrodt B, Luca A et al. Early use of TIPS in patients with cirrhosis and variceal bleeding. N Engl J Med. 2010; 362(25):2370–2379.
81. Hubmann R, Bodlaj G, Czompo M, Benko L, Pichler P, Al Kathib S et al. The use of self-expanding metal stents to treat acute esophageal variceal bleeding. Endoscopy 2006; 38(9):896–901.
82. Wright G, Lewis H, Hogan B, Burroughs A, Patch D, O'Beirne J. A self-expanding metal stent for complicated variceal hemorrhage: experience at a single center. Gastrointest Endosc 2010; 71(1):71–78.
83. Gournay J, Masliah C, Martin T, Perrin D, Galmiche JP. Isosorbide mononitrate and propranolol compared with propranolol alone for the prevention of variceal rebleeding. Hepatology 2000; 31:1239–1245.
84. Lo GH, Chen WC, Lin CK, Tsai WL, Chan HH, Chen TA et al. Improved survival in patients receiving medical therapy as compared with banding ligation for the prevention of esophageal variceal rebleeding. Hepatology 2008; 48(2):580–587.
85. Gonzalez R, Zamora J, Gomez-Camarero J, Molinero LM, Banares R, Albillos A. Meta-analysis: Combination endoscopic and drug therapy to prevent variceal rebleeding in cirrhosis. Ann Intern Med 2008; 149(2):109–122.
86. Lo GH, Lai KH, Cheng JS, Chen MH, Huang HC, Hsu PI et al. Endoscopic variceal ligation plus nadolol and sucralfate compared with ligation alone for the prevention of variceal rebleeding: a prospective, randomized trial. Hepatology 2000; 32:461–465.
87. de la PJ, Brullet E, Sanchez-Hernandez E, Rivero M, Vergara M, Martin-Lorente JL et al. Variceal ligation plus nadolol compared with ligation for prophylaxis of variceal rebleeding: a multicenter trial. Hepatology 2005; 41(3):572–578.
88. Villanueva C, Minana J, Ortiz J, Gallego A, Soriano G, Torras X et al. Endoscopic ligation compared with combined treatment with nadolol and isosorbide mononitrate to prevent recurrent variceal bleeding. N Engl J Med 2001; 345:647–655.
89. Patch D, Goulis J, Gerunda G, Greenslade L, Merkel C, Burroughs AK. A randomized controlled trial of medical therapy versus endoscopic ligation for the prevention of variceal rebleeding in patients with cirrhosis. Gastroenterology 2002; 123: 1013–1019.
90. Lo G-H, Chen W-C, Chen M-H, Hsu P-I, Lin C-K, Tsai W-L et al. A prospective, randomized trial of endoscopic variceal ligation versus nadolol and isosorbide mononitrate for the prevention of esophageal variceal rebleeding. Gastroenterology 2002; 123:728–734.
91. Romero G, Kravetz D, Argonz J, Vulcano C, Suarez A, Fassio E et al. Comparative study between nadolol and 5-isosorbide mononitrate vs. endoscopic band ligation plus sclerotherapy in the prevention of variceal rebleeding in cirrhotic patients: a randomized controlled trial. Aliment Pharmacol Ther 2006; 24(4):601–611.
92. Garcia-Pagan JC, Villanueva C, Albillos A, Banares R, Morillas R, Abraldes JG et al. Nadolol plus isosorbide mononitrate alone or associated with band ligation in the prevention of variceal rebleeding: A multicenter randomized controlled trial. Gut 2009; 58(8):1144–1150.
93. Kumar A, Jha SK, Sharma P, Dubey S, Tyagi P, Sharma BC et al. Addition of propranolol and isosorbide mononitrate to endoscopic variceal ligation does not reduce variceal rebleeding incidence. Gastroenterology 2009; 137(3):892–901, 901.
94. Luca A, D'Amico G, LaGalla R, Midiri M, Morabito A, Pagliaro L. TIPS for prevention of recurrent bleeding in patients with cirrhosis: meta-analysis of randomized clinical trials. Radiology 1999; 212: 411–421.
95. Papatheodoridis GV, Goulis J, Leandro G, Patch D, Burroughs AK. Transjugular intrahepatic portsystemic shunt compared with endoscopic treatment for prevention of variceal rebleeding. A meta-analysis. Hepatology 1999; 30:612–622.
96. Villanueva C, Aracil C, Colomo A, Lopez-Balaguer JM, Piqueras M, Gonzalez B et al. Clinical trial: a randomized controlled study on prevention of variceal rebleeding comparing nadolol + ligation vs. hepatic venous pressure gradient-guided pharmacological therapy. Aliment Pharmacol Ther 2009; 29(4): 397–408.
97. La Mura V, Abraldes JG, Raffa S, Retto O, Berzigotti A, Garcia-Pagan JC et al. Prognostic value of acute hemodynamic response to i.v. propranolol in patients with cirrhosis and portal hypertension. J Hepatol 2009; 51(2):279–287.

Portal Vein Thrombosis

12

Dominique-Charles Valla

Abstract

Portal vein obstruction is a common finding at necropsy where it is usually related to cirrhosis or malignancy of abdominal organs. Noncirrhotic, nonmalignant portal vein thrombosis is uncommon. The main risk factors for noncirrhotic nonmalignant portal vein thrombosis are inflammatory foci in the abdomen, abdominal surgery (particularly splenectomy), myeloproliferative diseases, and factor II gene mutation. Acute portal vein thrombosis usually manifests itself with abdominal pain and a systemic inflammatory reaction. In the most severe forms of acute portal vein thrombosis intestinal infarction may occur. Chronic portal thrombosis is characterized by cavernomatous transformation, and is associated with portal hypertension. Diagnosis is based on a high degree of clinical suspicion, and findings at imaging with CT or Doppler ultrasound. Recognition of underlying myeloproliferative disease has been facilitated by testing for V617F JAK2 mutation in peripheral blood. Therapy for acute portal vein thrombosis is based on early anticoagulation, which prevents extension of the thrombus in most patients, but achieves recanalization in less than 40% of them. Treatment for chronic portal vein thrombosis consists of pharmacological or endoscopic prophylaxis of bleeding from portal hypertension. Surgery can also be done in selected cases. Anticoagulation is logical in patients with underlying high-risk thrombophilia. Some findings suggest that anticoagulation could be of clinical benefit without increasing the risk of bleeding from portal hypertension.

Keywords

Venous thrombosis • Myeloproliferative disorders • Blood coagulation disorders • Anticoagulants.

Introduction

Portal vein thrombosis (PVT) is the development of a thrombus in the main portal vein or its right or left branches or the development of sequelae

D.-C. Valla (✉)
Hépatologie, Hopital Beaujon, APHP;
Université Denis, Diderot-Paris 7; and INSERM U773,
100 Bvd Leclerc, 92118 Clichy, France
e-mail: dominique.valla@bjn.ap-hop-paris.fr

L.D. DeLeve and G. Garcia-Tsao (eds.), *Vascular Liver Disease: Mechanisms and Management*,
DOI 10.1007/978-1-4419-8327-5_12, © Springer Science+Business Media, LLC 2011

of PVT, such as portal cavenomatosis. Generally, the early stage of recent thrombosis is referred to as "acute PVT," while the stage in which only sequelae are observed is referred to as "chronic PVT." As a rule, in the chronic stage the thrombus is no longer recognizable. Therefore, the term "extrahepatic portal vein obstruction" is preferred to chronic PVT [1]. The terms "portal cavernoma," or "carvernomatous transformation of the portal vein," which depict the multiple venous channels that develop as a consequence of portal vein obstruction, are equivalent to chronic PVT or to extrahepatic portal vein obstruction. However, it is recognized that mechanisms other than thrombosis might explain obstruction of the portal vein and development of a cavernoma, particularly in children. Invasion of the portal venous lumen by a malignant tumor is often referred to as "malignant thrombus" or "tumor thrombus," improper terminology that will not be used here.

Epidemiology, Demographics and Etiology

Prevalence

Although generally regarded as a rare disease, PVT was found to affect 1.0% of the general population between 1970 and 1982 in a Swedish autopsy registry [2]. PVT was associated with hepatobiliary malignancy in almost half the patients, and with cirrhosis in a quarter of patients. A strong association with malignancy or with cirrhosis has also been found in a large multicenter study of unselected Dutch patients admitted for PVT between 1984 and 1997 [3], and in a recent report from India [4]. These studies do not distinguish between mere thrombosis associated with malignancy and malignant invasion of the portal vein with certainty, an issue of practical importance.

In developing countries in the late nineties, extrahepatic portal vein obstruction accounted for more than half the children with portal hypertension and for 85% of those with gastrointestinal bleeding [5].

Demographics

In adults, males and females appear to be almost equally affected [2, 3, 6]. The average age was about 70 years in the necropsy registry [2], 50 years in unselected hospitalized patients [3], and only 40 years in patients without cirrhosis or malignant invasion [6].

Etiology

Among malignant diseases, primary tumors of the liver, bile ducts or pancreas, and adenocarcinoma metastatic to the liver are most commonly associated with portal venous obstruction [2, 3]. Studies in patients with hepatocellular carcinoma indicate that malignant invasion of the lumen accounts for most, but not all, cases of obstruction of the portal vein, the rest being related to mere thrombosis [7]. A contribution of genetic risk factors to the development of PVT in patients with hepatocellular carcinoma has been recently suggested [8].

Cirrhosis, in the absence of hepatocellular carcinoma, appears to facilitate the development of PVT by decreasing portal venous flow [9]. Underlying genetic risk factors for thrombosis, particularly the prothrombin gene mutation, likely exacerbate the potential for PVT in cirrhotic patients [10–14]. The association with decreased portal blood flow likely underlies the well-established relationship between the incidence of PVT and the severity of liver disease. The role of changes in the levels of coagulation inhibitors and antiphospholipid antibodies secondary to liver disease remains unclear. In patients with cirrhosis, surgery, portosystemic shunting, splenectomy and endoscopic therapy have been incriminated. However, it is difficult to ascertain whether these interventions are direct causal factors or only reflect the severity of portal hypertension and decreased portal blood flow [10, 11]. Patients with noncirrhotic intrahepatic portal hypertension [15, 16] or with Budd–Chiari syndrome [17] are at a high risk of PVT, which is probably related both to decreased portal blood flow and to the underlying causes for these conditions, such as prothrombotic disorders [16].

In the absence of cirrhosis and malignant tumors, PVT is associated with general prothrombotic conditions and with local factors for thrombosis. Myeloproliferative diseases represent the most common of these general conditions, accounting for about 25% of the cases in the absence of cirrhosis and malignant invasion [18–20]. The availability of V617F JAK2 mutation testing in circulating granulocytes has represented a major advance for diagnosing the myeloproliferative disease in a context where portal hypertension and hypersplenism mask the usual features of myeloproliferation in peripheral blood [18–20]. However, in patients with a negative test for the V617F JAK2 mutation, a myeloproliferative disease is still possible and a bone marrow biopsy is needed for diagnosis [18–20]. Among inherited prothrombotic disorders, the strongest and best documented association is with the prothrombin gene mutation and, less strongly, with factor V Leiden mutation [13]. The association with inherited protein C, protein S or antithrombin deficiency, or hyperhomocysteinemia has been difficult to assess because PVT per se induces changes in the plasma levels of these substances even in the absence of obvious liver disease [21–24]. Homozygous M677T polymorphism in the methylene tetrahydrofolate reductase gene appears to play a limited or no role [14, 22]. Increased factor VIII levels are likely implicated, independent of an inflammatory state [25]. In contrast to their impact on hepatic vein thrombosis or venous thromboembolism, oral contraceptives have not been found to be a significant risk factor for PVT [22–24]. The concurrence of several prothrombotic disorders in a patient with PVT is more frequent than expected in the general population [22, 24]. Thus, the identification of a single risk factor for thrombosis does not exclude other factors.

Local factors for PVT mainly comprise inflammatory conditions (such as appendicitis, diverticulitis, pancreatitis, inflammatory bowel disease [26] or acute cytomegalovirus hepatitis [27]), trauma, and surgery, particularly when these factors affect intraperitoneal organs [28, 29]. However, local factors are found in only about 25–35% of patients with PVT unrelated to cirrhosis or malignancy, even when they are investigated at the early stage [28, 30]. Thus, in 70% of the patients, the reason for thrombosis development in the portal vein remains unexplained. Splenectomy is a particularly high risk for PVT when the operation is performed in patients with hemolytic anemia or myeloproliferative disease [31]. General risk factors for venous thrombosis are present in a majority of patients developing PVT after laparoscopic surgery; it remains unknown whether the risk of postoperative PVT with the laparoscopic approach differs from open laparotomy [32]. Septic pylephlebitis, characterized by an infected thrombus, is usually associated with *Bacteroides* or *Fusobacterium* bacteremia even in the absence of detectable local inflammatory focus [28, 33, 34].

Work-Up for Causes

The data summarized above have formed the basis for the following AASLD practice guideline recommendations [35]. Search for a local factor, including cirrhosis, malignancy and inflammatory focus, should be the first step in elucidating the cause for PVT. For this purpose, taking a history and reviewing CT scan or sonographic images is crucial. In patients with abnormal liver tests or a dysmorphic liver at imaging [36, 37], a diagnosis of cirrhosis can be difficult to rule out without performing a liver biopsy. Obliterative portal venopathy or related microvascular changes should always be considered [16]. In the absence of advanced cirrhosis or cancer, multiple, concurrent risk factors for thrombosis should be checked in all patients as indicated in Table 12.1. A diagnosis of myeloproliferative disease should not be ruled out solely on the basis of normal or low peripheral blood cell counts. When coagulation factor levels are decreased, low levels of protein C, protein S or antithrombin, should be considered as a possible consequence of liver dysfunction [35].

Table 12.1 Proposed work-up for investigating causes of portal vein thrombosis

In all patients
Personal and familial history of recurrent spontaneous deep vein thrombosis
Personal history of abdominal disease and operation
CT scan of the abdomen and pelvis for detection of inflammatory foci or tumors; or hepatic, biliary, or pancreatic disease
V617F JAK 2 mutation in peripheral blood granulocytes. When the mutation is undetected, bone marrow biopsy looking for clusters of dystrophic megacaryocytes (myeloproliferative diseases)
Flow cytometry for CD55 and CD59 deficient blood cells (paroxysmal nocturnal hemoglobinuria)
Activated protein C resistance. When available, molecular test for Factor V Leiden mutation
Molecular test for G20210A prothrombin gene mutation
Lupus anticoagulant, antibeta2 glycoprotein-1 antibodies, anticardiolipin antibodies (antiphospholipid syndrome)
In patients without marked liver dysfunction (normal prothrombin level)
Protein C, protein S and antithrombin plasma levels
Plasma homocysteine levels
In patients with familial or personal history of recurrent spontaneous deep vein thrombosis: refer to blood coagulation specialist for a detailed study

PVT Unrelated to Cirrhosis or Malignancy

Manifestations, Course and Diagnosis

The proportion of patients in whom the disease is recognized at the early stage of acute PVT has steadily increased with time [28]. This is obviously due to the increased availability of accurate imaging studies (sonography and CT scan) that can be performed on an emergency basis in the workup of abdominal pain.

Acute Portal Vein Thrombosis

There is some evidence that the severity of manifestations is related to the extent of the thrombus in the mesenteric veins. Furthermore, acute mesenteric arterial vasoconstriction that accompanies the abrupt interruption of mesenteric venous flow [38] likely plays a role in causing intestinal ischemia and infarction.

Clinical Features

Acute PVT can probably develop with no or with nonspecific signs and symptoms, as the disease has been frequently diagnosed fortuitously only at the chronic stage [29]. Abdominal pain and the systemic inflammatory syndrome are most characteristic [30]. Pain is of abrupt or progressive onset, usually severe, and lasts for several days in the absence of treatment, often radiating to the back. The absence of guarding contrasting with the severity of pain suggests acute PVT. Features of the inflammatory syndrome (fever, increased CRP) are very common even in the absence of an inflammatory focus. A spiking fever with chills suggests associated bacteremia. Abdominal distention due to ileus is usual. When a local factor is present (e.g., pancreatitis, appendicitis, diverticulitis or recent surgery), its manifestations may or may not be easily distinguished from those of acute PVT.

When the disease progresses to a more severe stage of intestinal ischemia, persistent and severe pain is associated with diarrhea and hematochezia. Frank ascites is often present. Further progression to the stage of intestinal necrosis is usually accompanied by signs of peritonitis and multiorgan failure. The mortality of intestinal infarction of venous origin is extremely high.

With current therapy (see below), the progression of thrombosis can be halted in most patients. It may take several days, however, for abdominal pain to abate, during which time high doses of narcotics may be needed. Spontaneous recanalization appears to be uncommon although there is scarce data on this crucial point [28, 39].

Laboratory Features

Except at the advanced stage, laboratory tests are often unremarkable or related to the underlying disease (e.g., myeloproliferative disease), and to the nonspecific inflammatory syndrome [30]. A transient moderate increase in serum aminotransferases can be seen in some patients. Blood cultures should be performed routinely, particularly, but not exclusively, for the isolation of *Bacteroides* or *Fusobacterium* species.

Imaging Features

Imaging with sonography, computed tomography (CT) or magnetic resonance (MR) is central to the diagnosis and management of acute PVT [40–46]. Sonography can show hyperechoic material in the vessel lumen with distension of the portal vein and its tributaries. Doppler imaging shows the absence of flow in part or all of the lumen. CT scan without contrast can show hyperattenuating material in the portal vein. After contrast, lack of luminal enhancement, increased hepatic enhancement in the arterial phase, and decreased hepatic enhancement in the portal phase are shown. For the assessment of thrombus extension within the portal venous system, CT or MR angiography are more sensitive techniques than Doppler sonography, because the mesenteric veins are more difficult to visualize ultrasonographically. Thinning of the intestinal wall, or lack of mucosal enhancement of a thickened intestinal wall after intravenous contrast injection, is further evidence of intestinal infarction. Enlargement of preexisting veins in the porta hepatis is seen as early as a few days after the onset of acute PVT. This is particularly conspicuous in the gallbladder wall, which is thickened and enhances after contrast injection, and which should not be confused with acute cholecystitis.

Diagnosis

A diagnosis of acute PVT should always be considered in a patient with persistent recent abdominal pain [35]. Only when the portal vein is clearly patent can the diagnosis be ruled out. Imaging can be based on CT, preferably with and without contrast, or Doppler sonography [35]. Progression to intestinal ischemia and infarction should be suspected with persistent pain, particularly when ascites is present [35].

Chronic Portal Vein Thrombosis

In the absence of early recanalization of the thrombosed portal vein, permanent obliteration ensues and a network of collateral hepatopetal veins develops and enlarges with time. This network connects the patent portions of the portal venous system upstream and downstream from the obstruction. It consists mainly of enlarged preexisting veins. Resistance of these collaterals is greater than that of the normal portal vein, thus causing portal hypertension when the main portal vein or both its left and right branches are occluded. Based on animal models [38] and clinical data, hepatic and mesenteric arterial blood flows increase thereby explaining the absence of significant liver injury.

Clinical Features

Gastrointestinal hemorrhage related to ruptured gastroesophageal varices had been the most frequent mode of presentation in the past. Variceal hemorrhage may occur as early as 1 year following acute PVT [39] and its natural history is unpredictable. It seems to be better tolerated than in other forms of portal hypertension probably because patients are usually younger and liver function is normal. In the absence of a bleeding episode, cirrhosis, or malignancy, symptoms are usually absent. Still, chronic abdominal pain has been described in association with intestinal stenosis (a likely sequela of a previous ischemic lesion) [47] and postprandial pain suggesting intestinal ischemia has also been reported [48].

Physical signs are usually limited to splenomegaly which is a finding that commonly leads to its diagnosis. Transient and easy-to-treat ascites or encephalopathy may occur following a bleeding episode. In asymptomatic patients, subclinical (minimal) encephalopathy and stage 1 ascites can be present [49, 50].

In patients with long standing cavernoma, portal cholangiopathy (also called portal biliopathy or portal hypertensive biliopathy) may develop [51–53]. This entity is characterized by stenosis and dilatation of intra- or extrahepatic bile ducts, related to the compression of bile ducts by the cavernomatous veins. While evidence of cholangiopathy is almost always present at imaging, clinical manifestations are rare. They consist mainly of biliary pain, cholecystitis and cholangitis; rarely with jaundice. An unusual form of portal cholangiopathy, so-called tumor-like cavernoma, may mimic cholangiocarcinoma and produce progressive cholestasis [51, 53].

Laboratory and Hemodynamic Features

Blood cell counts are variably altered, while some patients demonstrate marked hypersplenism others have normal blood cell counts. In the latter, a diagnosis of underlying myeloproliferative disease should be strongly considered when there is splenomegaly and evidence of portal hypertension [54]. A fortuitous finding of hypersplenism has become a common reason in the identification of the disease.

Liver tests are typically normal in patients with chronic PVT. However, a mild to moderate decrease in the levels of coagulation factors and inhibitors is common and likely related to subtle liver dysfunction [21, 22]. Features of cholestasis should raise a suspicion of portal cholangiopathy/biliopathy, but the absence of cholestatic features does not rule out this condition.

Patients with prehepatic portal hypertension manifest a hyperkinetic circulatory syndrome similar to the one present in patients with cirrhosis [55]. In patients without underlying liver disease, hepatic venous pressure gradient is characteristically normal [56]. In India, hepatopulmonary syndrome was found to affect only 2% of patients, compared to 11% of patients with cirrhosis [57].

Imaging and Endoscopic Features

The typical features of portal cavernoma on Doppler sonography, CT scan or MRI are serpiginous structures in the area of the portal vein, with lack of visualization of the main portal vein and/or its main branches [43, 58, 59]. Hepatic arteries are usually enlarged. Even in the absence of cirrhosis, there might be an enlarged caudate lobe and an atrophic left lateral segment or right lobe of the liver [36, 37]. Typically, the umbilical vein is not dilated as it connects to the left portal vein branch downstream of the obstruction. In some patients a large, prominent collateral vein at the porta hepatis can be mistaken for a normal portal vein. A cavernoma develops in the pancreatic area when the confluence of the splenic vein and the superior mesenteric vein is obstructed, which might be confused with an enlarged pancreas [60]. Portal cholangiopathy/biliopathy, which mimics the bead-like appearance of primary sclerosing cholangitis [52] is much more commonly seen on biliary tract imaging than clinical or laboratory features of biliary disease would suggest [51, 53]. A tumor-like cavernoma is characterized by tiny collateral channels forming a mass that encases the main bile duct, and enhances at the portal phase of contrast injection [51]. Endosonography, MR angiography, and cholangiography may help in the differential diagnoses [61, 62].

Endoscopy shows the usual features of portal hypertension. Gastroesophageal varices may develop as early as 1 month after the initial episode of acute PVT [39]. At a mean follow-up of about 4 years after the initial episode, 65% of patients have developed varices [39].

Diagnosis

The classical presentation with variceal hemorrhage is currently uncommon in Western countries [6], whereas it remains frequent in India [4]. Most Western patients are diagnosed following a fortuitous finding of an enlarged spleen, decreased blood cell counts, gastroesophageal varices, or a portal cavernoma at an unrelated abdominal imaging. A diagnosis of chronic PVT should be considered in any patient with portal hypertension. Collateral veins are easily recognized by Doppler sonography or triphasic CT scan with and without contrast, particularly when an experienced operator is aware of the suspected diagnosis [35]. MRI, with and without contrast, is an alternative to CT scan. Abnormal liver morphology may occur in the absence of underlying liver disease, and a liver biopsy may be necessary to rule out not only cirrhosis, but also obliterative portal venopathy or other uncommon conditions.

In patients with biliary symptoms or cholestasis, MR cholangiography is the procedure of choice to establish a diagnosis of portal cholangiopathy/biliopathy [53]. In rare patients, when a tumor of the bile duct or pancreas cannot be ruled out, endosonography is needed.

Course and Prognosis

The most common complication of chronic PVT is variceal hemorrhage [3, 6, 29, 39]. Risk factors are similar to those identified in portal hypertension related to cirrhosis: previous bleeding [6, 29] and size of gastroesophageal varices [6]. The second most common complication is recurrent thrombosis, affecting extrasplanchnic or splanchnic veins [6, 29, 39]. An underlying prothrombotic disorder is a risk factor for recurrent thrombosis [6, 29, 39]. Biliary disease is much less common than the former two complications and its risk increases over time after diagnosis [51, 53]. Late intestinal stenoses appear to be uncommon [47]. Encephalopathy (even in patients with a minimal form at baseline) and ascites develop uncommonly [39, 50].

In Western series dating back to the end of the last millennium, overall outcome has been good in the absence of cirrhosis and malignancy [3, 6, 29]. Extension to the superior mesenteric vein is the only prognostic factor directly related to PVT [3, 29]. Otherwise, the underlying conditions, whether or not the cause of PVT, are the main prognostic factors [3, 6, 29, 39]. In this regard, the most common cause, myeloproliferative diseases, has the potential for transformation that jeopardizes the late outcome in affected patients [54].

Treatment

Except for treatment of the underlying disease, management of PVT differs according to whether the patient is seen at an acute or chronic stage. The discussion of treatment options for underlying blood disorders or local factors is beyond the scope of this chapter, although this aspect is of utmost importance. In many situations, close interaction with hematologists is required for optimal management. Some underlying prothrombotic diseases are amenable to specific treatment whereas others are controlled with antithrombotic or anticoagulant therapy. It is reasonable to assume that, as a rule, these treatments should be undertaken as soon as possible.

Acute Portal Vein Thrombosis

In this context, the recognition of a local factor should be considered an emergency and its treatment should be considered in conjunction with specific therapy for thrombosis, on an individual basis. Immediate consideration should also be given to the possible presence of sepsis. Indeed, recanalization of septic pylephlebitis has been reported with antibiotic therapy alone [63, 64].

Early anticoagulation therapy is recommended in recent expert consensus statements [65] and practice guidelines [35] based on limited retrospective data. In a recent prospective multicenter study, 95 patients with recent PVT were given anticoagulation, mostly heparin-based [30]. Data showed that early anticoagulation effectively prevented clot extension with recanalization occurring in only 30–40% of the patients [30]. Only two patients experienced a mesenteric infarction, which was nonlethal and required limited intestinal resection. There were five patients with nonlethal variceal hemorrhage requiring transfusion or specific therapy. One-year recanalization rate was 38% for the portal vein, 61% for the superior mesenteric vein and 54% for the splenic vein. At the end of follow-up, 40% of patients had developed a cavernoma. Factors predicting lack of recanalization were the combination of baseline splenic vein thrombosis and presence of abdominal fluid at baseline imaging. In their absence, recanalization occurred in 60% of patients. Thus these data support the recommendation for early anticoagulation in order to prevent thrombus extension. The virtual absence of recanalization reported in the limited number of patients not given anticoagulation also supports routine anticoagulation [28, 39]. High recanalization rates have also been reported in patients given anticoagulation therapy for post-splenectomy PVT [31] or for acute thrombosis involving the superior mesenteric vein [28, 63, 66, 67]. Early anticoagulation and low number of underlying prothrombotic conditions have been found to predict recanalization [39], although not in the prospective cohort [30]. The duration of anticoagulation therapy remains unsettled. While the portal vein does not appear to recanalize beyond 6 months of anticoagulation, it does occur in splenic and superior mesenteric vein thrombosis [30]. The rate of recanalization is not related to duration of anticoagulation [30]. Current recommendations are to maintain anticoagulation for at least 3 months [35, 65]. The presence of a permanent underlying prothrombotic condition should be taken into consideration in the decision to continue anticoagulation beyond 3 months [35, 65].

There is a clear need for a more effective therapy to achieve recanalization, particularly in patients predictably nonresponsive to anticoagulation. However, alternatives to anticoagulation therapy are currently limited. Thrombolytic therapy, delivered intraportally or in the superior mesenteric artery, does not appear to be more effective than systemic anticoagulation, but seems to be much riskier, with several reports of procedure-related death [68–71]. TIPS insertion with mechanical disruption of thrombi has been used [72], but more data are necessary.

When clinical and radiological features indicate that a patient has intestinal infarction, emergency laparotomy for resection of necrotic gut should be performed. The risk of postoperative malabsorption is related to the extent of intestinal resection. Moreover, the extent of irreversible lesions can be overestimated at gross inspection. Therefore, various procedures have been proposed to limit the extent of intestinal resection while addressing the risk of necrosis after operation [73]. This aspect is beyond the scope of the present chapter. Surgical thrombectomy can be performed at the time of the resection/laparotomy. Anticoagulation therapy appears to improve the survival of patients who undergo surgery.

Chronic Portal Vein Thrombosis

Therapy for chronic PVT consists of two different, and apparently conflicting, aspects, namely prevention of variceal hemorrhage and prevention of recurrent thrombosis. Treatment options for portal cholangiopathy/biliopathy will also be considered.

Prevention of Portal Hypertension-Related Bleeding

Randomized controlled trials are lacking. However, retrospective studies have shown a reduction in first or recurrent hemorrhage or even an improved survival when recommendations for cirrhotic portal hypertension are followed in this setting [6, 74–76]. Beta-blockers should be useful given the favorable hemodynamic effects of beta-adrenergic blockade in the rat model of prehepatic portal hypertension (partial portal vein ligation) [77–79]. In fact, in patients with prehepatic portal hypertension, where hepatic venous pressure gradient cannot be used to assess portosystemic pressure gradient, favorable effects of beta-blockers on azygos blood flow have been documented [80].

Endoscopic sclerotherapy has achieved eradication of varices and a reduction in the number of bleeding episodes in uncontrolled surveys [74, 76]. Data on endoscopic ligation are lacking and, even though variceal ligation is superior to sclerotherapy in cirrhotic portal hypertension, it is uncertain which therapy, ligation or beta-blockers, would be superior for the primary prophylaxis of variceal hemorrhage in chronic PVT.

Regarding prevention of recurrent hemorrhage, contrasting findings have been reported regarding the feasibility and outcome of surgical portosystemic shunting, which suggests differences in patient selection or referral [81, 82]. Data on splenectomy and devascularization are limited. There are reports of successful TIPS insertion in patients with a portal cavernoma in the absence of cirrhosis [72, 83]. However, this procedure is not technically feasible in most patients.

Thus, it has recently been recommended that in patients with chronic PVT guidelines for the management of portal hypertension in cirrhosis should be followed [35].

Prevention of Recurrent Thrombosis

Again, there has been no randomized controlled trial to study prevention of recurrent thrombosis in this rare condition. Most available data derive from a retrospective study of 136 adult patients, in which multivariate analysis was used to identify risk factors for bleeding and thrombosis [6]. Although results should be taken cautiously, this study showed that in patients receiving anticoagulation therapy, as compared to the other patients, the risk of recurrent thrombosis was significantly decreased while the risk for bleeding was not significantly increased [6]. Moreover, the severity of bleeding, as assessed by hemoglobin on admission, number of transfused units and length of hospital stay did not differ significantly between patients receiving and not receiving anticoagulants [6]. These findings have been supported in other retrospective studies that included a smaller number of patients [39, 84] and in which multivariate analysis could not be used [29]. A study showed a significant decrease in mortality univariate analysis in patients receiving warfarin for chronic portomesenteric venous thrombosis [75]. These consistent data provide support, although not firm evidence, to recent AASLD recommendations to consider long-term anticoagulation therapy in patients with chronic PVT without cirrhosis and with a permanent risk factor for venous thrombosis that cannot be corrected otherwise, provided there is no major contraindication. In patients with gastroesophageal varices, anticoagulation is to be initiated only after adequate prophylaxis for variceal bleeding has been instituted. More data are needed on this delicate issue, preferably from a randomized clinical trial.

Portal Cholangiopathy/Biliopathy

Data on this rare entity have been recently reviewed [53]. Only patients with symptoms clearly attributable to the biliary disease require treatment. Surgical [85], endoscopic [51, 86] and radiological [51, 86] interventions have been proposed. Patients in whom symptoms are related to stones and debris are best treated with endoscopic techniques, although care should be taken not to precipitate massive bleeding [87, 88]. In patients with a dominant stenosis that does not respond to prolonged endostenting, decompression should be attempted either through TIPS placement (which is rarely feasible [86]), or a surgical shunt (preferably spenorenal [85]). Although data are lacking in adults, the mesenterico-left portal vein bypass increasingly used in children would theoretically be an optimal solution to cope with simultaneous portal and biliary decompression.

Extrahepatic Portal Vein Obstruction in Children

Extrahepatic portal vein obstruction in this age group may not always result from thrombosis [1, 89]. The prevalence of underlying prothrombotic diseases was high in most, but not all, studies [90–96]. Primary protein C, protein S or antithrombin deficiency may be overdiagnosed, as these inhibitors are nonspecifically decreased in many affected children with a negative family screening [90, 92]. These low plasma levels are further decreased by portosystemic shunting [90], but corrected by surgical restoration of portal venous inflow [97]. Occult myeloproliferative diseases have not been assessed in this age group. Umbilical cannulation, omphalitis and abdominal infections are the most commonly incriminated factors. However, the risk of a properly placed, uninfected umbilical catheter, in the absence of underlying thrombophilia [91], is probably minimal. In this situation, a portal vein thrombus occurs frequently but full portal vein patency is restored in most infants. The probability of full recanalization is inversely related to the size of the thrombus [98]. There are few features of extrahepatic portal vein obstruction that are specific for children. It is unclear whether growth retardation occurs in the absence of recurrent bleeding [99].

Band ligation of esophageal varices may be the optimal therapy to prevent first bleed or recurrent bleeding [100]. Surgical shunts, when a central vein (mesenteric or splenic vein) is available, have achieved good results [81, 101], in contrast to other, atypical shunts, which have invariably thrombosed [82]. Recently, mesenteric-to-left portal vein bypass has been reported by several groups with good results in terms of feasibility, prevention of rebleeding, restoration of portal inflow and hepatic function and improvement in cognitive function [97, 102]. However, prior attempts at portosystemic shunts or mesenteric embolization negatively impact the results of mesenteric-to-left portal vein bypass [103]. Anticoagulation has rarely been considered in children with extrahepatic portal vein obstruction. Outcome may be mostly jeopardized by cholangiopathy in patients whose recurrent bleeding is well controlled with endoscopic therapy [52].

PVT in Cirrhotic Patients

PVT in cirrhotic patients is often accompanied by gastrointestinal bleeding, ascites, or encephalopathy [104, 105]. In many patients, the thrombus is partial and changes in appearance and location at follow-up imaging. When the thrombus extends to the superior mesenteric vein, the risk of intestinal infarction is high [104].

Endoluminal growth of hepatocellular carcinoma should always be considered, especially when serum alpha fetoprotein levels are increased, when the portal vein is larger than 23 mm in diameter, when endoluminal material enhances during the arterial phase of contrast injection [106], or when an arterial-like pulsatile flow is seen on Doppler ultrasound [107]. Needle biopsy of an obstructed intrahepatic portal vein is specific but relatively insensitive for diagnostic purposes [108].

Data on anticoagulation for PVT in cirrhotic patients are almost completely lacking. There is limited information on anticoagulation therapy in patients who develop PVT while awaiting liver transplantation. While recanalization of portal vein occurred in 10 of 19 patients who received anticoagulation, this did not occur in any of the 10 historical controls who did not receive anticoagulation [109]. Posttransplant outcome may be compromised by pretransplant complete PVT [109]. Discussion of the techniques that can be employed to deal with complete PVT at transplantation is beyond the scope of this chapter. At present, some experts strongly support considering anticoagulation in all cirrhotic patients with PVT [110]. However, data are insufficient to adequately assess the risk–benefit ratio. Therefore, decisions should be made on a case-by-case basis taking into account liver transplant candidacy, likelihood of adherence to therapy and surveillance, risk of bleeding (including portal hypertension related bleeding), the presence of underlying permanent prothrombotic conditions, and extension to the superior mesenteric vein.

Conclusions

PVT is a highly heterogeneous entity regarding its underlying risk factors and the stage at which diagnosis is established. Although significant advances have been made in the field of portal vein thrombosis in recent decades, many important questions remain unanswered. Perhaps the most critical issue that requires assessment in future studies is the risk–benefit ratio of permanent anticoagulation in different groups of patients.

References

1. Sarin SK, Sollano JD, Chawla YK, Amarapurkar D, Hamid S, Hashizume M, et al. Consensus on extrahepatic portal vein obstruction. Liver Int. 2006;26:512–9.
2. Ogren M, Bergqvist D, Bjorck M, Acosta S, Eriksson H, Sternby NH. Portal vein thrombosis: prevalence, patient characteristics and lifetime risk: a population study based on 23, 796 consecutive autopsies. World J Gastroenterol. 2006;12:2115–9.
3. Janssen HL, Wijnhoud A, Haagsma EB, van Uum SH, van Nieuwkerk CM, Adang RP, et al. Extrahepatic portal vein thrombosis: aetiology and determinants of survival. Gut. 2001;49:720–4.
4. Jain P, Nijhawan S. Portal vein thrombosis: etiology and clinical outcome of cirrhosis and malignancy-related non-cirrhotic, non-tumoral extrahepatic portal venous obstruction. World J Gastroenterol. 2007;13:5288–9.
5. Poddar U, Thapa BR, Rao KL, Singh K. Etiological spectrum of esophageal varices due to portal hypertension in Indian children: is it different from the West? J Gastroenterol Hepatol. 2008;23:1354–7.
6. Condat B, Pessione F, Hillaire S, Denninger MH, Guillin MC, Poliquin M, et al. Current outcome of portal vein thrombosis in adults: risk and benefit of anticoagulant therapy. Gastroenterology. 2001;120:490–7.

7. Sorrentino P, D'Angelo S, Tarantino L, Ferbo U, Bracigliano A, Vecchione R. Contrast-enhanced sonography versus biopsy for the differential diagnosis of thrombosis in hepatocellular carcinoma patients. World J Gastroenterol. 2009;15:2245–51.
8. D'Amico M, Pasta L, Sammarco P. MTHFR C677TT, PAI1 4G-4G, V Leiden Q506, and prothrombin G20210A in hepatocellular carcinoma with and without portal vein thrombosis. J Thromb Thrombolysis. 2009;28:70–3.
9. Zocco MA, Stasio ED, Cristofaro RD, Novi M, Ainora ME, Ponziani F, et al. et al. Thrombotic risk factors in patients with liver cirrhosis: Correlation with MELD scoring system and portal vein thrombosis development. J Hepatol; 2009.
10. Amitrano L, Brancaccio V, Guardascione MA, Margaglione M, Iannaccone L, D'Andrea G, et al. Inherited coagulation disorders in cirrhotic patients with portal vein thrombosis. Hepatology. 2000;31:345–8.
11. Amitrano L, Brancaccio V, Guardascione MA, Margaglione M, Sacco M, Martino R, et al. Portal vein thrombosis after variceal endoscopic sclerotherapy in cirrhotic patients: role of genetic thrombophilia. Endoscopy. 2002;34:535–8.
12. Amitrano L, Guardascione MA, Ames PR, Margaglione M, Iannaccone L, Brancaccio V, et al. Increased plasma prothrombin concentration in cirrhotic patients with portal vein thrombosis and prothrombin G20210A mutation. Thromb Haemost. 2006;95:221–3.
13. Dentali F, Galli M, Gianni M, Ageno W. Inherited thrombophilic abnormalities and risk of portal vein thrombosis. A meta-analysis. Thromb Haemost. 2008;99:675–82.
14. Erkan O, Bozdayi AM, Disibeyaz S, Oguz D, Ozcan M, Bahar K, et al. Thrombophilic gene mutations in cirrhotic patients with portal vein thrombosis. Eur J Gastroenterol Hepatol. 2005;17:339–43.
15. Chang PE, Miquel R, Blanco JL, Laguno M, Bruguera M, Abraldes JG, et al. Idiopathic portal hypertension in patients with HIV infection treated with highly active antiretroviral therapy. Am J Gastroenterol. 2009;104:1707–14.
16. Hillaire S, Bonte E, Denninger MH, Casadevall N, Cadranel JF, Lebrec D, et al. Idiopathic non-cirrhotic intrahepatic portal hypertension in the West: a re-evaluation in 28 patients. Gut. 2002;51:275–80.
17. Darwish Murad S, Valla DC, de Groen PC, Zeitoun G, Haagsma EB, Kuipers EJ, et al. Pathogenesis and treatment of Budd–Chiari syndrome combined with portal vein thrombosis. Am J Gastroenterol. 2006; 101:83–90.
18. Fiorini A, Chiusolo P, Rossi E, Za T, De Ritis DG, Ciminello A, et al. Absence of the JAK2 exon 12 mutations in patients with splanchnic venous thrombosis and without overt myeloproliferative neoplasms. Am J Hematol. 2009;84:126–7.
19. Kiladjian JJ, Cervantes F, Leebeek FW, Marzac C, Cassinat B, Chevret S, et al. The impact of JAK2 and MPL mutations on diagnosis and prognosis of splanchnic vein thrombosis: a report on 241 cases. Blood. 2008;111:4922–9.
20. Primignani M, Barosi G, Bergamaschi G, Gianelli U, Fabris F, Reati R, et al. Role of the JAK2 mutation in the diagnosis of chronic myeloproliferative disorders in splanchnic vein thrombosis. Hepatology. 2006;44: 1528–34.
21. Fisher NC, Wilde JT, Roper J, Elias E. Deficiency of natural anticoagulant proteins C, S, and antithrombin in portal vein thrombosis: a secondary phenomenon? Gut. 2000;46:534–9.
22. Denninger MH, Chait Y, Casadevall N, Hillaire S, Guillin MC, Bezeaud A, et al. Cause of portal or hepatic venous thrombosis in adults: the role of multiple concurrent factors. Hepatology. 2000;31:587–91.
23. Primignani M, Martinelli I, Bucciarelli P, Battaglioli T, Reati R, Fabris F, et al. Risk factors for thrombophilia in extrahepatic portal vein obstruction. Hepatology. 2005;41:603–8.
24. Janssen HL, Meinardi JR, Vleggaar FP, van Uum SH, Haagsma EB, van Der Meer FJ, et al. Factor V Leiden mutation, prothrombin gene mutation, and deficiencies in coagulation inhibitors associated with Budd–Chiari syndrome and portal vein thrombosis: results of a case-control study. Blood. 2000;96:2364–8.
25. Martinelli I, Primignani M, Aghemo A, Reati R, Bucciarelli P, Fabris F, et al. High levels of factor VIII and risk of extra-hepatic portal vein obstruction. J Hepatol. 2009;50:916–22.
26. Di Fabio F, Obrand D, Satin R, Gordon PH. Intra-abdominal venous and arterial thromboembolism in inflammatory bowel disease. Dis Colon Rectum. 2009;52:336–42.
27. Ladd AM, Goyal R, Rosainz L, Baiocco P, Difabrizio L. Pulmonary embolism and portal vein thrombosis in an immunocompetent adolescent with acute cytomegalovirus hepatitis. J Thromb Thrombolysis. 2008; 28(4):496–9.
28. Condat B, Pessione F, Helene Denninger M, Hillaire S, Valla D. Recent portal or mesenteric venous thrombosis: increased recognition and frequent recanalization on anticoagulant therapy. Hepatology. 2000;32: 466–70.
29. Amitrano L, Guardascione MA, Scaglione M, Pezzullo L, Sangiuliano N, Armellino MF, et al. Prognostic factors in noncirrhotic patients with splanchnic vein thromboses. Am J Gastroenterol. 2007;102:2464–70.
30. Plessier A, Darwish Murad S, Hernandez-Guerra M, Consigny Y, Fabris F, Trebicka I, et al. Acute portal vein thrombosis unrelated to cirrhosis: a prospective multicenter follow-up study. Hepatology. 2009;51(1): 210–8.
31. Krauth MT, Lechner K, Neugebauer EA, Pabinger I. The postoperative splenic/portal vein thrombosis after splenectomy and its prevention – an unresolved issue. Haematologica. 2008;93:1227–32.
32. James AW, Rabl C, Westphalen AC, Fogarty PF, Posselt AM, Campos GM. Portomesenteric venous thrombosis after laparoscopic surgery: a systematic literature review. Arch Surg. 2009;144:520–6.

33. Bultink IE, Dorigo-Zetsma JW, Koopman MG, Kuijper EJ. Fusobacterium nucleatum septicemia and portal vein thrombosis. Clin Infect Dis. 1999;28:1325–6.
34. Hamidi K, Pauwels A, Bingen M, Simo AC, Medini A, Jarjous N, et al. Recent portal and mesenteric venous thrombosis associated with *Fusobacterium bacteremia*. Gastroenterol Clin Biol. 2008;32: 734–9.
35. DeLeve LD, Valla DC, Garcia-Tsao G. Vascular disorders of the liver. Hepatology. 2009;49:1729–64.
36. Vilgrain V, Condat B, Bureau C, Hakime A, Plessier A, Cazals-Hatem D, et al. Atrophy-hypertrophy complex in patients with cavernous transformation of the portal vein: CT evaluation. Radiology. 2006;241: 149–55.
37. Tublin ME, Towbin AJ, Federle MP, Nalesnik MA. Altered liver morphology after portal vein thrombosis: not always cirrhosis. Dig Dis Sci. 2008;53:2784–8.
38. Sikuler E, Kravetz D, Groszmann RJ. Evolution of portal hypertension and mechanisms involved in its maintenance in a rat model. Am J Physiol. 1985;248:G618–25.
39. Turnes J, Garcia-Pagan JC, Gonzalez M, Aracil C, Calleja JL, Ripoll C, et al. Portal hypertension-related complications after acute portal vein thrombosis: impact of early anticoagulation. Clin Gastroenterol Hepatol. 2008;6:1412–7.
40. Rahmouni A, Mathieu D, Golli M, Douek P, Anglade MC, Caillet H, et al. Value of CT and sonography in the conservative management of acute splenoportal and superior mesenteric venous thrombosis. Gastrointest Radiol. 1992;17:135–40.
41. Bach AM, Hann LE, Brown KT, Getrajdman GI, Herman SK, Fong Y, et al. Portal vein evaluation with US: comparison to angiography combined with CT arterial portography. Radiology. 1996;201:149–54.
42. Haddad MC, Clark DC, Sharif HS, al Shahed M, Aideyan O, Sammak BM. MR, CT, and ultrasonography of splanchnic venous thrombosis. Gastrointest Radiol. 1992;17:34–40.
43. Kreft B, Strunk H, Flacke S, Wolff M, Conrad R, Gieseke J, et al. Detection of thrombosis in the portal venous system: comparison of contrast-enhanced MR angiography with intraarterial digital subtraction angiography. Radiology. 2000;216:86–92.
44. Tessler FN, Gehring BJ, Gomes AS, Perrella RR, Ragavendra N, Busuttil RW, et al. Diagnosis of portal vein thrombosis: value of color Doppler imaging. AJR Am J Roentgenol. 1991;157:293–6.
45. Van Gansbeke D, Avni EF, Delcour C, Engelholm L, Struyven J. Sonographic features of portal vein thrombosis. AJR Am J Roentgenol. 1985;144:749–52.
46. Wiersema MJ, Chak A, Kopecky KK, Wiersema LM. Duplex Doppler endosonography in the diagnosis of splenic vein, portal vein, and portosystemic shunt thrombosis. Gastrointest Endosc. 1995;42:19–26.
47. Eugene C, Valla D, Wesenfelder L, Fingerhut A, Bergue A, Merrer J, et al. Small intestinal stricture complicating superior mesenteric vein thrombosis. A study of three cases. Gut. 1995;37:292–5.
48. Cardot F, Borg JY, Guedon C, Lerebours E, Colin R. Syndromes of venous mesenteric ischemia: infarction and transient ischemia. Gastroentérol Clin Biol. 1992;16:644–8.
49. Minguez B, Garcia-Pagan JC, Bosch J, Turnes J, Alonso J, Rovira A, et al. Noncirrhotic portal vein thrombosis exhibits neuropsychological and MR changes consistent with minimal hepatic encephalopathy. Hepatology. 2006;43:707–14.
50. Sharma P, Sharma BC, Puri V, Sarin SK. Natural history of minimal hepatic encephalopathy in patients with extrahepatic portal vein obstruction. Am J Gastroenterol. 2009;104:885–90.
51. Condat B, Vilgrain V, Asselah T, O'Toole D, Rufat P, Zappa M, et al. Portal cavernoma-associated cholangiopathy: a clinical and MR cholangiography coupled with MR portography imaging study. Hepatology. 2003;37:1302–8.
52. Khuroo MS, Yattoo GN, Zargar SA, Javid G, Dar MY, Khan BA, et al. Biliary abnormalities associated with extrahepatic portal venous obstruction. Hepatology. 1993;17:807–13.
53. Dhiman RK, Behera A, Chawla YK, Dilawari JB, Suri S. Portal hypertensive biliopathy. Gut. 2007;56: 1001–8.
54. Chait Y, Condat B, Cazals-Hatem D, Rufat P, Atmani S, Chaoui D, et al. Relevance of the criteria commonly used to diagnose myeloproliferative disorder in patients with splanchnic vein thrombosis. Br J Haematol. 2005;129:553–60.
55. Jha SK, Kumar A, Sharma BC, Sarin SK. Systemic and pulmonary hemodynamics in patients with extrahepatic portal vein obstruction is similar to compensated cirrhotic patients. Hepatol Int. 2009;3:384–91.
56. Lebrec D, Bataille C, Bercoff E, Valla D. Hemodynamic changes in patients with portal venous obstruction. Hepatology. 1983;3:550–3.
57. Gupta D, Vijaya DR, Gupta R, Dhiman RK, Bhargava M, Verma J, et al. Prevalence of hepatopulmonary syndrome in cirrhosis and extrahepatic portal venous obstruction. Am J Gastroenterol. 2001;96:3395–9.
58. Mathieu D, Vasile N, Grenier P. Portal thrombosis: dynamic CT features and course. Radiology. 1985;154:737–41.
59. Ueno N, Sasaki A, Tomiyama T, Tano S, Kimura K. Color Doppler ultrasonography in the diagnosis of cavernous transformation of the portal vein. J Clin Ultrasound. 1997;25:227–33.
60. Vilgrain V, Condat B, O'Toole D, Plessier A, Ruszniewski P. Valla DC. Pancreatic portal cavernoma in patients with cavernous transformation of the portal vein: MR findings. Eur Radiol; 2009.
61. Dumortier J, Vaillant E, Boillot O, Poncet G, Henry L, Scoazec JY, et al. Diagnosis and treatment of biliary obstruction caused by portal cavernoma. Endoscopy. 2003;35:446–50.
62. Palazzo L, Hochain P, Helmer C, Cuillerier E, Landi B, Roseau G, et al. Biliary varices on endoscopic ultrasonography: clinical presentation and outcome. Endoscopy. 2000;32:520–4.

63. Baril N, Wren S, Radin R, Ralls P, Stain S. The role of anticoagulation in pylephlebitis. Am J Surg. 1996; 172:449–52; discussion 452–3.
64. Plemmons RM, Dooley DP, Longfield RN. Septic thrombophlebitis of the portal vein (pylephlebitis): diagnosis and management in the modern era. Clin Infect Dis. 1995;21:1114–20.
65. de Franchis R. Evolving consensus in portal hypertension. Report of the Baveno IV consensus workshop on methodology of diagnosis and therapy in portal hypertension. J Hepatol. 2005;43:167–76.
66. Lagasse JP, Bahallah ML, Salem N, Debillon G, Labarriere D, Serve MP, et al. [Acute thrombosis of the portal system. Treatment with alteplase and heparin or with heparin alone in 10 patients]. Gastroentérol Clin Biol. 1997;21:919–23.
67. Sheen CL, Lamparelli H, Milne A, Green I, Ramage JK. Clinical features, diagnosis and outcome of acute portal vein thrombosis. QJM. 2000;93:531–4.
68. Smalberg JH, Spaander MV, Jie KS, Pattynama PM, van Buuren HR, van den Berg B, et al. Risks and benefits of transcatheter thrombolytic therapy in patients with splanchnic venous thrombosis. Thromb Haemost. 2008;100:1084–8.
69. Hollingshead M, Burke CT, Mauro MA, Weeks SM, Dixon RG, Jaques PF. Transcatheter thrombolytic therapy for acute mesenteric and portal vein thrombosis. J Vasc Interv Radiol. 2005;16:651–61.
70. Grisham A, Lohr J, Guenther JM, Engel AM. Deciphering mesenteric venous thrombosis: imaging and treatment. Vasc Endovascular Surg. 2005;39:473–9.
71. Malkowski P, Pawlak J, Michalowicz B, Szczerban J, Wroblewski T, Leowska E, et al. Thrombolytic treatment of portal thrombosis. Hepatogastroenterology. 2003;50:2098–100.
72. Senzolo M, Patch D, Miotto D, Ferronato C, Cholongitas E, Burroughs AK. Interventional treatment should be incorporated in the algorithm for the management of patients with portal vein thrombosis. Hepatology. 2008;48:1352–3.
73. Brunaud L, Antunes L, Collinet-Adler S, Marchal F, Ayav A, Bresler L, et al. Acute mesenteric venous thrombosis: case for nonoperative management. J Vasc Surg. 2001;34:673–9.
74. Kahn D, Krige JE, Terblanche J, Bornman PC, Robson SC. A 15-year experience of injection sclerotherapy in adult patients with extrahepatic portal venous obstruction. Ann Surg. 1994;219:34–9.
75. Orr DW, Harrison PM, Devlin J, Karani JB, Kane PA, Heaton ND, et al. Chronic mesenteric venous thrombosis: evaluation and determinants of survival during long-term follow-up. Clin Gastroenterol Hepatol. 2007;5:80–6.
76. Vleggaar FP, van Buuren HR, Schalm SW. Endoscopic sclerotherapy for bleeding oesophagogastric varices secondary to extrahepatic portal vein obstruction in an adult Caucasian population. Eur J Gastroenterol Hepatol. 1998;10:81–5.
77. Cales P, Braillon A, Girod C, Lebrec D. Acute effect of propranolol on splanchnic circulation in normal and portal hypertensive rats. J Hepatol. 1985;1:349–57.
78. Hillon P, Blanchet L, Lebrec D. Effect of propranolol on hepatic blood flow in normal and portal hypertensive rats. Clin Sci (Lond). 1982;63:29–32.
79. Pizcueta MP, de Lacy AM, Kravetz D, Bosch J, Rodes J. Propranolol decreases portal pressure without changing portocollateral resistance in cirrhotic rats. Hepatology. 1989;10:953–7.
80. Braillon A, Moreau R, Hadengue A, Roulot D, Sayegh R, Lebrec D. Hyperkinetic circulatory syndrome in patients with presinusoidal portal hypertension. Effect of propranolol. J Hepatol. 1989;9:312–8.
81. Orloff MJ, Orloff MS, Girard B, Orloff SL. Bleeding esophagogastric varices from extrahepatic portal hypertension: 40 years' experience with portal-systemic shunt. J Am Coll Surg. 2002;194:717–28; discussion 728–30.
82. Warren WD, Henderson JM, Millikan WJ, Galambos JT, Bryan FC. Management of variceal bleeding in patients with noncirrhotic portal vein thrombosis. Ann Surg. 1988;207:623–34.
83. Senzolo M, Tibbals J, Cholongitas E, Triantos CK, Burroughs AK, Patch D. Transjugular intrahepatic portosystemic shunt for portal vein thrombosis with and without cavernous transformation. Aliment Pharmacol Ther. 2006;23:767–75.
84. Kitchens CS, Weidner MH, Lottenberg R. Chronic oral anticoagulant therapy for extrahepatic visceral thrombosis is safe. J Thromb Thrombolysis. 2007; 23(3):223–8.
85. Vibert E, Azoulay D, Aloia T, Pascal G, Veilhan LA, Adam R, et al. Therapeutic strategies in symptomatic portal biliopathy. Ann Surg. 2007;246:97–104.
86. Htun Oo Y, Olliff S, Haydon G, Thorburn D. Symptomatic portal biliopathy: a single centre experience from the UK. Eur J Gastroenterol Hepatol. 2009;21:206–3.
87. Sharma M, Ponnusamy RP. Is balloon sweeping detrimental in portal biliopathy? A report of 3 cases. Gastrointest Endosc. 2009;70:171–3.
88. Layec S, D'Halluin PN, Pagenault M, Bretagne JF. Massive hemobilia during extraction of a covered self-expandable metal stent in a patient with portal hypertensive biliopathy. Gastrointest Endosc. 2009;70:555–6; discussion 556.
89. Shinohara T, Ando H, Watanabe Y, Seo T, Harada T, Kaneko K. Extrahepatic portal vein morphology in children with extrahepatic portal hypertension assessed by 3-dimensional computed tomographic portography: a new etiology of extrahepatic portal hypertension. J Pediatr Surg. 2006;41:812–6.
90. Dubuisson C, Boyer-Neumann C, Wolf M, Meyer D, Bernard O. Protein C, protein S and antithrombin III in children with portal vein obstruction. J Hepatol. 1997;27:132–5.
91. Heller C, Schobess R, Kurnik K, Junker R, Gunther G, Kreuz W, et al. Abdominal venous thrombosis in neonates and infants: role of prothrombotic risk factors – a multicentre case-control study. For the Childhood Thrombophilia Study Group. Br J Haematol. 2000;111:534–9.

92. Balta G, Altay C, Gurgey A. PAI-1 gene 4G/5G genotype: a risk factor for thrombosis in vessels of internal organs. Am J Hematol. 2002;71:89–93.
93. El-Karaksy H, El-Koofy N, El-Hawary M, Mostafa A, Aziz M, El-Shabrawi M, et al. Prevalence of factor V Leiden mutation and other hereditary thrombophilic factors in Egyptian children with portal vein thrombosis: results of a single-center case-control study. Ann Hematol. 2004;83:712–5.
94. Pinto RB, Silveira TR, Rosling L, Bandinelli E. Thrombophilic disorders in children and adolescents with portal vein thrombosis. J Pediatr (Rio J). 2003;79:165–72.
95. Yachha SK, Aggarwal R, Sharma BC, Misra RN, Aggarwal A, Naik SR. Functional protein C and anticardiolipin antibody in children with portal vein thrombosis. Indian J Gastroenterol. 2001;20:47–9.
96. Abd El-Hamid N, Taylor RM, Marinello D, Mufti GJ, Patel R, Mieli-Vergani G, Davenport M, et al. Aetiology and management of extrahepatic portal vein obstruction in children: King's College Hospital experience. J Pediatr Gastroenterol Nutr. 2008;47:630–4.
97. Mack CL, Superina RA, Whitington PF. Surgical restoration of portal flow corrects procoagulant and anticoagulant deficiencies associated with extrahepatic portal vein thrombosis. J Pediatr. 2003;142:197–9.
98. Morag I, Epelman M, Daneman A, Moineddin R, Parvez B, Shechter T, et al. Portal vein thrombosis in the neonate: risk factors, course, and outcome. J Pediatr. 2006;148:735–9.
99. Bellomo-Brandao MA, Morcillo AM, Hessel G, Cardoso SR, Servidoni Mde F, da-Costa-Pinto EA. Growth assessment in children with extra-hepatic portal vein obstruction and portal hypertension. Arq Gastroenterol. 2003;40:247–50.
100. Zargar SA, Javid G, Khan BA, Yattoo GN, Shah AH, Gulzar GM, et al. Endoscopic ligation compared with sclerotherapy for bleeding esophageal varices in children with extrahepatic portal venous obstruction. Hepatology. 2002;36:666–72.
101. Pande GK, Reddy VM, Kar P, Sahni P, Berry M, Tandon BN, et al. Operations for portal hypertension due to extrahepatic obstruction: results and 10 year follow up. Br Med J (Clin Res Ed). 1987;295:1115–7.
102. Superina R, Bambini DA, Lokar J, Rigsby C, Whitington PF. Correction of extrahepatic portal vein thrombosis by the mesenteric to left portal vein bypass. Ann Surg. 2006;243:515–21.
103. Chin AC, Thow F, Superina RA. Previous portal hypertension surgery negatively affects results of mesenteric to left portal vein bypass. J Pediatr Surg. 2008;43:114–9; discussion 119.
104. Amitrano L, Guardascione MA, Brancaccio V, Margaglione M, Manguso F, Iannaccone L, et al. Risk factors and clinical presentation of portal vein thrombosis in patients with liver cirrhosis. J Hepatol. 2004;40:736–41.
105. Nonami T, Yokoyama I, Iwatsuki S, Starzl TE. The incidence of portal vein thrombosis at liver transplantation. Hepatology. 1992;16:1195–8.
106. Tublin ME, Dodd 3rd GD, Baron RL. Benign and malignant portal vein thrombosis: differentiation by CT characteristics. AJR Am J Roentgenol. 1997;168:719–23.
107. Rossi S, Rosa L, Ravetta V, Cascina A, Quaretti P, Azzaretti A, et al. Contrast-enhanced versus conventional and color Doppler sonography for the detection of thrombosis of the portal and hepatic venous systems. AJR Am J Roentgenol. 2006;186:763–73.
108. Tarantino L, Francica G, Sordelli I, Esposito F, Giorgio A, Sorrentino P, et al. Diagnosis of benign and malignant portal vein thrombosis in cirrhotic patients with hepatocellular carcinoma: color Doppler US, contrast-enhanced US, and fine-needle biopsy. Abdom Imaging. 2006;31:537–44.
109. Francoz C, Belghiti J, Vilgrain V, Sommacale D, Paradis V, Condat B, et al. Splanchnic vein thrombosis in candidates for liver transplantation: usefulness of screening and anticoagulation. Gut. 2005;54:691–7.
110. Senzolo M, Ferronato C, Burra P, Sartori MT. Anticoagulation for portal vein thrombosis in cirrhotic patients should be always considered. Intern Emerg Med. 2009;4:161–2; author reply 163–4.

Budd-Chiari Syndrome

13

Susana Seijo-Ríos, Puneeta Tandon,
Jaime Bosch, and Juan Carlos García-Pagán

Abstract

The Budd-Chiari syndrome (BCS) is an uncommon and life-threatening disorder defined as the obstruction of hepatic venous outflow regardless of its causative mechanism or level of obstruction. The clinical presentation of BCS is highly variable and can range from asymptomatic cases to fulminant hepatic failure with encephalopathy. In the vast majority of cases, it is possible to identify an inherited or acquired prothrombotic risk factor as the underlying cause of thrombosis being chronic myeloproliferative diseases the most frequent etiological cause of BCS. In many cases, multiple factors are present. Anticoagulation is mandatory in patients with BCS. The need for an additional intervention, such as hepatic vein angioplasty, thrombolysis, transjugular intrahepatic portosystemic shunt, surgical shunts, or liver transplantation, depends on the severity of symptoms and response to treatment.

Keywords

Chronic myeloproliferative disease • *JAK2*V617F mutation • Prothrombotic disorder • Anticoagulation • Surgical shunt • Transjugular intrahepatic portosystemic shunt • Liver transplantation

Introduction

The Budd-Chiari syndrome (BCS) is an uncommon and life-threatening disorder defined as the obstruction of hepatic venous outflow regardless of its causative mechanism or level of obstruction. This obstruction can be traced from the small hepatic venules up to the entrance of the inferior vena cava (IVC) into the right atrium [1]. Hepatic outflow obstruction related to cardiac disease, pericardial disease, or sinusoidal obstruction syndrome is excluded from this definition [2].

The BCS is classified as primary or secondary depending on the cause of the obstruction: primary, when it originates from the vein, such as thrombosis or phlebitis; and secondary, when the cause of obstruction originates outside the vein (compression or invasion by tumors, abscess) [2, 3]. Obstruction leads to sinusoidal congestion,

J.C. García-Pagán (✉)
Hepatic Hemodynamic Laboratory, Liver Unit,
Hospital Clinic Barcelona-CIBERehd-IDIBAPS-Institut Clinic de Malalties Digestives I Metaboliques,
Villarroel 170 street, Barcelona 08036, Spain
e-mail: jcgarcia@clinic.ub.es

L.D. DeLeve and G. Garcia-Tsao (eds.), *Vascular Liver Disease: Mechanisms and Management*,
DOI 10.1007/978-1-4419-8327-5_13, © Springer Science+Business Media, LLC 2011

followed by ischemia and hepatocellular necrosis. This can result in centrilobular fibrosis, nodular regenerative hyperplasia, and finally cirrhosis [4].

In the vast majority of cases, it is possible to identify an inherited or acquired prothrombotic risk factor as the underlying cause of thrombosis. Furthermore, in many patients a combination of several risk factors is present.

The clinical presentation of BCS is highly variable and can range from asymptomatic cases to fulminant hepatic failure with encephalopathy [1, 5]. Typical symptoms are the triad of abdominal pain, hepatomegaly, and ascites. The diagnosis can only be established upon unequivocal radiological confirmation of hepatic venous outflow obstruction.

Anticoagulation is mandatory in all patients with BCS. The need for an additional intervention, such as hepatic vein (HV) angioplasty, thrombolysis, TIPS, surgical shunts, or liver transplantation depends on the severity of symptoms and response to treatment.

Epidemiology

There are limited data available regarding the prevalence and incidence of BCS. Interestingly, it varies according to geographic distribution with wealthy countries demonstrating much lower incidence rates [2, 3]. For example, studies from France and Spain have shown incidence rates of 1 in 2.5 million inhabitants per year [6], and 0.41 per million inhabitants per year [7], respectively. Conversely, BCS is the leading cause of hospitalization due to liver disease in third world countries [8, 9].

These geographic differences between developing and developed countries also apply to the type and level of obstruction to hepatic outflow. In Asia a pure IVC or combined IVC/HV block predominates, often related to membrane–web occlusion, that is thought to be the consequence of a previous thrombus [10, 11]; whereas in the West, pure HV block caused by HV thrombosis is most common [2, 3].

Differences also exist according to gender and age. While there is a slight male predominance in Asia, with a median age at diagnosis of 45 years, in Europe, BCS has a greater female prevalence [3] and a younger median age (35–38 years) at diagnosis [7]. This female predominance has decreased in recent BCS series [7, 12], attributed, at least in part, to the lower estrogen content of newer oral contraceptives.

Etiology

The BCS can be classified into primary or secondary disease. Given the different therapeutic and prognostic implications of secondary BCS, in the present review we will refer only to primary BCS.

In approximately 90% of BCS patients, at least one predisposing thrombophilic factor is identified. In 25–46% of cases, several factors coexist [7, 13–15]. Therefore, it is advisable to perform a complete etiological study even after a candidate thrombophilic factor has been identified [7]. Prothrombotic causes can be acquired or inherited (Table 13.1).

Acquired

Chronic myeloproliferative diseases (MPD) are the most frequent etiological cause of BCS, found in up to 50% of cases [7, 14, 16]. The characteristic increase of blood cells in MPD is often, however, masked by the presence of portal hypertension with its consequent expansion of plasma volume [17] and hypersplenism [18]. Hence, all patients with BCS should be evaluated for MPD, even in the absence of typical clinical findings. The diagnosis of MPD has recently been facilitated by genetic testing for the V617F mutation of the *JAK2* gene. This is recognized as a diagnostic criterion of MPD according to the most recent World Health Organization guidelines [19]. By including the analysis of this mutation in the etiological workup of patients with BCS, the probability of diagnosing underlying MPD increases by up to 20% [20]. However, even though over 90% of patients with polycythemia vera, 50–70% of

Table 13.1 Risk factors associated with primary and secondary Budd-Chiari syndrome [2, 7, 13–16, 23, 83–86]

Primary Budd-Chiari syndrome			
Inherited conditions	Prevalence (%)	Acquired conditions	Prevalence (%)
Factor V Leiden mutation	6–32	*Myeloproliferative diseases* Polycythemia vera Essential thrombocytemia Myelofibrosis	28–49
Prothrombin gene G20210A mutation	3–7	Antiphospholipid syndrome	4–25
Protein C deficiency	0–30	Paroxysmal nocturnal hemoglobinuria (PNH)	0–19
Protein S deficiency	0–20	Behçet disease	0–33
Antithrombin deficiency	0–23	*External factors*[a] Recent pregnancy Oral contraceptives	 0–12 6–60
C677T MTHFR gene mutations	13–52	Hyperhomocysteinemia	0–37
Secondary Budd-Chiari syndrome			
Hepatocellular carcinoma Renal adenocarcinoma Adrenal adenocarcinoma Hepatic or IVC angiosarcoma Right atrial myxoma		Hepatic cysts and abscess Post-OLT or hepatic resection Blunt abdominal trauma Polycystic hepatic disease Others	

[a] These factors are frequently associated with other prothrombotic factors

patients with essential thrombocytosis and 40–50% of patients with primary myelofibrosis carry the V617F mutation of *JAK2* gene [16, 18], the presence of this mutation does not define the phenotype of MPD. Hence, it is often necessary to perform additional hematological studies, including morphological evaluation of the bone marrow. Figure 13.1 details the proposed diagnostic algorithm for MPD in BCS.

Pregnancy and the use of oral contraceptives are recognized prothrombotic risk factors in patients with BCS [21]. The prevalence of oral contraceptive use in BCS patients is estimated at up to 50–60%. Although common, both of these risk factors are weak and therefore almost always occur in conjunction with another predisposing thrombophilic condition [21, 22]. Apparently, pregnancy and contraceptive use are not sufficient to induce BCS in the absence of an underlying prothrombotic factor. Therefore, they behave as triggers or facilitators of thrombosis in these cases. Hence, both should be considered as risk factors for thrombotic diseases but not as primary prothrombotic disorders [23].

Less commonly acquired diseases (e.g., antiphospholipid syndrome, paroxysmal nocturnal hemoglobinuria, Behçet disease, hypereosinophilic syndrome, granulomatous venulitis, etc.) have also been associated with BCS [2, 24].

Inherited

Other inherited prothrombotic disorders have been identified as candidate causes of BCS including factor V Leiden mutation, G20210A prothrombin gene mutation, and protein C, S, or antithrombin III deficiencies [13, 14]. The diagnosis of protein C, protein S, and antithrombin III deficiencies can be complicated by impaired synthesis due to hepatic dysfunction. In this situation, one diagnostic strategy is to compare the levels of the candidate deficient factor with the levels of other vitamin K-dependent factors. If these levels are globally reduced, it is reasonable to assume that the deficiency is secondary to hepatic dysfunction. Family history or genetic testing of relatives can be helpful to determine whether a specific deficit is primary or secondary.

The measurement of anticardiolipin antibodies and homocysteine levels are also affected by liver disease as they are commonly elevated in these patients, regardless of the etiology of hepatic dysfunction [25, 26]. Hyperhomocysteinemia is a

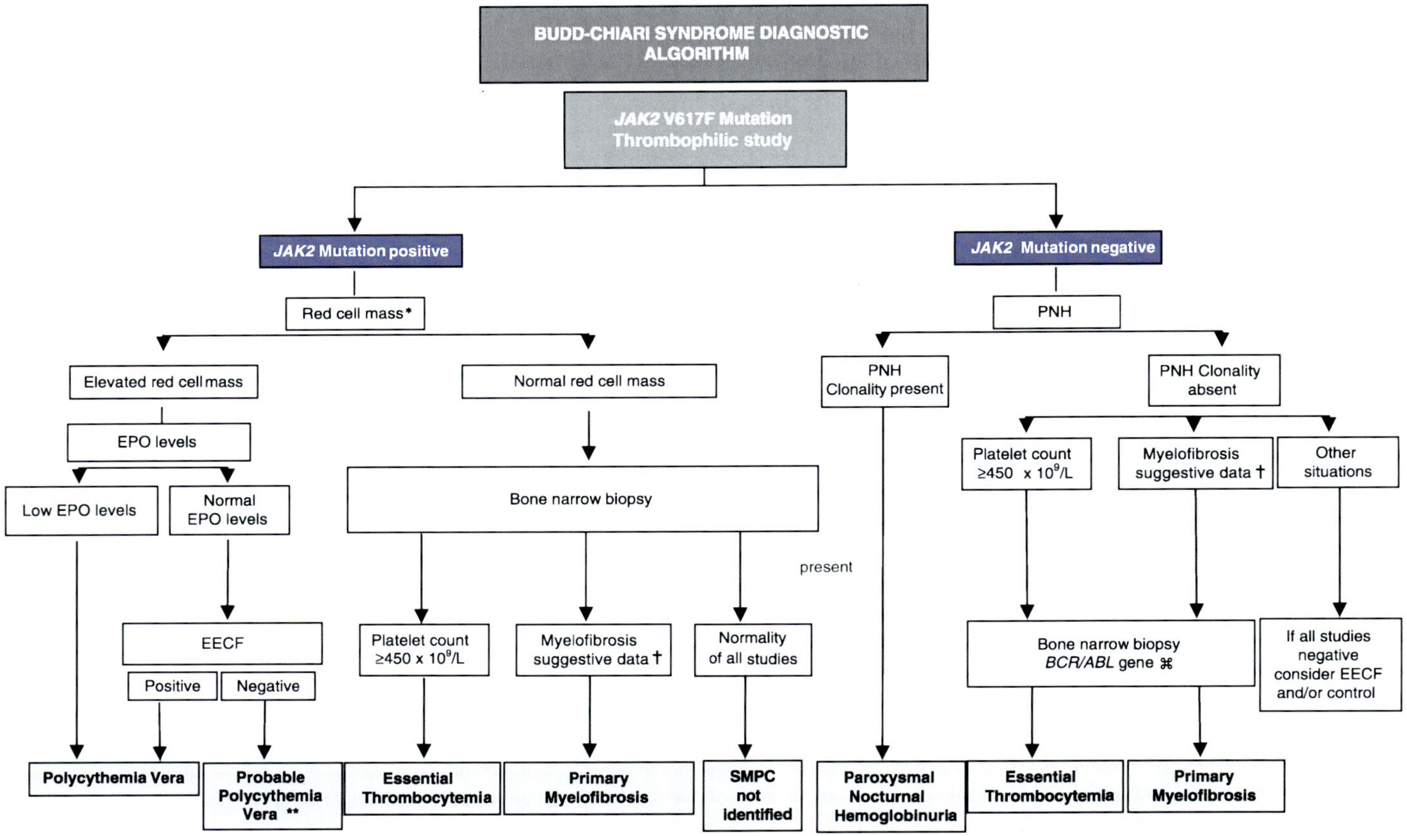

* Hemoglobin>18.5g/dL in men and >16.5 g/dL in women are considered increased red cell mass and it is unnecessary tested by isotopic methods
** PV highly probably: consider perform bone narrow biopsy in order to complete WHO criteria
† Cytopenias, leukoerythroblastic syndrome and/or dacryocytes or elevated lactate dehydrogenase levels.
⌘ Requires the absence of *BCR/ABL*

MPD: Myeloproliferative diseases
EPO: Serum erythropoietin levels
PNH: Paroxysmal nocturnal hemoglobinuria
EECF: Endogenous erythroid colony formation in vitro

Fig. 13.1 Diagnostic algorithm of myeloproliferative disorders in Budd-Chiari syndrome relatively weak risk factor for thrombosis [18] and, in most cases, homocysteine levels are highly influenced by diet and by vitamin B12 or folic acid deficiencies [2].

Recently, genetic variations in the gene inhibitor of thrombin-activated fibrinolysis (TAFI) [27] and the plasminogen activator inhibitor 1 (PAI-1) [28] have been described as candidate etiological factors associated with both portal vein thrombosis (PVT) and BCS. Further studies are needed to assess the possible etiological role of these factors before their inclusion in routine diagnostic algorithms of BCS can be considered.

Clinical Manifestations

The clinical presentation of BCS is extremely heterogeneous and can range from the absence of symptoms to the development of fulminant hepatic failure with encephalopathy [1, 5]. The classical clinical triad of BCS consists of abdominal pain, hepatomegaly, and ascites. In a recent multicenter prospective European study of 163 patients with BCS, ascites was present at diagnosis in 83% of patients, hepatomegaly in 67%, and abdominal pain in 61% [7]. Esophageal varices were present at diagnostic endoscopy in 58% of these patients and gastrointestinal bleeding in 5% of cases [7].

The severity of presentation of BCS is influenced by (1) the number and type of affected veins; (2) the extension of thrombosis; and (3) the efficiency of compensatory mechanisms (hepatic collaterals and spontaneous intrahepatic portocaval shunts) [3, 29, 30]. An asymptomatic presentation occurs in anywhere from 3 [7] to 15–20% of patients [3, 29] and is often associated with the presence of hepatic venous collaterals [29].

In other cases thrombosis is extensive and develops rapidly, leading to more severe symptoms and in rare cases to presentation with acute liver failure leading to renal impairment, coagulopathy, and death. Fever, jaundice, edema of lower limbs, hepatic encephalopathy, and hepatorenal syndrome, although infrequent, are other possible symptoms. When BCS is associated with thrombosis of the IVC collateral circulation, nephrotic syndrome may appear (proteinuria and edema in lower limbs).

In approximately 15% of cases, BCS and PVT occur simultaneously [7, 31]. In these patients there is a higher prevalence of multiple etiologies (58% of cases), the number increasing significantly with the extent of thrombosis [31]. Prognosis is worse than that for isolated PVT (5-year survival 59% vs. 85%, respectively). Likewise, therapeutic options and prognosis tend to be worse in BCS-PVT patients with additional splenic and/or superior mesenteric vein thrombosis compared to those without (5-year survival 48% vs. 76%, respectively) [31]. Therefore, patients with BCS and portal venous system thrombosis constitute an exceptional group with limited therapeutic options.

Another clinical finding in 60–80% of patients with BCS is the presence of benign hepatic regenerative nodules [4, 32]. The reported time for detection ranges between 1 and 14 years from diagnosis [33]. On computed tomography (CT) or magnetic resonance (MR) imaging, these nodules are characteristically small, in most cases under 4 cm in diameter, multiple (frequently more than 10 lesions), hypervascularized, and disseminated throughout the liver, with a periportal distribution [33]. Although there is no pathognomonic pattern, these nodules are frequently homogeneous; hyperechogenic on ultrasound, hyperattenuating on unenhanced CT [33]; markedly and homogeneously hyperattenuating on arterial phase and slightly hyperattenuating on portal-venous phase images [34]. On MR images benign nodules are characteristically bright on unenhanced T1-weighted and enhance strongly following endovenous administration of gadolinium-based contrast agents [35]. On T2-weighted images they are predominantly isointense or hypointense relative to the normal liver [35]. Histologically, nodules are composed of moderately enlarged hepatocyte plates without nuclear atypia [33]. The presence of a central scar, found in less than 50% of patients, is a characteristic feature in nodules larger than 1 cm in diameter [36]. The pathogenesis of these nodules remains unclear, but they seem to be the result of focal defects of portal perfusion combined with hypervascularized areas of preserved venous outflow. A recent study conducted in BCS patients using serial multiphase contrast-enhanced multidetector CT has shown that benign hepatic nodules may increase in number and size over time [37].

Since the radiological characteristics of these benign hepatic nodules may be very similar to those found in hepatocellular carcinomas (HCC) nodules, imaging criteria for the diagnosis of HCC recommended in the AASLD-EASL guidelines are not applicable to patients with BCS [38, 39]. The distinction between benign nodules and HCC is especially relevant, because in a recent study by Valla et al., the cumulative incidence of HCC in BCS patients was 4% (after a median follow-up of 5 years) [40]. In this study, male gender, presence of factor V Leiden mutation, and IVC thrombosis were the most frequent factors associated with HCC [40]. Biopsy was suggested in patients with less than or equal to three nodules, nodules with a diameter more than or equal to 3 cm, heterogeneity or washout on the venous phase, changes in two consecutive imaging techniques, or increase in AFP levels [40]. Furthermore, an AFP above a cutoff value of 15 ng/mL had a positive predictive value of 100% and a negative predictive value of 90% for the diagnosis of HCC [40]. These findings need to be validated in larger cohort studies. It must also be kept in mind that liver biopsy in this population could be complicated by the risk of bleeding with ongoing anticoagulation therapy and with the risk of thrombotic events after discontinuation of anticoagulation.

Diagnosis

In most cases, the diagnosis of BCS can be established with noninvasive radiological techniques (e.g., Doppler ultrasound, computerized tomography – CT, and magnetic resonance – MRI) (Chap. 9). Doppler ultrasound has a diagnostic sensitivity of more than 75% and should be the first line of investigation [1]. The absence of retrograde flow in the first phase of the triphasic HV waveform, failure to visualize HV, presence of intrahepatic or subcapsular collaterals, or obstruction of the intrahepatic IVC are the main sonographic findings in BCS (Fig. 13.2). As suggested by recent guidelines, MRI and CT evaluation can be considered for the purpose of diagnostic confirmation or if an experienced sonographer is not available [2]. In addition to obstruction of the hepatic venous outflow tract, both CT and MRI may demonstrate caudate lobe hypertrophy (75% of patients), rapid clearance of dye from the caudate lobe, and patchy hepatic enhancement due to uneven portal perfusion [2].

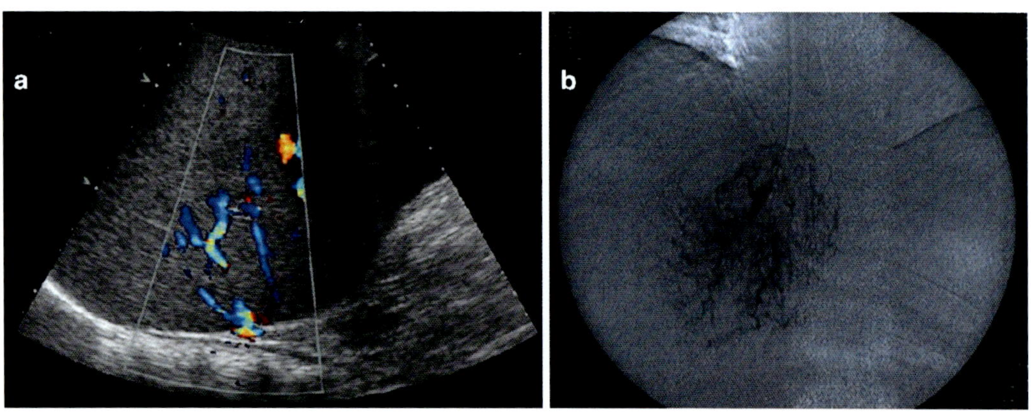

Fig. 13.2 (**a**) Doppler ultrasound studies of a BCS patient showing the presence of multiple venous intrahepatic and subcapsular collaterals. Also note the absence of visualization of the hepatic veins. The association of both features is a distinctive characteristic of BCS, and it is present in 80% of cases. (**b**) Hepatic venography of another BCS patient demonstrating a fine spider-web network pattern without filling hepatic veins

Due to the increasing sophistication of these noninvasive radiological techniques, invasive diagnostic methods (e.g., venography of the IVC and HV) are nowadays limited to a small number of patients. As per recent guidelines, this gold standard technique is recommended if the diagnosis remains uncertain despite the above investigations or for the characterization of anatomy prior to treatment [2]. Venography classically demonstrates a spiderweb pattern formed by a rich collateral circulation between the tributaries of the HV [41] (see Fig. 13.2). Liver biopsy is infrequently required in the diagnostic algorithm for BCS. Its utility is hampered by sample variation and the risk of delaying therapeutic anticoagulation. Guidelines suggest that biopsy should be considered when imaging has failed to demonstrate obstruction of the large HVs and IVC but the diagnosis of BCS remains suspect [2].

Hemodynamic studies in patients with BCS demonstrate a normal cardiac index and normal mean systemic and cardiopulmonary pressures. Despite this, these patients have activation of the neurohumoral vasoactive systems, as evidenced by increased plasma renin activity, aldosterone and norepinephrine levels, and plasma volume expansion [17].

During pregnancy, in cases where a definitive diagnosis remain unclear after Doppler ultrasound, gadolinium MRI may be used, according to the guidelines of the European Society of Radiology, based on the probable safety of gadolinium during the pregnancy and importance of diagnosis for the mother's health [22].

Treatment

The management of BCS rests on three pillars: (1) supportive care, (2) anticoagulation and control of the underlying thrombophilic disease, and (3) correction of hepatic venous outflow obstruction. Unfortunately, to date there are no prospective randomized controlled clinical trials comparing different treatment options in BCS. Therefore, recommendations are based on retrospective cohorts and prospective series of patients. Figure 13.3 summarizes the currently accepted therapeutic algorithm of BCS [2, 3].

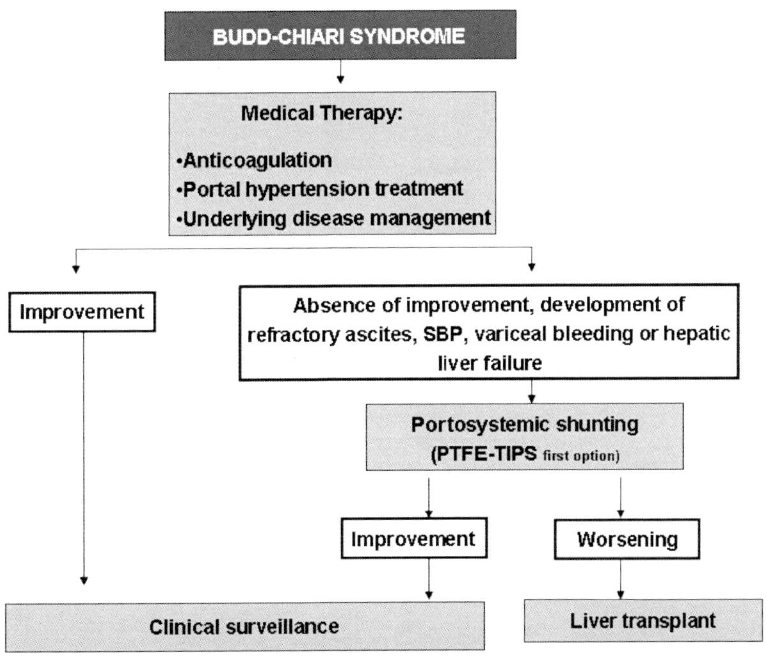

Fig. 13.3 Proposed therapeutic algorithm in Budd-Chiari syndrome

Supportive Care

Patients with BCS will often require therapy for ascites and varices. Since there are no specific guidelines for the management of portal hypertension in BCS patients, it is reasonable to follow the same treatment recommendations as for portal hypertension in cirrhosis.

Anticoagulation and Control of Underlying Thrombotic Disorders

All patients with BCS, even those without an underlying prothrombotic condition (<10%), and those who are asymptomatic, should receive anticoagulant therapy as soon as possible and for an indefinite period of time [42]. This recommendation aims to reduce the risk of clot extension and new thrombotic episodes. Although there are no prospective randomized controlled studies evaluating the efficacy of anticoagulants, indirect evidence suggests that this practice has significantly improved the prognosis of the disease [43, 44]. After initial management with low molecular weight heparin, treatment with coumarin derivatives (acenocoumarol or warfarin) is recommended [2]. Although there has been little research into the optimal level for chronic anticoagulation in patients with BCS, most studies aim for an international normalized ratio (INR) between 2 and 3, the conventional target for thrombosis in other vascular beds [2]. In addition, any supplemental therapies for coexisting MPD should be initiated and underlying prothrombotic risk factors such as oral contraceptives should be avoided.

Correction of Hepatic Venous Outflow Obstruction

Thrombolysis

The experience of thrombolysis in BCS is limited. Recombinant tissue plasminogen activator, streptokinase, or urokinase have been used. These agents can be instilled through a peripheral vein or locally after catheterization of the thrombosed vein. There are no studies comparing the efficacy of local vs. systemic infusion. A review by Sharma et al. indicates that the best results are achieved in patients with a recent and incomplete thrombosis who are treated with local and early infusion combined with another interventional procedure (e.g., angioplasty, stenting) to restore venous outflow [45]. Complications of thrombolysis can be fatal. Hence, this therapeutic option is contraindicated in patients with a potentially hemorrhagic condition, or patients who have had an invasive procedure, including paracentesis, in the previous 24 h. In summary, thrombolysis should only be attempted in select cases with acute or subacute BCS, and at experienced centers.

Angioplasty/Stenting of Short-Length Hepatic Veins Stenosis

Partial or segmental stenosis is present in 60% of patients with IVC obstruction and 25–30% of those with HV obstruction [46]. Since angioplasty or stenting of this short-length stenosis could reestablish the physiological drainage of portal and sinusoidal blood through the HVs [47], their existence must be properly evaluated in all patients with BCS. Postangioplasty, restenosis may occur that necessitates subsequent angioplasties. Restenosis appears to occur more frequently when angioplasty is performed alone as in comparison to in combination with a stent [2]. As misplacement of a stent may compromise the subsequent performance of a portosystemic intrahepatic shunt, these procedures should only be attempted by highly experienced personnel.

Portosystemic Shunt

For many years surgical procedures, together with liver transplantation, have been the only therapeutic alternative for patients with BCS who have not responded to medical treatment or have not been candidates for angioplasty/stenting. The aim of these derivative techniques is to transform the portal system into the outflow tract [48]. The most frequent shunt performed is the mesocaval shunt with a calibrated 8–10 mm polytetrafluoroethylene stent or autologous jugular vein interposition. It is preferable to a portocaval side-to-side shunt because it is easier to perform when hypertrophy of the caudate lobe is present [49]. Surgical shunts are ineffective if there is associated IVC thrombosis or severe compression of the IVC by an enlarged liver. In the setting of IVC compression, the presence of an infrahepatic caval pressure of greater than 20 mmHg or a gradient between it and the right atrium of 15 mmHg is predictive of inadequate shunt function unless the stenosis/compression of the IVC is simultaneously corrected with the placement of a stent [1, 50]. In the setting of IVC thrombosis or severe stenosis not amenable to standard shunts, some groups have performed a mesoatrial shunt. The utility of this remains limited; however, as it is quite challenging and is associated with considerable morbidity and occlusion risk [51].

Overall, surgical shunts are associated with significant mortality (close to 25% of patients) and have not demonstrated an independent survival advantage in large cohorts of patients [52, 53]. This is likely related to the high inherent mortality rate of the patient population with severe BCS who meet criteria for this treatment as well as to the high rate of dysfunction/thrombosis of the shunts (approximately 30% of cases) [51, 54, 55]. In support of this concept, it has been shown that patients who survive a surgical procedure and who maintain shunt patency have excellent long-term outcomes [55, 56]. Regardless, since the introduction of the transjugular intrahepatic portosystemic shunt (TIPS), surgical shunts are considered a second line derivative alternative.

Transjugular Intrahepatic Portosystemic Shunt (TIPS)

In experienced hands, TIPS is an extremely useful therapy for most BCS patients in whom medical treatment or recanalization have failed [57]. TIPS has a lower morbidity and mortality than surgery, and, contrary to surgical shunts, it is feasible in most patients with IVC obstruction and in those with severe IVC stenosis. A recent multicenter European study that included 124 BCS patients treated with TIPS showed excellent 1- and 5-year OLT-free survival (88 and 78%, respectively [57]). Furthermore, TIPS is even feasible in pregnant patients, because the radiation received by the fetus during TIPS placement is below the threshold to induce fetal deleterious effects [22].

Early stent thrombosis is not uncommon, even during the release of the prosthesis. Therefore, a sodium heparin infusion should be initiated immediately after the puncture of the portal vein [58]. To reduce the recurrence of postprocedure TIPS obstruction or dysfunction due to stent occlusion, PTFE covered stents are suggested. Recent data has shown a primary patency rate of 67% at 1 and 2 years in PTFE-covered stents compared to 19% at 1 year and 9% at 2 years in bare stents [57, 59].

In some patients, TIPS obstruction is not accompanied by the reappearance of symptoms of portal hypertension due to the formation of collaterals during the time that it was permeable [58, 59].

The use of TIPS instead of OLT in patients in whom angioplasty/stenting is not an option can avoid the risk of long-term immunosuppression and potentially increase the number of donor organs available to transplant centers [57].

Orthotopic liver transplantation (OLT) remains an alternative in those cases in which TIPS fails to improve the clinical evolution. Although it has been suggested that previous TIPS placement can jeopardize OLT [50, 60], recent studies have shown that TIPS did not worsen prognosis after OLT in BCS patients [57, 61]. TIPS placement does, however, require specialized training and it can be significantly more complex than in patients with cirrhosis alone. In more than 45% of cases, a transcaval approach (direct puncture from the intrahepatic inferior vena cava) may be required due to complete thrombosis of the HVs [57]. It is therefore highly recommended to refer such patients to centers with expertise in this technique [57].

Orthotropic Liver Transplantation (OLT)

The BCS represents 1% of all OLT cases in American and European databases [62] and should be restricted to those patients in whom TIPS has failed (see Fig. 13.3) (Chap. 17). OLT in BCS patients is a technical challenge for the surgical team because of the presence of retroperitoneal fibrosis related to HV thrombosis and also because the liver is often large, firm, and difficult to mobilize during hepatectomy. In addition, the classical "piggyback" technique for anastomosis becomes more challenging due to the increased size of the caudate lobe and occlusion of the HV ostia. Living donor liver transplantation (LDLT) is technically even more difficult and thus far, the only experience is in Asian centers [63, 64].

Disease recurrence after OLT is variable and ranges from 0 to 11% in different series [44, 65–69]. Other postoperative thrombotic complications are also frequent [66] but may be prevented by initiating heparin in the first 6 hours after surgery. Although there is insufficient evidence, indefinite anticoagulation is recommended. An exception would be those patients in whom OLT is performed for antithrombin III, protein C or S deficiencies, or a factor V mutation, as all of these disorders are corrected by OLT [70].

The natural history of MPD must also be considered in the posttransplant course. There is a risk of myelofibrosis or leukemic transformation that increases over time, estimated at between 10% and 25% at 15 and 25 years, respectively [71]. Although isolated cases of leukemic transformation after OLT in MPD patients have been reported [66, 68, 72], the rate of malignant transformation of MPD over a 10-year posttransplant period is comparable to that of nontransplant patients [3, 66]. Posttransplant recurrence of BCS in patients with paroxysmal nocturnal hemoglobinuria may occur and has been shown to affect up to 40% of patients [73]. The combination of two underlying thrombophilic disease further increases the risk of recurrence.

Five-year posttransplant survival in patients with BCS ranges from 45 to 95% [44, 50, 60–68, 74–76]. This wide range is likely due to the high heterogeneity in the type of BCS patients listed for OLT. A recent European study showed an actuarial overall survival of 76, 71, and 68% at 1, 5, and 10 years, respectively [65], similar to the survival rates reported using TIPS (88 and 78% at 1 and 5-year OLT-free survival, respectively) [57]. The overall mortality rate has been estimated at up to 25% [65, 66] with approximately half of the patients dying within the first 2 months after OLT as a result of surgical complications, infections, or rejection. In addition, there have been some cases of early mortality associated with early recurrence of BCS. These have been attributed to inadequate anticoagulation in the immediate posttransplant period [44, 67, 69]. Late mortality is typically associated with recurrence or progression of the underlying disease. In summary, it is clear that careful, multidisciplinary management of these patients, including appropriate treatment for hematological disease, is essential.

Budd-Chiari and Pregnancy

The majority of patients with BCS in Western countries are at child-bearing age, and many express their desire to become pregnant. For this reason it is important to understand the evolution and the possible consequences of pregnancy on BCS, and vice versa.

Management of Budd-Chiari Syndrome Established Prior to Pregnancy

Anticoagulation should be maintained during pregnancy. Oral anticoagulants are associated with a high risk of miscarriage (14.6–56%) and congenital malformations (30%) [22]. Therefore, although it is not necessary to change to heparin before conception, clinical practice guidelines recommend a pregnancy test as early as possible to confirm pregnancy, and then a switch to heparin [77]. Low molecular weight heparins (LMWH) such as enoxaparin, dalteparin, or tinzaparin are recommended (all three are approved by the FDA for use during pregnancy). During pregnancy, increased glomerular filtration, increased plasma distribution volume, and the presence of placental heparinase may necessitate increasing doses of heparin, and therefore periodic monitoring of anti-Xa activity should also be carried out [22].

Epidural anesthesia is contraindicated if the last dose of LMWH was administrated less than 12 h before. Prophylactic anticoagulation must be restarted within the first 24 h after delivery and, if there are no contraindications, therapeutic doses in the first 48 h.

Impact on the Course of Pregnancy

A recent multicenter retrospective study that evaluated the impact of BCS on pregnancy demonstrated an excellent maternal outcome provided that patients were compensated with well-controlled disease. Fetal outcome was, however, concerning with a 29% rate of pregnancy loss before week 20 of gestation, as compared to a rate of 16.2% in age-matched controls [78]. Pregnancies reaching week 20 of gestation were associated with an acceptable fetal prognosis even though 76% had preterm delivery [78].

Vaginal delivery is recommended in the setting of BCS as cesarean sections may be complicated by the presence of ascites, bleeding from pelvic collaterals, and a higher rate of postoperative thromboembolic disease [78]. All women with BCS who wish to become pregnant should therefore be properly informed of maternal and fetal risks and prognosis and should be considered high-risk pregnancies.

Prognosis

Due to recent therapeutic advances, the survival of BCS patients has improved to over 80% at 5 years [2]. Hepatocellular carcinoma, portal vein axis thrombosis, and aggravation or leukemic transformation of myeloproliferative disease are relevant factors that may overshadow outcome in this complex group of patients [2, 3].

There have been various attempts to determine parameters or combinations of parameters that may predict prognosis in BCS patients. The first BCS-specific prognostic index was described in 1999 by Zeitoun et al. and showed that age, serum creatinine, refractory ascites, and the Child-Pugh score were inversely related independent factors that allowed the differentiation of patients with good and poor prognoses (95% vs. 62% 5-year survival) [52]. A revised index by the same group incorporated a novel clinicopathological classification and identified age, the Child-Pugh score, ascites, serum creatinine, and the presence of features indicating acute injury superimposed on chronic lesions as independent prognostic indicators. This stratified patients into "low" and "high risk" had an excellent correlation with short- and long-term survival [79]. Subsequently, Murad et al. proposed the Rotterdam score, a model based on the presence of hepatic encephalopathy, ascites, prothrombin time and bilirubin, classifying patients into three groups with an estimated 5-year survival of 89, 74, and 42%, respectively [80]. It must be kept in mind that all of these prognostic indices were developed in the pre-TIPS era. They remain useful to identify patients with a poor prognosis on anticoagulation and supportive care who should be considered for TIPS. Indeed, with the introduction of TIPS into the current therapeutic algorithm, the prognosis of BCS patients has improved.

Some patients, however, are too sick for TIPS and require early OLT. To identify this group, a new prognostic index has been developed, called the BCS-TIPS prognostic index score [57]. A BCS-TIPS prognostic index score over 7 correlates with a sensitivity and specificity of 99% for death or OLT 1 year after TIPS [57]. Other prognostic indices such as the Child-Pugh score and model for end-stage liver disease (MELD) score have also been used, but exhibit a suboptimal prognostic accuracy [81]. Accordingly, a recent study published by Ratou et al. suggests that although all of these prognostic indices are valid for the assessment of transplant-free survival and invasive therapy-free survival, their predictive accuracy is suboptimal for use in individual patients in day-to-day clinical practice [82].

Acknowledgments Thanks to Dr. Cervantes, Dr. Reverter, Dra. Gilabert, and Dra. García-Criado for their precious and helpful collaboration. SSR is founded by "Río Hortega" Instituto de Salud Carlos III (CM08/00161). This work is supported in part by grants from Instituto de Salud Carlos III, Ministerio de Ciencia e Innovación (FIS 06/0623, FIS 09/01261 and SAF 07/61298). CIBERehd is funded by the Instituto de Salud Carlos III.

References

1. Janssen HL, Garcia-Pagan JC, Elias E, Mentha G, Hadengue A, Valla DC. Budd-Chiari syndrome: a review by an expert panel. J Hepatol. 2003;38:364–71.
2. DeLeve LD, Valla DC, Garcia-Tsao G. Vascular disorders of the liver. Hepatology. 2009;49:1729–64.
3. Plessier A, Valla DC. Budd-Chiari syndrome. Semin Liver Dis. 2008;28:259–69.
4. Tanaka M, Wanless IR. Pathology of the liver in Budd-Chiari syndrome: portal vein thrombosis and the histogenesis of veno-centric cirrhosis, veno-portal cirrhosis, and large regenerative nodules. Hepatology. 1998;27:488–96.
5. Hernandez-Guerra M, Garcia-Pagan JC. Recommendations for the diagnosis and treatment of patients with Budd-Chiari syndrome. Gastroenterol Hepatol. 2004;27:473–9.
6. Valla DC. Hepatic venous outflow tract obstruction etiopathogenesis: Asia versus the West. J Gastroenterol Hepatol. 2004;19:S204–11.
7. Darwish MS, Plessier A, Hernandez-Guerra M, Fabris F, Eapen CE, Bahr MJ, et al. Etiology, management, and outcome of the Budd-Chiari syndrome. Ann Intern Med. 2009;151:167–75.
8. Shrestha SM, Okuda K, Uchida T, Maharjan KG, Shrestha S, Joshi BL, et al. Endemicity and clinical picture of liver disease due to obstruction of the hepatic portion of the inferior vena cava in Nepal. J Gastroenterol Hepatol. 1996;11:170–9.
9. Amarapurkar DN, Punamiya SJ, Patel ND. Changing spectrum of Budd-Chiari syndrome in India with special reference to non-surgical treatment. World J Gastroenterol. 2008;14:278–85.
10. Horton JD, San Miguel FL, Membreno F, Wright F, Paima J, Foster P, et al. Budd-Chiari syndrome: illustrated review of current management. Liver Int. 2008;28:455–66.
11. Okuda K. Inferior vena cava thrombosis at its hepatic portion (obliterative hepatocavopathy). Semin Liver Dis. 2002;22:15–26.
12. Valla DC. Primary Budd-Chiari syndrome. J Hepatol. 2009;50:195–203.
13. Denninger MH, Chait Y, Casadevall N, Hillaire S, Guillin MC, Bezeaud A, et al. Cause of portal or hepatic venous thrombosis in adults: the role of multiple concurrent factors. Hepatology. 2000;31:587–91.
14. Janssen HL, Meinardi JR, Vleggaar FP, van Uum SH, Haagsma EB, Der Meer FJ, et al. Factor V Leiden mutation, prothrombin gene mutation, and deficiencies in coagulation inhibitors associated with Budd-Chiari syndrome and portal vein thrombosis: results of a case-control study. Blood. 2000;96:2364–8.
15. Primignani M, Barosi G, Bergamaschi G, Gianelli U, Fabris F, Reati R, et al. Role of the JAK2 mutation in the diagnosis of chronic myeloproliferative disorders in splanchnic vein thrombosis. Hepatology. 2006;44:1528–34.
16. Bittencourt PL, Couto CA, Ribeiro DD. Portal vein thrombosis and Budd-Chiari syndrome. Clin Liver Dis. 2009;13:127–44.
17. Hernandez-Guerra M, Lopez E, Bellot P, Piera C, Turnes J, Abraldes JG, et al. Systemic hemodynamics, vasoactive systems, and plasma volume in patients with severe Budd-Chiari syndrome. Hepatology. 2006;43:27–33.
18. Primignani M, Mannucci PM. The role of thrombophilia in splanchnic vein thrombosis. Semin Liver Dis. 2008;28:293–301.
19. Tefferi A, Thiele J, Orazi A, Kvasnicka HM, Barbui T, Hanson CA, et al. Proposals and rationale for revision of the World Health Organization diagnostic criteria for polycythemia vera, essential thrombocythemia, and primary myelofibrosis: recommendations from an ad hoc international expert panel. Blood. 2007;110:1092–7.
20. Kiladjian JJ, Cervantes F, Leebeek FW, Marzac C, Cassinat B, Chevret S, et al. The impact of JAK2 and MPL mutations on diagnosis and prognosis of splanchnic vein thrombosis: a report on 241 cases. Blood. 2008;111:4922–9.
21. Valla D, Le MG, Poynard T, Zucman N, Rueff B, Benhamou JP. Risk of hepatic vein thrombosis in relation to recent use of oral contraceptives. A case-control study. Gastroenterology. 1986;90:807–11.
22. Perarnau JM, Bacq Y. Hepatic vascular involvement related to pregnancy, oral contraceptives, and estrogen replacement therapy. Semin Liver Dis. 2008;28:315–27.
23. Briere JB. Budd-Chiari syndrome and portal vein thrombosis associated with myeloproliferative disorders: diagnosis and management. Semin Thromb Hemost. 2006;32:208–18.
24. Hoekstra J, Leebeek FW, Plessier A, Raffa S, Murad SD, Heller J, et al. Paroxysmal nocturnal hemoglobinuria in Budd-Chiari Syndrome: Findings from a cohort study. J Hepatol. 2009;51:696–706.
25. Mangia A, Margaglione M, Cascavilla I, Gentile R, Cappucci G, Facciorusso D, et al. Anticardiolipin antibodies in patients with liver disease. Am J Gastroenterol. 1999;94:2983–7.
26. Bosy-Westphal A, Ruschmeyer M, Czech N, Oehler G, Hinrichsen H, Plauth M, et al. Determinants of hyperhomocysteinemia in patients with chronic liver disease and after orthotopic liver transplantation. Am J Clin Nutr. 2003;77:1269–77.
27. de Bruijne EL, Darwish MS, de Maat MP, Tanck MW, Haagsma EB, van HB, et al. Genetic variation in thrombin-activatable fibrinolysis inhibitor (TAFI) is

associated with the risk of splanchnic vein thrombosis. Thromb Haemost. 2007;97:181–5.
28. Hoekstra J, Leebeek FW, Guimaraes A, Murad S, Malfliet J, Plessier A, et al. Impaired fibrinolysis as risk factor for Budd-Chiari syndrome. Blood. 2010; 115:388–95.
29. Hadengue A, Poliquin M, Vilgrain V, Belghiti J, Degott C, Erlinger S, et al. The changing scene of hepatic vein thrombosis: recognition of asymptomatic cases. Gastroenterology. 1994;106:1042–7.
30. Valla D. Hepatic vein thrombosis (Budd-Chiari syndrome). Semin Liver Dis. 2002;22:5–14.
31. Darwish MS, Valla DC, de Groen PC, Zeitoun G, Haagsma EB, Kuipers EJ, et al. Pathogenesis and treatment of Budd-Chiari syndrome combined with portal vein thrombosis. Am J Gastroenterol. 2006; 101:83–90.
32. Wanless IR. Benign liver tumors. Clin Liver Dis. 2002;6:513–26, ix.
33. Vilgrain V, Lewin M, Vons C, Denys A, Valla D, Flejou JF, et al. Hepatic nodules in Budd-Chiari syndrome: imaging features. Radiology. 1999;210: 443–50.
34. Brancatelli G, Vilgrain V, Federle MP, Hakime A, Lagalla R, Iannaccone R, et al. Budd-Chiari syndrome: spectrum of imaging findings. AJR Am J Roentgenol. 2007;188:W168–76.
35. Erden A, Erden I, Karayalcin S, Yurdaydin C. Budd-Chiari syndrome: evaluation with multiphase contrast-enhanced three-dimensional MR angiography. AJR Am J Roentgenol. 2002;179:1287–92.
36. Maetani Y, Itoh K, Egawa H, Haga H, Sakurai T, Nishida N, et al. Benign hepatic nodules in Budd-Chiari syndrome: radiologic-pathologic correlation with emphasis on the central scar. AJR Am J Roentgenol. 2002;178:869–75.
37. Flor N, Zuin M, Brovelli F, Maggioni M, Tentori A, Sardanelli F, et al. Regenerative nodules in patients with chronic Budd-Chiari syndrome: A longitudinal study using multiphase contrast-enhanced multidetector CT. Eur J Radiol. 2010;73:588–93.
38. Bruix J, Sherman M. Management of hepatocellular carcinoma. Hepatology. 2005;42:1208–36.
39. Bruix J, Sherman M, Llovet JM, Beaugrand M, Lencioni R, Burroughs AK, et al. Clinical management of hepatocellular carcinoma. Conclusions of the Barcelona-2000 EASL conference. European Association for the Study of the Liver. J Hepatol. 2001;35:421–30.
40. Moucari R, Rautou PE, Cazals-Hatem D, Geara A, Bureau C, Consigny Y, et al. Hepatocellular carcinoma in Budd-Chiari syndrome: characteristics and risk factors. Gut. 2008;57:828–35.
41. Kamath PS. Budd-Chiari syndrome: radiologic findings. Liver Transpl. 2006;12:S21–2.
42. Valla DC. The diagnosis and management of the Budd-Chiari syndrome: consensus and controversies. Hepatology. 2003;38:793–803.
43. Campbell Jr DA, Rolles K, Jamieson N, O'Grady J, Wight D, Williams R, et al. Hepatic transplantation with perioperative and long term anticoagulation as treatment for Budd-Chiari syndrome. Surg Gynecol Obstet. 1988;166:511–8.
44. Halff G, Todo S, Tzakis AG, Gordon RD, Starzl TE. Liver transplantation for the Budd-Chiari syndrome. Ann Surg. 1990;211:43–9.
45. Sharma S, Texeira A, Texeira P, Elias E, Wilde J, Olliff SP. Pharmacological thrombolysis in Budd Chiari syndrome: a single centre experience and review of the literature. J Hepatol. 2004;40: 172–80.
46. Valla D, Hadengue A, El Younsi M, Azar N, Zeitoun G, Boudet MJ, et al. Hepatic venous outflow block caused by short-length hepatic vein stenoses. Hepatology. 1997;25:814–9.
47. Fisher NC, McCafferty I, Dolapci M, Wali M, Buckels JAC, Olliff SP, et al. Managing Budd-Chiari syndrome: a retrospective review of percutaneous hepatic vein angioplasty and surgical shunting (see comments). Gut. 1999;44:568–74.
48. Tilanus HW, Metselaar HJ, Lameris JS. Budd-Chiari syndrome (see comments). Ned Tijdschr Geneeskd. 1995;139:161–5.
49. Mitchell MC, Boitnott JK, Kaufman S, Cameron JL, Maddrey WC. Budd-Chiari syndrome: etiology, diagnosis and management. Medicine (Baltimore). 1982;61:199–218.
50. Shaked A, Goldstein RM, Klintmalm GB, Drazan K, Husberg B, Busuttil RW. Portosystemic shunt versus orthotopic liver transplantation for the Budd-Chiari syndrome. Surg Gynecol Obstet. 1992;174: 453–9.
51. Hemming AW, Langer B, Greig P, Taylor BR, Adams R, Heathcote EJ. Treatment of Budd-Chiari syndrome with portosystemic shunt or liver transplantation. Am J Surg. 1996;171:176–80.
52. Zeitoun G, Escolano S, Hadengue A, Azar N, El Younsi M, Mallet A, et al. Outcome of Budd-Chiari syndrome: a multivariate analysis of factors related to survival including surgical portosystemic shunting. Hepatology. 1999;30:84–9.
53. Langlet P, Valla D. Is surgical portosystemic shunt the treatment of choice in Budd-Chiari syndrome? Acta Gastroenterol Belg. 2002;65:155–60.
54. Panis Y, Belghiti J, Valla D, Benhamou JP, Fekete F. Portosystemic shunt in Budd-Chiari syndrome: long-term survival and factors affecting shunt patency in 25 patients in Western countries. Surgery. 1994;115: 276–81.
55. Bachet JB, Condat B, Hagege H, Plessier A, Consigny Y, Belghiti J, et al. Long-term portosystemic shunt patency as a determinant of outcome in Budd-Chiari syndrome. J Hepatol. 2007;46:60–8.
56. Madsen MS, Petersen TH, Sommer H. Segmental portal hypertension. Ann Surg. 1986;204(1):72–7.
57. Garcia-Pagan JC, Heydtmann M, Raffa S, Plessier A, Murad S, Fabris F, et al. TIPS for Budd-Chiari syndrome: long-term results and prognostics factors in 124 patients. Gastroenterology. 2008;135: 808–15.

58. Perello A, Garcia-Pagan JC, Gilabert R, Suarez Y, Moitinho E, Cervantes F, et al. TIPS is a useful long-term derivative therapy for patients with Budd-Chiari syndrome uncontrolled by medical therapy. Hepatology. 2002;35:132–9.
59. Hernandez-Guerra M, Turnes J, Rubinstein P, Olliff S, Elias E, Bosch J, et al. PTFE-covered stents improve TIPS patency in Budd-Chiari syndrome. Hepatology. 2004;40:1197–202.
60. Turnes J, Garcia-Pagan JC, Gonzalez-Abraldes J, Real M, Moitinho E, Gilabert R, et al. Stenosis of the suprahepatic inferior vena cava as a complication of transjugular intrahepatic portosystemic shunt in Budd-Chiari patients. Liver Transpl. 2001;7:649–51.
61. Segev DL, Nguyen GC, Locke JE, Simpkins CE, Montgomery RA, Maley WR, et al. Twenty years of liver transplantation for Budd-Chiari syndrome: a national registry analysis. Liver Transpl. 2007;13: 1285–94.
62. Adam R, McMaster P, O'Grady JG, Castaing D, Klempnauer JL, Jamieson N, et al. Evolution of liver transplantation in Europe: report of the European Liver Transplant Registry. Liver Transp. 2003;9: 1231–43.
63. Yamada T, Tanaka K, Ogura Y, Ko S, Nakajima Y, Takada Y, et al. Surgical techniques and long-term outcomes of living donor liver transplantation for Budd-Chiari syndrome. Am J Transplant. 2006;6: 2463–9.
64. Yan L, Li B, Zeng Y, Wen T, Zhao J, Wang W, et al. Living donor liver transplantation for Budd-Chiari syndrome using cryopreserved vena cava graft in retrohepatic vena cava reconstruction. Liver Transpl. 2006;12:1017–9.
65. Mentha G, Giostra E, Majno PE, Bechstein WO, Neuhaus P, O'Grady J, et al. Liver transplantation for Budd-Chiari syndrome: a European study on 248 patients from 51 centres. J Hepatol. 2006;44: 520–8.
66. Cruz E, Ascher NL, Roberts JP, Bass NM, Yao FY. High incidence of recurrence and hematologic events following liver transplantation for Budd-Chiari syndrome. Clin Transplant. 2005;19:501–6.
67. Ringe B, Lang H, Oldhafer KJ, Gebel M, Flemming P, Georgii A, et al. Which is the best surgery for Budd-Chiari syndrome: venous decompression or liver transplantation? A single-center experience with 50 patients. Hepatology. 1995;21:1337–44.
68. Srinivasan P, Rela M, Prachalias A, Muiesan P, Portmann B, Mufti GJ, et al. Liver transplantation for Budd-Chiari syndrome. Transplantation. 2002;73: 973–7.
69. Melear JM, Goldstein RM, Levy MF, Molmenti EP, Cooper B, Netto GJ, et al. Hematologic aspects of liver transplantation for Budd-Chiari syndrome with special reference to myeloproliferative disorders. Transplantation. 2002;74:1090–5.
70. Karasu Z, Nart D, Lebe E, Demirbas T, Memis A, Kilic M, et al. Liver transplantation in a patient with Budd-Chiari Syndrome secondary to factor V Leiden mutation. Transplant Proc. 2003;35(8):3008–10.
71. Ganguli SC, Ramzan NN, McKusick MA, Andrews JC, Phyliky RL, Kamath PS. Budd-Chiari syndrome in patients with hematological disease: a therapeutic challenge. Hepatology. 1998;27:1157–61.
72. Au WY, Fung A, Liu CL, Fan ST, Ma SK, Liang R, et al. Serial analysis of JAK2 mutation in a patient who developed essential thrombocythemia after orthotopic liver transplantation. Am J Hematol. 2006;81:880–2.
73. Bahr MJ, Schubert J, Bleck JS, Tietge UJ, Boozari B, Schmidt RE, et al. Recurrence of Budd-Chiari syndrome after liver transplantation in paroxysmal nocturnal hemoglobinuria. Transpl Int. 2003;16:890–4.
74. Jamieson NV, Williams R, Calne RY. Liver transplantation for Budd-Chiari syndrome, 1976-1990. Ann Chir. 1991;45:362–5.
75. Rao AR, Chui AK, Gurkhan A, Shi LW, Al-Harbi I, Waugh R, et al. Orthotopic liver transplantation for treatment of patients with Budd-Chiari syndrome: a Singe-center experience. Transplant Proc. 2000;32:2206–7.
76. Ulrich F, Steinmuller T, Lang M, Settmacher U, Muller AR, Jonas S, et al. Liver transplantation in patients with advanced Budd-Chiari syndrome. Transplant Proc. 2002;34:2278.
77. Bates SM, Greer IA, Pabinger I, Sofaer S, Hirsh J. Venous thromboembolism, thrombophilia, antithrombotic therapy, and pregnancy: American College of Chest Physicians Evidence-Based Clinical Practice Guidelines (8th Edition). Chest. 2008;133: 844S–86.
78. Rautou PE, Angermayr B, Garcia-Pagan JC, Moucari R, Peck-Radosavljevic M, Raffa S, et al. Pregnancy in women with known and treated Budd-Chiari syndrome: maternal and fetal outcomes. J Hepaol. 2009;51:47–54.
79. Langlet P, Escolano S, Valla D, Coste-Zeitoun D, Denie C, Mallet A, et al. Clinicopathological forms and prognostic index in Budd-Chiari syndrome. J Hepatol. 2003;39:496–501.
80. Murad SD, Valla DC, de Groen PC, Zeitoun G, Hopmans JA, Haagsma EB, et al. Determinants of survival and the effect of portosystemic shunting in patients with Budd-Chiari syndrome. Hepatology. 2004;39:500–8.
81. Darwish MS, Kim WR, de Groen PC, Kamath PS, Malinchoc M, Valla DC, et al. Can the model for end-stage liver disease be used to predict the prognosis in patients with Budd-Chiari syndrome? Liver Transpl. 2007;13:867–74.
82. Rautou PE, Moucari R, Escolano S, Cazals-Hatem D, Denie C, Chagneau-Derrode C, et al. Prognostic indices for Budd-Chiari syndrome: valid for clinical studies but insufficient for individual management. Am J Gastroenterol. 2009;104:1140–6.
83. Mohanty D, Shetty S, Ghosh K, Pawar A, Abraham P. Hereditary thrombophilia as a cause of Budd-Chiari syndrome: a study from Western India. Hepatology. 2001;34:666–70.

84. Mahmoud AE, Elias E, Beauchamp N, Wilde JT. Prevalence of the factor V Leiden mutation in hepatic and portal vein thrombosis [see comments]. Gut. 1997;40:798–800.
85. Bhattacharyya M, Makharia G, Kannan M, Ahmed RP, Gupta PK, Saxena R. Inherited prothrombotic defects in Budd-Chiari syndrome and portal vein thrombosis: a study from North India. Am J Clin Pathol. 2004; 121:844–7.
86. Bayraktar Y, Balkanci F, Bayraktar M, Calguneri M. Budd-Chiari syndrome: a common complication of Behcet's disease. Am J Gastroenterol. 1997;92:858–62.

14 Congenital Hepatic Vascular Malformations

Guadalupe Garcia-Tsao

Abstract

Congenital hepatic vascular malformations are rare entities that result in abnormal shunting of blood through the liver. Three different types of shunting can occur: arteriovenous (hepatic artery to hepatic vein), arterio-portal (hepatic artery to portal vein) and portovenous (portal vein to hepatic vein). Malformations result from alterations in the formation of blood vessels during fetal development and can occur as an isolated abnormality or form a part of a systemic illness, such as hereditary hemorrhagic telangiectasia in which all three types of shunting coexist. Clinical features depend on the type and extent of shunting.

Keywords

Hepatic vascular malformations • Arteriohepatic shunt • Arterioportal shunt • Portosystemic shunt • Hereditary hemorrhagic telangiectasia

Congenital hepatic vascular malformations (HVMs) are rare entities that result in abnormal shunting of blood through the liver. Given the dual blood supply to the liver (hepatic artery and portal vein), three different patterns of abnormal vascular communications can occur between the hepatic artery and the hepatic vein (arterio-venous), between the hepatic artery and the portal vein (arterioportal) and between the portal vein and the hepatic vein (portovenous). Congenital HVMs result from alterations in the formation of blood vessels during fetal development [1] and can occur as an isolated abnormality or form a part of a systemic illness, such as hereditary hemorrhagic telangiectasia (HHT) [2].

HVMs can be discovered fortuitously at the time of abdominal imaging studies performed for other reasons or they can be diagnosed in a symptomatic patient. Symptoms depend mostly on the type and extent of the intrahepatic shunt. Symptoms of HVMs in the setting of HHT do not occur in children [3]; therefore when compatible symptoms present in children they are usually due to a vascular tumor or an isolated abnormality of a single type (arteriovenous,

G. Garcia-Tsao(✉)
Section of Digestive Diseases, Yale University School of Medicine, 333 Cedar Street, LMP 1080, New Haven, CT 06520, USA
and
Section of Digestive Diseases, VA Connecticut Health Care System, West Haven, CT, USA
e-mail: guadalupe.garcia-tsao@yale.edu

L.D. DeLeve and G. Garcia-Tsao (eds.), *Vascular Liver Disease: Mechanisms and Management*,
DOI 10.1007/978-1-4419-8327-5_14, © Springer Science+Business Media, LLC 2011

arterioportal *or* portosystemic). In HVMs associated with HHT, all three types of shunts may coexist and therefore this entity will be considered separately.

Congenital Hepatic Arteriovenous Malformations (HAVM)

These consist of hepatic artery to hepatic vein shunts. Although congenital hepatic vascular neoplasms, such as hemangioendothelioma, account for the large majority of hepatic arteriovenous shunting in infants [4], they cannot be considered AVMs [1, 5] and are therefore not considered in this chapter (see Chap. 17). Congenital HAVMs occur in less than 1:100,000 live births [6]. They are usually discrete, localized in one lobe of the liver and, unlike AVMs associated with vascular tumors they do not grow or regress [1].

Pathophysiology

In HAVMs, blood from the high-pressure artery is shunted to a low-pressure vein (the hepatic vein), thereby decreasing systemic vascular resistance. This results in a compensatory increase in the heart rate and stroke volume, and total plasma volume is increased, i.e., a hyperdynamic circulatory state develops that, over time, leads to heart failure (Fig. 14.1).

Clinical Presentation

The usual clinical presentation is that of high-output heart failure occurring in the first 6 months of life (mean 2.2 months). Other presenting features include hepatomegaly, "fetal hydrops" (anasarca), consumptive coagulopathy and features of pulmonary hypertension [6]. Congenital HAVM carry a mortality rate that is 50–90% higher than that of hemangioendothelioma [4]. The presence of multiple feeder vessels is a poor prognostic sign.

Diagnosis

Sonographically, AVMs characteristically appear as echopenic dilated vascular channels replacing

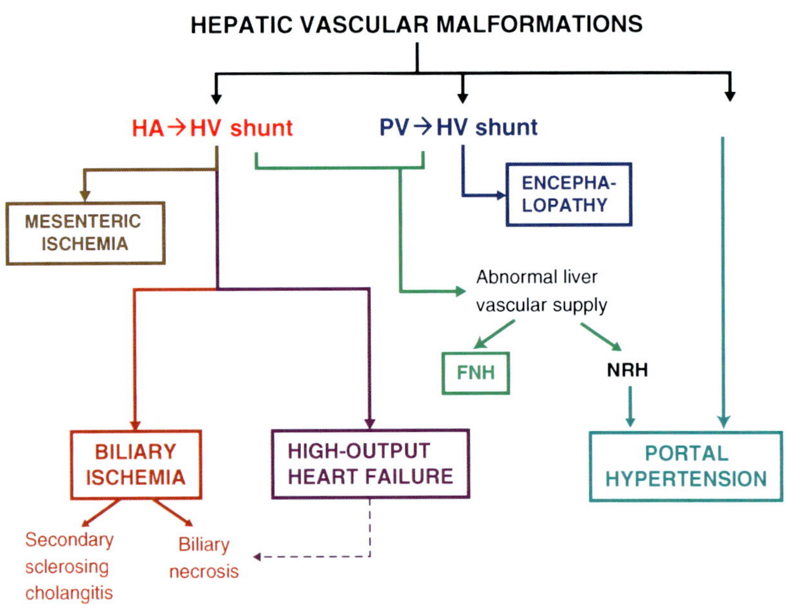

Fig. 14.1 Pathogenesis of different clinical presentations of hepatic vascular malformations. *VMs* vascular malformations; *HA* hepatic artery; *HV* hepatic vein; *PV* portal vein; *FNH* focal nodular hyperplasia; *NRH* nodular regenerative hyperplasia. Adapted from ref. [2]

liver parenchyma that, on Doppler ultrasonography (DUS), show a high flow with lack of arterial pulsation [7]. Prenatal (in utero) diagnosis is possible when sonography detects multiple engorged vascular channels in the fetal liver [7].

The main differential is with proliferating liver tumors that have a more solid homogeneous or slightly heterogeneous appearance and are less echogenic than the surrounding tissue [7]. Magnetic resonance imaging (MRI) is the most useful tool to make the differential diagnosis.

Treatment

Treatment initially consists of the conservative medical management of heart failure. In patients who fail to respond to this therapy, embolization or surgical ligation of the feeder vessel is the most effective therapy, particularly in patients with a single HAVM.

Orthotopic liver transplant may be the only recourse for those infants with HAVM and multiple feeder vessels who do not respond to transcatheter embolization and whose lesion is not amenable to surgical resection.

Congenital Hepatic Arterioportal Malformations (HAPM)

These represent shunting from the hepatic artery to the portal vein and are also called intrahepatic arterioportal fistulae. Congenital HAPM represent less than 10% of all arterioportal fistulae, most of which are acquired, resulting mostly from trauma [8]. Diffuse, or multiple, HAPM are virtually always congenital, while acquired fistulae are usually solitary. Congenital HAPM are a rare but treatable cause of portal hypertension in infancy and early childhood.

Pathophysiology

The main consequence of this type of HVM is portal hypertension. The most obvious cause of portal hypertension is shunting of blood from the hepatic artery to the portal vein (see Fig. 14.1). However, with abnormal hepatic flow, nodular regenerative hyperplasia, and/or hepatoportal sclerosis and fibrosis of the portal radicles develop, further contributing to the increased portal pressure. Therefore the condition should be suspected early on and treated as soon as it is diagnosed before it progresses to an irreversible stage.

Clinical Presentation

The diagnosis should be suspected in an infant or child with recurrent and severe upper gastrointestinal bleeding, failure to thrive, hepatic bruit and splenomegaly or ascites [9, 10]. Congenital HAPM can be classified as (a) unilateral (supplied by either the right, the left or the main hepatic artery), (b) bilateral in which arterial blood is supplied from both the left and right hepatic arteries or their branches, and (c) complex lesions that consist typically of a plexiform vascular nidus with multiple feeding arteries, including supply from arteries other than the hepatic arteries (e.g., gastric artery) [10]. A review of the literature shows that the unilateral presentation is present in slightly over half of the patients. Three quarters present by 2 years of age, with a mean age of approximately 3 years (range, 1 week to 16 years), with cases of unilateral HAPM presenting considerably later than bilateral or complex cases [10, 11].

Diagnosis

DUS is the single most useful diagnostic method [1, 9]. The key diagnostic finding is a pulsatile (inverted) flow in the portal vein [10, 12]. Hepatic angiography is useful to confirm the diagnosis and to accurately delineate the vascular anatomy as this will allow for treatment planning.

Treatment

Transarterial embolization is the mainstay of treatment for children with noncomplex congenital HAPM. Single (unilateral) arterioportal shunts are usually resolved by embolization of the feeding artery. Complex congenital HAPM are prone to collateralization and/or recurrence after radiological intervention. Hence, they may be difficult to treat without a combination of surgery and embolization [10]. In fact, a surgical approach should be considered for fistulae that do not resolve after several trials of embolization and should be considered as the initial treatment of patients with complex HAPM [10]. Liver transplantation is a therapeutic option if embolization is unsuccessful or unfeasible [12]. Transplantation may be complicated because of the presence of portal vein arterialization and previous HA ligation. Portosystemic shunts should not be undertaken in the treatment of portal hypertension secondary to HAPM, as they may precipitate heart failure by rerouting arterialized portal blood directly into the systemic venous circulation [10].

Congenital Portosystemic Shunts (CPSS)

CPSS represent shunts between the portal vein and the systemic circulation (i.e., portosystemic shunts). They are very rare anomalies that occur in the absence of portal hypertension and result from developmental abnormalities of the portal venous system. Until 2007 there had only been approximately 107 cases of CPSS reported in the literature [13]. Anatomically, CPSS are divided into extra- and intrahepatic shunts [9, 14].

Congenital *extrahepatic* portosystemic shunts (CEPS) were first described by Abernethy in 1793 and are therefore called Abernethy malformations. Two anatomical subtypes of CEPS have been described: in type 1, there is "absence" (or severe hypoplasia) of the portal vein with total shunting of blood from the mesenteric and splenic veins into the systemic circulation, while in type 2 the portal vein (or intrahepatic branches) is patent but some of its flow is diverted into a systemic vein through an extrahepatic communication (partial shunt) [15]. Type 1 CEPS predominates in females, is diagnosed at a median age of 10 years (range 31 weeks of intrauterine life to 76 years) and is associated with multiple other malformations, such as polysplenia, malrotation, complex congenital heart abnormalities, biliary atresia, skeletal and renal abnormalities. Type 2 is even rarer with no gender preference and its diagnosis is established at a median age of 18 months (range 28 weeks of intrauterine life to 69 years) [16].

Intrahepatic portosystemic shunts are abnormal intrahepatic connections between a branch of the portal vein and the hepatic vein, including patent ductus venosus. These shunts have also been further subclassified into different anatomical types [17]. As CEPS, they can also be associated with congenital anomalies, particularly cardiac malformations. Some congenital intrahepatic portosystemic venous shunts close spontaneously in infancy.

Clinical Presentation

The clinical presentation of CPSS varies widely. When present, symptoms are similar between the two types of CPSS and are secondary to shunting of blood away from the liver.

With the widespread use of ultrasound, extrahepatic PSS have been increasingly discovered in otherwise healthy patients or as part of the workup of cardiac anomalies [1]. In some countries, they are diagnosed during routine newborn screening for hypergalactosemia. Occasionally, shunts are detected as the cause of psychiatric disturbance or mental retardation secondary to chronic hyperammonemia [18].

Patients with symptomatic CPSS exhibit abnormalities of neuropsychological tests, magnetic resonance spectroscopy and response to oral glutamine challenge similar to those observed in patients with cirrhosis and minimal hepatic encephalopathy [18]. Overt encephalopathy is present in a minority (about 15%) of congenital PSS cases [16] and usually occurs in adults. An age-dependent decrease in the tolerance of the central nervous system to hyperammonemia has been implicated [19], although more compelling data indicate that the presence of encephalopathy may be more dependent on the degree of portosystemic shunting [20, 21]. Parkinsonism has been described as an evidence of encephalopathy in a patient with intrahepatic PSS [22]. Unlike hepatic encephalopathy, where in addition to portosystemic shunting there is an element of liver insufficiency, in CPSS encephalopathy is due solely to portosystemic shunting (real portosystemic encephalopathy) and it therefore belongs to the recently defined type B (bypass) encephalopathy [23].

Interestingly, CPSS (both intra and extrahepatic) are frequently (up to 40% of the cases) associated with hepatic tumors (including focal nodular hyperplasia (FNH), adenoma and hepatocellular carcinoma) and the development of at least some of these (e.g., FNH) may be related to an uneven liver vascular perfusion [16, 24, 25].

Other complications related to shunting and/or chronic hyperammonemia have been described such as nephrolithiasis and hepatopulmonary syndrome [26].

Diagnosis

DUS is the most useful in the diagnosis of CPSS and also in determining the shunt ratio (obtained by dividing the total flow volume in the shunt by that in the portal vein). Of note, spontaneous closure of patent ductus venosus may occur within the first 2 years of life and thus close follow-up is warranted because most of them are asymptomatic.

Treatment

Treatment is restricted to symptomatic patients and should be initially conservative and follow the same guidelines as in encephalopathy secondary to cirrhosis [27].

Treatment in symptomatic patients that do not respond to conservative treatment consists of surgical or laparoscopic ligation of the shunt or obliteration by interventional radiology using metallic coils. A key factor affecting the outcome after shunt occlusion is the patency (or lack of patency) of the portal vein and the consequent degree of increase in portal pressure after shunt ligation [16]. Preoperative evaluation of portal pressure and determination of the type of CPSS by angiography is crucial. Ligation/occlusion of the CPSS is an option when there is portal patency. In cases of severely hypoplastic intra- and extrahepatic portal system, liver transplantation should be considered [19].

Hereditary Hemorrhagic Telangiectasia

HHT, or Rendu-Osler-Weber disease, is a genetic disease with an autosomal dominant inheritance pattern, characterized by widespread vascular malformations that can involve the skin, mucous membranes, lung, brain, the gastrointestinal tract and/or liver. It has an estimated prevalence of 1 in 5,000–8,000 [28, 29]. Vascular malformations range in size from "pinpoint" telangiectases smaller than one millimeter (consisting of dilatation of preexisting postcapillary venules) to larger (1–2 mm) lesions (real arterio-venous communications) [30, 31] to malformations that can be larger than 5 cm, such as those that occur in the lung.

Pathophysiology of HHT

Most cases of HHT are due to heterozygous mutations in one of two genes: (a) the transforming growth factor β (TGF-β) type III receptor, *endoglin*, located in chromosome 9 and responsible for the more severe HHT type 1 phenotypic pattern with predominant involvement of pulmonary vasculature [32–35], or (b) the TGF-β type I receptor, *activin receptor-like kinase type 1 (ALK-1 or ACVRL1)*, located in chromosome 12 and responsible for the more frequent HHT type 2 phenotype [35–37]. Another identified mutation is the SMAD4 mutation, associated with a syndrome of combined juvenile polyposis and HHT [38]. Approximately 20% of families with typical HHT phenotype do not have mutations in any of these three genes [39]. Loci on chromosomes 5 and 7 have been associated with HHT in two families [40, 41], but genes associated with these loci have not been identified and testing is therefore not available.

The development of vascular malformations in HHT has been attributed to defective TGF-β activation by endothelial cells together with increased vascular endothelial growth factor (VEGF) production [42]. Reports of growth and spontaneous regression of cerebral AVMs [43–45] with endothelial proliferation on histology indicate that active angiogenesis may play a role in the growth and regression of AVMs in HHT [46]. In fact, anecdotal reports of antiangiogenic drugs such as interferon, bevacizumab (an anti-VEGF drug), and, more recently, thalidomide have been associated with an improvement in nosebleeds [42, 47], a reduction in gastrointestinal bleeding [48, 49] and amelioration of heart failure [49, 50]. Amelioration of epistaxis by thalidomide is apparently not the result of direct inhibition of endothelial cell proliferation and migration, but is rather due to increased mural cell coverage of the vasculature, through increased platelet-derived growth factor (PDGF) expression, making vessels less prone to bleeding [42]. Studies using these drugs, rather than indicating a clinical use, are essential to expand the knowledge of the molecular pathways that regulate mechanisms of vascular stabilization and should eventually lead to rational and safer therapies in the treatment of different VMs present in HHT [51].

Hepatic Vascular Malformations in HHT

HVMs are more common in HHT-2, the type associated with ALK-1 mutations. Overall, 77% (217/281) of HVMs and all but one of 31 symptomatic HVMs have been described in patients with ALK-1 mutation [52].

HVMs are widespread throughout the liver and include both microscopic and macroscopic vascular malformations of variable size, ranging from tiny telangiectases to discrete arteriovenous malformations [53–55]. Large prospective studies, in which sensitive Doppler ultrasound and/or multidetector computed tomography (CT) have been performed systematically in HHT-affected subjects, have demonstrated imaging abnormalities compatible with HVMs in up to 84% of patients with HHT [56–59]. The presence of HVMs appear to be age-dependent, with HVMs present in ~10% of patients younger than 40 years, compared to 50% in patients >40 years [59]. As mentioned previously, symptoms related to HVM do not occur in children. The three types of shunting (arteriohepatic, arterioportal and portovenous) likely occur concomitantly, but usually one of them predominates functionally and clinically.

Pathophysiology

The predominant type and the extent of shunting determine the clinical presentation (see Fig. 14.1).

Arteriovenous shunting (as described above for CAVM) leads to a chronically increased cardiac output and, eventually, to high-output heart failure. Notably, FNH, an asymptomatic focal mass of regenerating hepatocytes, is ten times more common in patients with HHT than in the general population (prevalence 2.9% vs. 0.3%) [60] and is most probably related to arteriovenous shunting with a greater arterial blood flow to that region compared to the adjacent parenchyma [61, 62]. Additionally, arteriovenous shunting in HHT can lead to shunting of blood away from the mesenteric circulation into the liver ("steal" syndrome) resulting in intestinal ischemia [63, 64].

Arterioportal shunting (as described above for CAPM) leads to portal hypertension that is further perpetuated by the development of nodular regenerative hyperplasia or portal venular fibrosis.

The biliary system derives its supply exclusively from the peribiliary plexus, which arises from the hepatic artery. Shunting of blood from the hepatic artery to either the hepatic or the portal vein leads to biliary hypoperfusion with subsequent development of biliary ischemia that in turn leads to biliary stricturing (with or without cholangitis) and biliary necrosis with cyst (biloma) formation. In its most severe form, biliary ischemia can lead to hepatic "disintegration" (also called acute biliary necrosis). This entity is characterized by disruption of liver structure, hepatocyte necrosis, hemorrhage and extravasation of bile [65].

Portovenous shunting (as described above for CPSS) leads to portosystemic encephalopathy, a rare presentation. Encephalopathy is the result of shunting from the portal vein to the hepatic vein and belongs to the recently defined type B (bypass) encephalopathy [23]. This type of shunt may also contribute to a high cardiac preload and heart failure.

Clinical Presentations

Only 5–8% of patients with HHT and HVMs are symptomatic [56, 57, 59, 66]. A recent review of the English literature spanning 29 years revealed only 89 unique patients with HHT and symptomatic HVMs [3].

The three most common and distinct clinical presentations are: high-output cardiac failure, biliary ischemia and portal hypertension [67]. Portosystemic encephalopathy and abdominal angina are rarer presentations that usually occur in the setting of other more common presentations [3].

High-Output Heart Failure

This is the most common presentation, corresponding to 63% of cases reported in the literature [3]. It occurs predominantly in females at a median age of around 52 years [3]. The presence of concomitant anemia and/or large AVMs elsewhere can worsen the hyperdynamic circulatory state. In younger patients, heart failure can be precipitated by pregnancy [68], which in itself is a hyperdynamic circulatory state. Patients present with exertional dyspnea, paroxysmal nocturnal dyspnea, orthopnea, ascites and/or peripheral edema. A liver bruit has been reported to be present in about half the cases [3]. Other signs on physical examination include systolic murmur and S3. Epistaxis worsens at the time of development of heart failure [69]. A recent study of 102 asymptomatic patients with HHT and HVMs showed that the size of the hepatic artery (as assessed by ultrasonography) and the presence of FNH were independent predictors of a high cardiac index [70].

Portal Hypertension

Seventeen percent of cases reported in the literature correspond to this clinical type [3]. In a prospective case series, this presentation was more common than the biliary presentation [67]. Portal hypertension presents equally in males and females at a median age of 62 years. Patients present with ascites, varices, and variceal hemorrhage. These symptoms, in the presence of a nodular liver (nodular regenerative hyperplasia), may reasonably lead to a misdiagnosis of cirrhosis, which may explain a probable under-reporting of this presentation in the literature. These patients also appear to be at an increased risk of bleeding from gastrointestinal AVMs [67].

Biliary Presentation

Nineteen percent of cases reported in the literature correspond to this clinical type [3]. It occurs almost exclusively in females at a median age of 39 years and is characterized by right upper quadrant pain and cholestasis with or without cholangitis [3]. Like heart failure, pregnancy can precipitate this presentation [71–74]. In some cases, pain resolves spontaneously, while in others it becomes chronic and resistant to treatment with narcotics [67]. In the most severe cases, the onset of pain is sudden with cholangitis, sepsis, liver failure and/or liver hemorrhage. These cases of "hepatic disintegration" have a very poor prognosis and represent the only emergency situation in HVMs related to HHT [65].

Portosystemic Encephalopathy

Portosystemic Encephalopathy is a rare presentation that has been described in 4% of patients with HVMs reported in the literature [3]. As in cirrhotic hepatic encephalopathy, a precipitating factor can sometimes be identified (e.g., blood in the gut).

Abdominal Angina

This is a rare presentation of HHT and its symptoms are those of mesenteric ischemia, typically postprandial generalized abdominal pain [63, 64].

Diagnosis

Screening of the lung and brain are recommended in patients with HHT to identify pulmonary and cerebral AVMs, given the availability of successful preventative treatment options and the risk of substantial morbidity and mortality in unscreened, untreated patients. Pulmonary AVMs may cause brain abscess, stroke, or hypoxemia due to right to left shunting while cerebral AVMs may cause brain hemorrhage and death. Since no standard therapy for asymptomatic HVMs exists to date, and as recently established by consensus [75, 76], screening (and surveillance) using DUS in patients with HHT should remain a research tool or be used to establish a diagnosis of "definite" HHT in patients who meet only 1–2 diagnostic criteria [77].

In patients with known HHT, the presence of symptoms of heart failure (dyspnea, orthopnea, paroxysmal nocturnal dyspnea, ascites or peripheral edema), portal hypertension (ascites, variceal hemorrhage), cholestasis (jaundice, increased alkaline phosphatase) with or without cholangitis and abdominal pain suggestive of mesenteric ischemia should suggest HVMs.

The diagnosis is difficult to make in patients with these symptoms who do not have a diagnosis of HHT and a higher degree of suspicion is necessary on the part of the clinician. In such patients a personal and/or family history of epistaxis, telangiectases (cutaneous or mucosal), heart failure, cerebrovascular accident, abscesses or liver disease should raise the suspicion of HHT with liver involvement.

Laboratory Tests

Most patients have elevated alkaline phosphatase and/or gamma-glutamyl transpeptidase serum levels. These elevations are usually mild, except in patients with the biliary presentation in which they can be quite elevated and associated with hyperbilirubinemia [67]. Despite extensive shunting, liver synthetic function is preserved and therefore albumin and prothrombin time are typically normal. Remarkably, platelet count is normal and actually somewhat elevated, even in patients with portal hypertension. This is further indication of a preserved liver synthetic function as thrombocytopenia in cirrhosis is partially due to deficient thrombopoietin synthesis from the cirrhotic liver [78].

Imaging Studies

Although angiography is the gold standard in establishing the presence of HVMs and the type of shunting, it is invasive and other less invasive modalities have now been shown to have a high sensitivity in detecting HVMs. Angiography is currently restricted to cases of abdominal angina in which the "steal" syndrome can be diagnosed based on superior mesenteric angiographic findings.

Currently, HVMs can be diagnosed by DUS [56, 79], CT [80, 81], or MRI [67], DUS, spiral and multidetector CT and MRI. The hallmark findings are intrahepatic hypervascularization (or telangiectases) and an enlarged common hepatic artery (Fig. 14.2).

A classification of the spectrum of HVMs on DUS has been proposed that includes earlier stages, prior to the development of hepatic arterial dilatation and thereby prior to the development of symptoms [56]. In such cases, the focus is on minor DUS signs of HVMs, such as peripheral hypervascularization and/or hepatic arterial increased flow velocity or decreased resistive index. However, while interobserver agreement is very good in determining the presence (or absence) of HVMs, it is only moderate for grading their severity [82]. In expert hands, DUS should be the screening test for HVMs because of its accuracy, noninvasiveness, availability and lower cost [75]. However, given the lack of therapy for asymptomatic HVMs, screening of asymptomatic patients is currently not warranted outside of research studies [76].

CT is arguably the most utilized noninvasive test for diagnosing HAVMs. All patients with symptomatic liver involvement have a markedly heterogeneous hepatic enhancement pattern and a markedly dilated hepatic artery [55, 81]. The type of shunting can be determined in over two-thirds of the patients by looking for early or differential enhancement of hepatic veins (arteriovenous shunting) or portal veins (arterioportal shunting) during various phases of imaging [81] (see

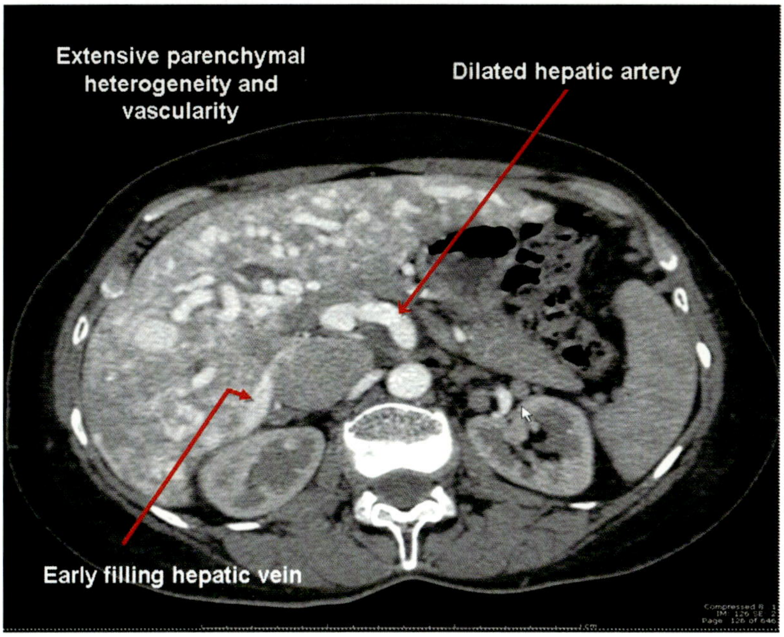

Fig. 14.2 Computed tomography showing the hallmark findings of HVMs in a patient with HHT. There is intrahepatic hypervascularization with heterogeneous liver perfusion, an enlarged common hepatic artery and early filling of the hepatic vein indicative of arteriovenous shunting

Fig. 14.2). Although arterioportal shunting is found significantly more frequently in patients with the portal hypertension clinical presentation, there is no real correlation between CT findings and the clinical presentation [81]. Portovenous shunts are rarely seen on imaging studies [55, 81].

Liver Biopsy

Liver biopsy is not indicated in patients suspected of hepatic involvement in HHT, not only because the procedure may be associated with an increased risk of bleeding given the presence of widespread VMs [75], but because histology is not helpful in making the diagnosis and may lead to confusion. A careful analysis of histological abnormalities in HHT reveals that common findings include ectatic vessels, changes compatible with nodular regenerative hyperplasia (with regeneration alternating with atrophic areas) and thick fibrous bands along ectatic vessels [67]. The combination of regeneration and fibrosis can lead to a misdiagnosis of cirrhosis, as had originally been described [83]. However, this is not true cirrhosis and has been termed "pseudocirrhosis" [84] as normal hepatocellular architecture is preserved within nodules, including central veins and portal areas.

Specific Tests Depending on Presentation

In patients with high-output heart failure, right heart catheterization is the gold standard for the diagnosis and determination of severity and may also be useful in determining response to therapy. Although cardiac output is increased in practically all patients with symptomatic HVMs (independent of type of presentation), the highest values are obtained in patients with the high-output heart failure presentation, with over 90% of them having a cardiac output >8 L/min or a cardiac index >6 L/min/m^2 (normal range is 2.5–4.0 L/min/m^2)[3]. Transthoracic Doppler echocardiogram has been proposed as an alternative to right heart catheterization in patients with heart failure but requires validation [52]. Mild elevations in pulmonary arterial pressure are observed in these patients (median 22 mmHg, range 19–35) [67] and are secondary to heart failure (and an increased pulmonary capillary wedged pressure). This is different from the primary pulmonary hypertension described in patients with

HHT in whom median pulmonary arterial pressure was 66 mmHg (range 45–120) [85, 86].

In patients with symptoms compatible with portal hypertension, portal pressure measurements by the hepatic venous pressure gradient (HVPG) demonstrate the presence of clinically significant portal hypertension, that is, an HVPG ≥10 mmHg [67].

Biliary abnormalities (by multidetector CT or magnetic resonance cholangiopancreatography or MRCP) include biliary strictures resembling sclerosing cholangitis, focal cystic dilatation resembling Caroli's disease and biliary cysts [87]. Notably, in patients with symptomatic HVMs, biliary abnormalities are the most common abnormality observed on CT, even in the absence of biliary symptoms [81]. This is in contrast to imaging studies of asymptomatic patients with HVMs in which biliary abnormalities are absent [57, 80]. This suggests that biliary ischemia occurs later in the disease process at a time when the degree of hepatic arterial shunting is greater. The diagnosis of active biliary ischemia/necrosis is established in a patient with right upper quadrant pain, worsening liver tests and the development and/or growth of biliary cysts. Endoscopic retrograde pancreatography (ERCP) should be avoided in these patients as it significantly increases the risk of cholangitis.

Treatment

Patients with HHT who do not have symptoms of hepatic involvement and in whom HVMs are discovered on imaging studies do not need any specific treatment or follow-up. In patients with a high cardiac output it may make sense to restrict sodium intake.

The following recommendations for patients with symptomatic HVMs are mostly based on expert opinion obtained and graded at consensus conferences [75, 76, 86, 88].

Symptomatic Therapy

Intensive medical treatment aimed at the predominant clinical presentation should be the first line of therapy.

High-output heart failure responds initially to intensive medical treatment with salt restriction, diuretics, beta-blockers, digoxin and angiotensin-converting enzyme inhibitors. In addition treatment should be focused on the correction of anemia and arrhythmias. Pregnant patients who develop high-output cardiac failure should be treated medically and delivered as expeditiously as possible given spontaneous regression of heart failure postpartum.

Treatment of portal hypertension and encephalopathy should follow the same guidelines recommended for patients with cirrhosis [27, 89, 90]. Notably, placement of transjugular intrahepatic portosystemic (TIPS) does not ameliorate bleeding from gastrointestinal AVMs [91]. However, in patients with intractable variceal hemorrhage, particularly if there is concomitant true cirrhosis, TIPS placement would be warranted [92].

Patients with right upper quadrant pain suggestive of biliary ischemia, without cholangitis, can be treated with analgesics. Use of ursodeoxycholic acid may be helpful although no data exist on its benefit. Patients with cholangitis need aggressive treatment with antibiotics. In patients with active biliary ischemia/necrosis with developing or growing biliary cysts, whose pain is not responding to analgesics and/or who develop signs of infection, biliary drainage should be considered with chronic administration of antibiotics [2].

Therapy of mesenteric ischemia is challenging and should initially be based on analgesics and small frequent meals.

Shunt Embolization/Ligation

Transarterial embolization or surgical ligation has been used most commonly in the treatment of high-output heart failure but has also been used in the treatment of a few patients with portal hypertension and mesenteric ischemia [2]. Although amelioration or resolution of symptoms has been reported in most of these cases, this effect is generally only transient and treatment is often associated with significant morbidity and mortality, mostly in the form of biliary and/or hepatic necrosis that can be associated with sepsis and death. In fact, of 23 cases reported in the literature in whom hepatic artery embolization/

ligation was performed for high-output heart failure, 7 (30%) developed complications that led to transplantation or death [93]. Gradual banding of the hepatic artery directed by intraoperative flow measurements has been recently described in two patients and may be a safer procedure [94].

Embolization or ligation of the hepatic artery will only worsen biliary ischemia and should therefore be proscribed in patients with evidence of biliary ischemia, even if this is associated with another clinical type. This is supported by two cases in the literature that had both high-output heart failure and biliary symptoms and were treated by transarterial embolization [95, 96]. In both cases, embolization resulted in ischemia of the biliary tree with recurrent episodes of cholangitis and sepsis that necessitated liver transplantation.

Liver Transplantation

As described in Chap. 17, in the largest series of liver transplantation in patients with HHT and symptomatic HVMs, excellent 1-, 5- and 10-year survival rates of 82.5% were observed [97]. The best results were obtained in patients with heart failure ($n=23$) with a median survival of 87% in a median follow-up period of 47 months and in those with the biliary presentation ($n=19$) with a median survival of 79% in a median follow-up period of 90 months [2]. Survival in the group transplanted for complications of portal hypertension ($n=9$) appeared to be the worst with an overall median survival of 63% in a median follow-up period of 47 months [2]. A more recent analysis of 12 patients transplanted in a single center showed a similar good outcome with a survival of 12/13 (92%) in a mean follow-up of 109 months. Interestingly in those with high-output heart failure, the cardiac index decreased significantly and nine patients experienced a dramatic improvement in epistaxis and quality of life [98].

Despite these encouraging results, definition of candidates for transplant and the best time to start transplant workup remain uncertain. Until natural history studies further clarify these issues, transplant candidacy is evaluated on a case-by-case basis and is mainly indicated in patients with intractable heart failure, mesenteric ischemia or biliary necrosis. Development of spontaneous biliary necrosis, particularly in patients with heart failure, carries the highest mortality (Young et al., unpublished observations), and emergent liver transplantation should be considered in these patients [99].

Experimental Therapy

A recent report showed that a 3-month course of bevacizumab, an anti-VEGF antibody, reversed the hemodynamic changes in a patient with HVMs and advanced heart failure with normalization of cardiac output from 10.2 to 5.1 L/min [50]. Another drug, thalidomide, was associated with a significant decrease in epistaxis [42]. Despite these exciting findings, these drugs should be used with extreme caution in humans, because they may also affect normal physiology and lead to potentially deleterious side effects. Rather than indicating a clinical use, future studies should elucidate the mechanism of action of these drugs so that their use or that of similar safer drugs can be targeted to specific patient populations [51].

References

1. Gallego C, Miralles M, Marin C, Muyor P, Gonzalez G, Garcia-Hidalgo E. Congenital hepatic shunts. Radiographics 2004; 24(3):755–772.
2. Khalid SK, Garcia-Tsao G. Hepatic vascular malformations in hereditary hemorrhagic telangiectasia. Sem Liv Dis 28, 247–258. 2008.Ref Type: Abstract
3. Garcia-Tsao G. Liver involvement in hereditary hemorrhagic telangiectasia (HHT). J Hepatol 2007; 46(3):499–507.
4. Boon LM, Burrows PE, Paltiel HJ, Lund DP, Ezekowitz RA, Folkman J et al. Hepatic vascular anomalies in infancy: a twenty-seven-year experience. J Pediatr 1996; 129(3):346–354.
5. Prokurat A, Kluge P, Chrupek M, Kosciesza A, Rajszys P. Hemangioma of the liver in children: proliferating vascular tumor or congenital vascular malformation? Med Pediatr Oncol 2002; 39(5):524–529.
6. Alexander CP, Sood BG, Zilberman MV, Becker C, Bedard MP. Congenital hepatic arteriovenous malformation: an unusual cause of neonatal persistent pulmonary hypertension. J Perinatol 2006; 26(5): 316–318.
7. Botha T, Rasmussen O, Carlan SJ, Greenbaum L. Congenital hepatic arteriovenous malformation: sonographic findings and clinical implications. Journal of Diagnostic Medical Sonography 2004; 20(17): 177–181.

8. Vauthey JN, Tomczak RJ, Helmberger T, Gertsch P, Forsmark C, Caridi J et al. The arterioportal fistula syndrome: clinicopathologic features, diagnosis, and therapy. Gastroenterology 1997; 113(4):1390–1401.
9. Gallego C, Velasco M, Marcuello P, Tejedor D, De Campo L, Friera A. Congenital and acquired anomalies of the portal venous system. Radiographics 2002; 22(1):141–159.
10. Norton SP, Jacobson K, Moroz SP, Culham G, Ng V, Turner J et al. The congenital intrahepatic arterioportal fistula syndrome: elucidation and proposed classification. J Pediatr Gastroenterol Nutr 2006; 43(2):248–255.
11. Kumar N, de GJ, V, Sharif K, McKiernan P, John P. Congenital, solitary, large, intrahepatic arterioportal fistula in a child: management and review of the literature. Pediatr Radiol 2003; 33(1):20–23.
12. Mallant MP, van den Berg FG, Verbeke JI, Bokenkamp A. Pulsatile hepatofugal flow in the portal vein: hallmark of a congenital hepatoportal arteriovenous fistula. J Pediatr Gastroenterol Nutr 2007; 44(1):143–145.
13. Witters P, Maleux G, George C, Delcroix M, Hoffman I, Gewillig M et al. Congenital veno-venous malformations of the liver: widely variable clinical presentations. J Gastroenterol Hepatol 2008; 23(8 Pt 2):e390-e394.
14. Stringer MD. The clinical anatomy of congenital portosystemic venous shunts. Clin Anat 2008; 21(2): 147–157.
15. Morgan G, Superina R. Congenital absence of the portal vein: two cases and a proposed classification system for portasystemic vascular anomalies. J Pediatr Surg 1994; 29(9):1239–1241.
16. Murray CP, Yoo SJ, Babyn PS. Congenital extrahepatic portosystemic shunts. Pediatr Radiol 2003; 33(9):614–620.
17. Park JH, Cha SH, Han JK, Han MC. Intrahepatic portosystemic venous shunt. AJR Am J Roentgenol 1990; 155(3):527–528.
18. Ortiz M, Cordoba J, Alonso J, Rovira A, Quiroga S, Jacas C et al. Oral glutamine challenge and magnetic resonance spectroscopy in three patients with congenital portosystemic shunts. J Hepatol 2004; 40(3): 552–557.
19. Wojcicki M, Haagsma EB, Gouw AS, Slooff MJ, Porte RJ. Orthotopic liver transplantation for portosystemic encephalopathy in an adult with congenital absence of the portal vein. Liver Transpl 2004; 10(9): 1203–1207.
20. Akahoshi T, Nishizaki T, Wakasugi K, Mastuzaka T, Kume K, Yamamoto I et al. Portal-systemic encephalopathy due to a congenital extrahepatic portosystemic shunt: three cases and literature review. Hepatogastroenterology 2000; 47(34):1113–1116.
21. Uchino T, Endo F, Ikeda S, Shiraki K, Sera Y, Matsuda I. Three brothers with progressive hepatic dysfunction and severe hepatic steatosis due to a patent ductus venosus. Gastroenterology 1996; 110(6):1964–1968.
22. da Rocha AJ, Braga FT, da Silva CJ, Maia AC, Jr., Mourao GS, Gagliardi RJ. Reversal of parkinsonism and portosystemic encephalopathy following embolization of a congenital intrahepatic venous shunt: brain MR imaging and 1H spectroscopic findings. AJNR Am J Neuroradiol 2004; 25(7):1247–1250.
23. Ferenci P, Lockwood A, Mullen KD, Tarter R, Weissenborn K, Blei AT et al. Hepatic encephalopathy - Definition, nomenclature, diagnosis, and quantification: Final report of the Working Party at the 11th World Congresses of Gastroenterology, Vienna, 1998. Hepatology 2002; 35:716–721.
24. Kim T, Murakami T, Sugihara E, Hori M, Wakasa K, Nakamura H. Hepatic nodular lesions associated with abnormal development of the portal vein. AJR Am J Roentgenol 2004; 183(5):1333–1338.
25. Wanless IR, Lentz JS, Roberts EA. Partial nodular transformation of liver in an adult with persistent ductus venosus. Review with hypothesis on pathogenesis. Arch Pathol Lab Med 1985; 109(5):427–432.
26. Cheung KM, Lee CY, Wong CT, Chan AK. Congenital absence of portal vein presenting as hepatopulmonary syndrome. J Paediatr Child Health 2005; 41(1-2): 72–75.
27. Garcia-Tsao G, Lim JK. Management and treatment of patients with cirrhosis and portal hypertension: recommendations from the Department of Veterans Affairs Hepatitis C Resource Center Program and the National Hepatitis C Program. Am J Gastroenterol 2009; 104(7):1802–1829.
28. Dakeishi M, Shioya T, Wada Y, Shindo T, Otaka K, Manabe M et al. Genetic epidemiology of hereditary hemorrhagic telangiectasia in a local community in the northern part of Japan. Hum Mutat 2002; 19(2):140–148.
29. Kjeldsen AD, Vase P, Green A. Hereditary haemorrhagic telangiectasia: a population-based study of prevalence and mortality in Danish patients. J Intern Med 1999; 245(1):31–39.
30. Braverman IM, Keh A, Jacobson BS. Ultrastructure and three-dimensional organization of the telangiectases of hereditary hemorrhagic telangiectasia. J Invest Dermatol 1990; 95(4):422–427.
31. Guttmacher AE, Marchuk DA, White RI. Hereditary hemorrhagic telangiectasia. New Eng J Med 1995; 333:918–924.
32. McAllister KA, Grogg KM, Johnson DW, Gallione CJ, Baldwin MA, Jackson CE et al. Endoglin, a TGF-beta binding protein of endothelial cells, is the gene for hereditary haemorrhagic telangiectasia type 1. Nat Genet 1994; 8(4):345–351.
33. McDonald MT, Papenberg KA, Ghosh S, Glatfelter AA, Biesecker BB, Helmbold EA et al. A disease locus for hereditary haemorrhagic telangiectasia maps to chromosome 9q33-34. Nat Genet 1994; 6(2): 197–204.
34. Shovlin CL, Hughes JM, Tuddenham EG, Temperley I, Perembelon YF, Scott J et al. A gene for hereditary haemorrhagic telangiectasia maps to chromosome 9q3. Nat Genet 1994; 6(2):205–209.
35. Lesca G, Olivieri C, Burnichon N, Pagella F, Carette MF, Gilbert-Dussardier B et al. Genotype-phenotype

correlations in hereditary hemorrhagic telangiectasia: data from the French-Italian HHT network. Genet Med 2007; 9(1):14–22.
36. Johnson DW, Berg JN, Gallione CJ, McAllister KA, Warner JP, Helmbold EA et al. A second locus for hereditary hemorrhagic telangiectasia maps to chromosome 12. Genome Res 1995; 5(1):21–28.
37. Vincent P, Plauchu H, Hazan J, Faure S, Weissenbach J, Godet J. A third locus for hereditary haemorrhagic telangiectasia maps to chromosome 12q. Hum Mol Genet 1995; 4(5):945–949.
38. Gallione CJ, Repetto GM, Legius E, Rustgi AK, Schelley SL, Tejpar S et al. A combined syndrome of juvenile polyposis and hereditary haemorrhagic telangiectasia associated with mutations in MADH4 (SMAD4). Lancet 2004; 363(9412):852–859.
39. Abdalla SA, Letarte M. Hereditary haemorrhagic telangiectasia: current views on genetics and mechanisms of disease. J Med Genet 2006; 43(2):97–110.
40. Cole SG, Begbie ME, Wallace GM, Shovlin CL. A new locus for hereditary haemorrhagic telangiectasia (HHT3) maps to chromosome 5. J Med Genet 2005; 42(7):577–582.
41. Bayrak-Toydemir P, McDonald J, Akarsu N, Toydemir RM, Calderon F, Tuncali T et al. A fourth locus for hereditary hemorrhagic telangiectasia maps to chromosome 7. Am J Med Genet A 2006; 140(20): 2155–2162.
42. Lebrin F, Srun S, Raymond K, Martin S, van den BS, Freitas C et al. Thalidomide stimulates vessel maturation and reduces epistaxis in individuals with hereditary hemorrhagic telangiectasia. Nat Med 2010; 16(4):420–428.
43. Cloft HJ. Spontaneous regression of cerebral arteriovenous malformation in hereditary hemorrhagic telangiectasia. AJNR Am J Neuroradiol 2002; 23(6): 1049–1050.
44. Leung KM, Agid R, terBrugge K. Spontaneous regression of a cerebral arteriovenous malformation in a child with hereditary hemorrhagic telangiectasia. Case report. J Neurosurg 2006; 105(5 Suppl):428–431.
45. Du R, Hashimoto T, Tihan T, Young WL, Perry V, Lawton MT. Growth and regression of arteriovenous malformations in a patient with hereditary hemorrhagic telangiectasia. Case report. J Neurosurg 2007; 106(3):470–477.
46. Hashimoto M, Tate E, Nishii T, Watarai J, Shioya T, White RI. Angiography of hepatic vascular malformations associated with hereditary hemorrhagic telangiectasia. Cardiovasc Intervent Radiol 2003; 26(2):177–180.
47. Wheatley-Price P, Shovlin C, Chao D. Interferon for metastatic renal cell cancer causing regression of hereditary hemorrhagic telangiectasia. J Clin Gastroenterol 2005; 39(4):344–345.
48. Massoud OI, Youssef WI, Mullen KD. Resolution of hereditary hemorrhagic telangiectasia and anemia with prolonged alpha-interferon therapy for chronic hepatitis C. J Clin Gastroenterol 2004; 38(4): 377–379.
49. Flieger D, Hainke S, Fischbach W. Dramatic improvement in hereditary hemorrhagic telangiectasia after treatment with the vascular endothelial growth factor (VEGF) antagonist bevacizumab. Ann Hematol 2006; 85(9):631–632.
50. Mitchell A, Adams LA, MacQuillan G, Tibballs J, vanden Driesen R, Delriviere L. Bevacizumab reverses need for liver transplantation in hereditary hemorrhagic telangiectasia. Liver Transpl 2008; 14(2): 210–213.
51. Akhurst RJ. Taking thalidomide out of rehab. Nat Med 2010; 16(4):370–372.
52. Garcia-Tsao G, Swanson KL. Hepatic vascular malformations in hereditary hemorrhagic telangiectasia: in search of predictors of significant disease. Hepatology 2008; 48(5):1377–1379.
53. Wanless IR, Gryfe A. Nodular transformation of the liver in hereditary hemorrhagic telangiectasia. Arch Pathol Lab Med 1986; 110:331–335.
54. Sawabe M, Arai T, Esaki Y, Tsuru M, Fukazawa T, Takubo K. Three-dimensional organization of the hepatic microvasculature in hereditary hemorrhagic telangiectasia. Arch Pathol Lab Med 2001; 125(9): 1219–1223.
55. Siddiki H, Doherty MG, Fletcher JG, Stanson AW, Vrtiska TJ, Hough DM et al. Abdominal findings in hereditary hemorrhagic telangiectasia: pictorial essay on 2D and 3D findings with isotropic multiphase CT. Radiographics 2008; 28(1):171–184.
56. Buscarini E, Danesino C, Olivieri C, Lupinacci G, De Grazia F, Reduzzi L et al. Doppler ultrasonographic grading of hepatic vascular malformations in hereditary hemorrhagic telangiectasia – results of extensive screening. Ultraschall Med 2004; 25(5):348–355.
57. Ianora AA, Memeo M, Sabba C, Cirulli A, Rotondo A, Angelelli G. Hereditary hemorrhagic telangiectasia: multi-detector row helical CT assessment of hepatic involvement. Radiology 2004; 230(1):250–259.
58. Memeo M, Stabile Ianora AA, Scardapane A, Buonamico P, Sabba C, Angelelli G. Hepatic involvement in hereditary hemorrhagic telangiectasia: CT findings. Abdom Imaging 2004; 29(2):211–220.
59. Buonamico P, Suppressa P, Lenato GM, Pasculli G, D'Ovidio F, Memeo M et al. Liver involvement in a large cohort of patients with hereditary hemorrhagic telangiectasia: Echo-color-Doppler vs multislice computed tomography study. J Hepatol 2008; 48(5): 811–812.
60. Buscarini E, Danesino C, Plauchu H, de Fazio C, Olivieri C, Brambilla G et al. High prevalence of hepatic focal nodular hyperplasia in subjects with hereditary hemorrhagic telangiectasia. Ultrasound Med Biol 2004; 30(9):1089–1097.
61. Wanless IR, Mawdsley C, Adams R. On the pathogenesis of focal nodular hyperplasia of the liver. Hepatology 1985; 5(6):1194–1200.
62. Bioulac-Sage P, Laumonier H, Cubel G, Saric J, Balabaud C. Over-expression of glutamine synthase in focal nodular hyperplasia (part 1): Early stages in the formation support the hypothesis of a focal

hyper-arterialisation with venous (portal and hepatic) and biliary damage. Comp Hepatol 2008; 7(1):2.
63. Odorico JS, Hakim MN, Becker YT, Van der Werf W, Musat A, Knechtle SJ et al. Liver transplantation as definitive therapy for complications after arterial embolization for hepatic manifestations of hereditary hemorrhagic telangiectasia. Liver Transplant Surg 1998; 4:483–490.
64. Caselitz M, Wagner S, Chavan A, Gebel M, Bleck JS, Wu A et al. Clinical outcome of transfemoral embolisation in patients with arteriovenous malformations of the liver in hereditary hemorrhagic telangiectasia (Weber-Rendu-Osler disease). Gut 1998; 42:123–126.
65. Blewitt RW, Brown CM, Wyatt JI. The pathology of acute hepatic disintegration in hereditary haemorrhagic telangiectasia. Histopathology 2003; 42(3): 265–269.
66. Buscarini E, Buscarini L, Danesino C, Piantanida M, Civardi G, Quaretti P et al. Hepatic vascular malformations in hereditary hemorrhagic telangiectasia: Doppler sonographic screning in a large family. J Hepatol 1997; 26:111–118.
67. Garcia-Tsao G, Korzenik JR, Young L, Henderson KJ, Byrd R, Pollak JS et al. Liver disease in patients with hereditary hemorrhagic telangiectasia. N Engl J Med 2000; 343:931–936.
68. Livneh A, Langevitz P, Morag B, Catania A, Pras M. Functionally reversible hepatic arteriovenous fistulas during pregnancy in patients with hereditary hemorrhagic telangiectasia. Southern Med J 1988; 81(8): 1047–1049.
69. Khalid SK, Pershbacher J, Makan M, Barzilai B, Goodenberger D. Worsening of nose bleeding heralds high cardiac output state in hereditary hemorrhagic telangiectasia. Am J Med 2009; 122(8):779.
70. Gincul R, Lesca G, Gelas-Dore B, Rollin N, Barthelet M, Dupuis-Girod S et al. Evaluation of previously nonscreened hereditary hemorrhagic telangiectasia patients shows frequent liver involvement and early cardiac consequences. Hepatology 2008; 48(5):1570–1576.
71. Bauer T, Britton P, Lomas D, Wight DGD, Friend PJ, Alexander G.J.M. Liver transplantation for hepatic arteriovenous malformation in hereditary hemorrhagic telangiectasia. J Hepatol 1995; 22:586–590.
72. McInroy B, Zajko AB, Pinna AD. Biliary necrosis due to hepatic involvement with hereditary hemorrhagic telangiectasia. AJR 1998; 170:413–415.
73. Boillot O, Bianco F, Viale J-P, Mion F, Mechet I, Gille D et al. Liver transplantation resolves the hyperdynamic circulation in hereditary hemorrhagic telangiectasia with hepatic involvement. Gastroenterology 1999; 116:187–192.
74. Hillert C, Broering DC, Gundlach M, Knoefel WT, Izbicki JR, Rogiers X. Hepatic involvement in hereditary hemorrhagic telangiectasia: an unusual indication for liver transplantation. Liver Transpl 2001; 7(3): 266–268.
75. Buscarini E, Plauchu H, Garcia-Tsao G., White RI, Jr., Sabba C, Miller F et al. Liver involvement in hereditary hemorrhagic telangiectasia: consensus recommendations. Liver Int 2006; 26(9):1040–1046.
76. Faughnan ME, Palda VA, Garcia-Tsao G, Geisthoff UW, McDonald J, Proctor DD et al. International Guidelines for the Diagnosis and Management of Hereditary Hemorrhagic Telangiectasia. J Med Genet 2009.
77. Shovlin CL, Guttmacher AE, Buscarini E, Faughnan ME, Hyland RH, Kjeldsen AD et al. Diagnostic criteria for hereditary hemorrhagic telangiectasia (Rendu-Osler-Weber syndrome). Am J Med Genetics 2000; 91:65–66.
78. Peck-Radosavljevic M, Zacher J, Meng YG, Pidlich J, Lipinski E, Langle F et al. Is inadequate thrombopoietin production a major cause of thrombocytopenia in cirrhosis of the liver? J Hepatol 1997; 27:127–131.
79. Caselitz M, Bahr MJ, Bleck JS, Chavan A, Manns MP, Wagner S et al. Sonographic criteria for the diagnosis of hepatic involvement in hereditary hemorrhagic telangiectasia (HHT). Hepatology 2003; 37(5):1139–1146.
80. Ravard G, Soyer P, Boudiaf M, Terem C, Abitbol M, Yeh JF et al. Hepatic involvement in hereditary hemorrhagic telangiectasia: helical computed tomography features in 24 consecutive patients. J Comput Assist Tomogr 2004; 28(4):488–495.
81. Wu JS, Saluja S, Garcia-Tsao G, Chong A, Henderson KJ, White RI. Liver involvement in hereditary hemorrhagic telangiectasia: CT and clinical findings do not correlate in symptomatic patients. AJR Am J Roentgenol 2006; 187:W399–405.
82. Buscarini E, Gebel M, Ocran K, Manfredi G, Del Vecchio BG, Stefanov R et al. Interobserver agreement in diagnosing liver involvement in hereditary hemorrhagic telangiectasia by Doppler ultrasound. Ultrasound Med Biol 2008.
83. Martini GA. The liver in hereditary haemorrhagic teleangiectasia: an inborn error of vascular structure with multiple manifestations: a reappraisal. Gut 1978; 19:531–537.
84. Cooney T, Sweeney EC, Coll R, Greally M. "Pseudocirrhosis" in hereditary hemorrhagic telangiectasia. J Clin Pathol 1977; 30:1134–1141.
85. Trembath RC, Thomson JR, Machado RD, Morgan NV, Atkinson C, Winship I et al. Clinical and molecular genetic features of pulmonary hypertension in patients with hereditary hemorrhagic telangiectasia. N Engl J Med 2001; 345:325–334.
86. Faughnan ME, Granton JT, Young LH. The pulmonary vascular complications of hereditary haemorrhagic telangiectasia. Eur Respir J 2009; 33(5): 1186–1194.
87. Lin E, Stall L. Spectrum of biliary abnormalities in hepatic hereditary hemorrhagic telangiectasia: demonstration by multidetector computed tomography. Emerg Radiol 2007; 14(6):461–463.
88. DeLeve LD, Valla DC, Garcia-Tsao G. Vascular disorders of the liver. Hepatology 2009; 49(5):1729–1764.
89. Garcia-Tsao G, Sanyal AJ, Grace ND, Carey W. Prevention and management of gastroesophageal

varices and variceal hemorrhage in cirrhosis. Hepatology 2007; 46(3):922–938.
90. Runyon BA. Management of adult patients with ascites due to cirrhosis. Hepatology 2004; 39(3):841–856.
91. Lee JY, Korzenik JR, DeMasi R, Lih-Brody L, White RI. Transjugular intrahepatic portosystemic shunts in patients with hereditary hemorrhagic telangiectasia: failure to palliate gastrointestinal bleeding. JVIR 1998; 9:994–997.
92. Chanson N, Carbonell N, Andreani T, Bellaiche G, Cluzel P, Serfaty L et al. TIPS in hereditary hemorrhagic telangiectasia: Never say never. J Hepatol 2008; 48(2):373–374.
93. Bourgeois N, Delcour C, Deviere J, Francois A, Lambert M, Cremer M et al. Osler-Weber-Rendu disease associated with hepatic involvement and high output heart failure. J Clin Gastroenterol 1990; 12(2):236–237.
94. Koscielny A, Willinek WA, Hirner A, Wolff M. Treatment of High Output Cardiac Failure by Flow-Adapted Hepatic Artery Banding (FHAB) in Patients with Hereditary Hemorrhagic Telangiectasia. J Gastrointest Surg 2007; %20.
95. Pfitzmann R, Heise M, Langrehr JM, Jonas S, Steinmuller T, Podrabsky P et al. Liver transplantation for treatment of intrahepatic Osler's disease: first experiences. Transplantation 2001; 72(2):237–241.
96. Thevenot T, Vanlemmens C, Di M, V, Becker MC, Denue PO, Kantelip B et al. Liver transplantation for cardiac failure in patients with hereditary hemorrhagic telangiectasia. Liver Transpl 2005; 11(7): 834–838.
97. Lerut J, Orlando G, Adam R, Sabba C, Pfitzmann R, Klempnauer J et al. Liver Transplantation for Hereditary Hemorrhagic Telangiectasia: Report of the European Liver Transplant Registry. Ann Surg 2006; 244(6):854–864.
98. Dupuis-Girod S, Chesnais AL, Ginon I, Dumortier J, Saurin JC, Finet G et al. Long-term outcome of patients with hereditary hemorrhagic telangiectasia and severe hepatic involvement after orthotopic liver transplantation: a single-center study. Liver Transpl 2010; 16(3):340–347.
99. Garcia-Tsao G, Gish RG, Punch J. MELD Exception for Hereditary Hemorrhagic Telangiectasia. Liver Transpl 2006.

Part III

Surgery and Interventional Radiology

15 Interventional Radiology in the Treatment of Portal Hypertension

Christophe Bureau, Philippe Otal, and Jean-Pierre Vinel

Abstract

Interventional radiology techniques, namely embolization and shunting, were developed mainly to deal with the failures of drug and/or endoscopic treatments. Among those techniques, the transjugular intrahepatic portosystemic shunt (TIPS) is the only that aims to normalize portal pressure and is therefore able to treat both refractory bleeding and intractable ascites.

Embolization of esophago-gastric or ectopic varices, balloon occluded retrograde transvenous obliteration of varices, or partial splenic embolization have been poorly evaluated. Severe complications may be observed and since portal hypertension is maintained or even increased, these procedures have only a transient effect with a high rebleeding rate. Their role should be explored in patients with uncontrolled variceal hemorrhage who have a contraindication for TIPS, such as pulmonary arterial hypertension, congestive heart failure, liver failure, or severe or recurrent encephalopathy.

Nowadays, TIPS should be performed using PTFE-covered prostheses, which were shown to decrease the rate of shunt dysfunction and improve clinical outcomes. TIPS has been found more effective than drug and/or endoscopic treatments in controlling active variceal bleeding as well as in preventing rebleeding, though survival was not improved and encephalopathy was more frequent. It can also be used for gastric or ectopic varices.

In refractory ascites, TIPS was shown to be more effective than large volume paracenteses. It has also been successfully used in hydrothorax.

Keywords

Interventional radiology • Embolization • TIPS • Variceal bleeding • Refractory ascites • Cirrhosis • Portal-hypertension

Variceal bleeding remains the most severe complication of portal hypertension, although within the last 2 decades, in-hospital death rate and rebleeding rates have decreased from 43 and 47% to 14.5 and 13%, respectively [1], mainly because of improved endoscopic and drug therapies.

J.-P. Vinel (✉)
Hepato-Gastro-Enterologie, University of Toulouse, CHU Toulouse-Purpan, Place du Dr Baylac, Toulouse 31059, France
e-mail: vinel.jp@chu-toulouse.fr

L.D. DeLeve and G. Garcia-Tsao (eds.), *Vascular Liver Disease: Mechanisms and Management*, DOI 10.1007/978-1-4419-8327-5_15,

However, despite these improvements, hemostasis cannot be achieved in a few patients. In some others, rebleeding cannot be effectively prevented. Nowadays, these failures are very seldom indications for surgery and can be dealt with by interventional radiology procedures. Such procedures can be classified into two categories: embolization and shunting. Among those techniques, the transjugular intrahepatic portosystemic shunt (TIPS) is the only one that aims to normalize portal pressure and is therefore able to treat both refractory bleeding and intractable ascites.

Embolization

Embolization of esophago-gastric varices was first described by Lunderquist and Vang in 1974 [2] using a percutaneous transhepatic route. Such an approach may prove deleterious in patients with poor general condition, gross coagulation defects, and a small hard shrunken liver, even if the puncture tract is embolized at the end of the procedure. To avoid those complications, a few groups used the transjugular approach, which proved much safer [3]. Bleeding varices can be obstructed by the injection of various materials, through a catheter advanced into the feeder vessel (Fig. 15.1). Sclerosing agents, glues such as histoacryl, gelfoam particles, coils, or, for large vessels, detachable balloons can be used. Three randomized controlled trials of embolization for acute variceal hemorrhage have been published (Table 15.1) [4–6]. Two found embolization to be more effective than sclerotherapy [5] or band ligation [6], with regards to both rebleeding and survival. However, the technique is a difficult one with a failure rate ranging from 20 [7] to 30% [8]. Hemostasis is achieved in 71 [4] to 94% [9] of the cases. This technique has also been used for bleeding duodenal [10], rectal [11], or esophagojejunal varices after total gastrectomy [12]. The main limitation of the method is that it does not reduce, and may actually increase, portal pressure [13] so that sooner or later new varices develop and bleeding recurs. In fact, rebleeding rates after embolization range from 30 [3] to 65% [4].

A specific technique is used mainly in Japan to obliterate gastric varices through a natural

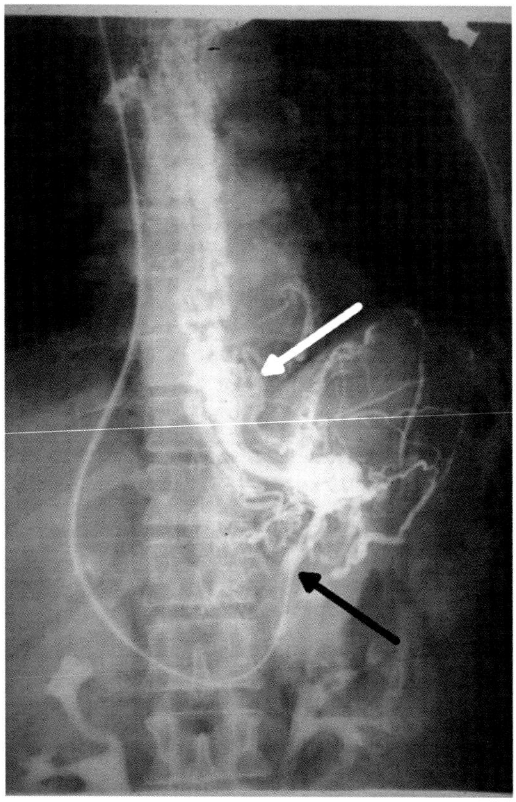

Fig. 15.1 Transjugular catheterization of the coronary vein (*black arrow*) with opacification of collaterals (*white arrow*) before embolization

gastro-renal shunt (BRTO for Balloon-occluded Retrograde Transvenous Obliteration of Varices). It was introduced by Kanagawa et al. in 1996 [14]. The shunt is occluded by a balloon and gastric varices are injected in a retrograde fashion with a sclerosing agent. The technique is reported to be highly effective. However, it has been poorly evaluated with only small uncontrolled series. Furthermore occlusion of the spontaneous gastro-renal shunt may aggravate preexisting esophageal varices, or lead to the development of new ones [15–17]. In a series of 19 patients, Tanihata et al. [18] observed a significant increase in portohepatic venous pressure gradient after BRTO. Endoscopy showed eradication of gastric varices in all patients with aggravation of preexisting esophageal varices in 58% of them. Cho et al. [17] reported a 12% failure rate among 49 patients, with enlargement of preexisting esophageal varices in 67% leading to variceal

Table 15.1 Randomized controlled trials of embolization of esophageal varices (EV) in patients with cirrhosis

References	Embolization	Control treatment	p
Smith-Laing et al. [4]		Conventional therapy	
N patients	29	25	
Outcome			NS
Terabayashi et al. [5]		Sclerotherapy	
N patients	33	33	
Overall rebleeding	6	21	<0.005
Rebleeding from EV	3	20	<0.005
Deaths	5	19	<0.054
Zhang et al. [6]		Band ligation	
N patients	52	50	
Rebleeding	8	21	0.004
Rebleeding from EV	3	12	0.012
Deaths	7	14	0.054

hemorrhage in 37%. Furthermore, the procedure proved far from safe with two procedural deaths, two cases of pulmonary thromboembolism, two portal vein thromboses, new or worsening ascites in 44% of the patients, and pleural effusion in 72%.

Partial splenic embolization (PSE) has been proposed to decrease portal pressure and reduce hypersplenism. In a recent review, Koconis et al. [19] pooled the results of available studies published in English from 1973 to 2005. The method has been very poorly evaluated with only one controlled, though not randomized, study comparing endoscopic band ligation alone to the combination of PSE and band ligation, which was found to be more effective [20]. Proponents of the technique claim that it improves liver function [21, 22], hematologic parameters (leukocyte, red blood cell, and platelet counts) [23, 24], and hepatic encephalopathy [25]. However, numerous serious complications have been described that are dependent on experience level and that increase with the volume of spleen that is infarcted [26]. The most significant complications are splenic abscess, portal vein thrombosis, pulmonary arterial embolism, and acute liver failure [19].

Finally, a few reports describe the use of embolization for arterio-portal fistulas [27]. These fistulas may be congenital, or secondary to liver biopsy, liver tumors, surgery, or trauma. They can be asymptomatic or lead to the development of portal hypertension and congestive heart failure. Embolization has been increasingly used in their treatment and is so successful that surgery has been relegated to the rare failures, mainly when the fistula is too large to be obstructed.

As a whole, available literature is inadequate to support hepatic artery embolization in patients with portal hypertension. Severe complications may be observed and since portal hypertension is maintained or even increased, these procedures have only a transient effect with a high rebleeding rate. With the advent of TIPS, this procedure lost popularity and is only seldom used in a few centers. Its role should be explored in patients with uncontrolled variceal hemorrhage who have a contraindication for TIPS, such as pulmonary arterial hypertension, congestive heart failure, liver failure, or severe or recurrent encephalopathy.

Transjugular Intrahepatic Portosystemic Shunt (TIPS)

Portocaval shunting has consistently been shown to be the most effective treatment for the complications of portal hypertension since it is the only procedure that normalizes portal pressure. However, surgical shunting was virtually abandoned because of a high rate of postshunt encephalopathy and a high mortality when performed in emergency conditions. In the last 20 years, shunting was popularized again owing to the development of TIPS. After W Hanafee and M Weiner described the percutaneous transjugular route to the liver to perform hepatic venography, cholangiography and liver biopsy, Rösch et al. [28] created the first intrahepatic portosystemic shunt in swine in 1969. Thirteen years later, Colapinto et al. reported their preliminary experience with intrahepatic portosystemic shunts in patients by dilating the intraparenchymal tract between the portal and the hepatic venous systems with a balloon catheter [29]. However, owing to the elasticity of the liver tissue, shunts occluded within a few days and several cases of liver capsule rupture with fatal intraperitoneal bleeds were reported. Palmaz et al. successfully maintained shunt patency in dogs using balloon expandable stents [30]. The first TIPS in humans was performed by Richter et al. [31] with a Palmaz stent. Thereafter, self-expandable stents and then, in 2002, polytetrafluoroethylene (PTFE) covered prostheses were made available. The use of the latter stent dramatically reduced the rate of shunt dysfunction and improved clinical outcomes [32]. These technical improvements must be kept in mind when evaluating the results of older studies.

Technique

The procedure involves multiple steps. Under ultrasonographic guidance, the jugular vein, usually the right internal one, is punctured. Then, under fluoroscopic control, a catheter is advanced through the right atrium and the inferior vena cava into a hepatic vein. The most demanding stage of the technique is the subsequent catheterization of a branch of the portal vein within the liver. Multiple methods can be used to facilitate this difficult step: ultrasonography (US), anatomical landmarks allowing localization of the portal vein in most patients [33, 34], or target catheters placed trans-cutaneously in the portal vein [31], which may be the only technique to localize the portal vein in patients with portal vein thrombosis. Currently, the most convenient and reliable method is retrograde portography through a wedged catheter in the hepatic vein. Because ruptures of the liver capsule have been reported with this technique [35], balloon occlusion of the hepatic vein is preferred with injection of carbon dioxide that results in better visualization of the portal vein, lower cost and absence of renal toxicity compared to iodinated contrast dye [36]. In order to achieve effective protection against the complications of portal hypertension, the portosystemic pressure gradient should be decreased by 50% of its initial value or below the threshold of 12 mmHg. Rarely, the portosystemic gradient remains higher than expected after TIPS and a second parallel shunt must be performed. The stent should be inserted from the ostium of the hepatic vein into the inferior vena cava to avoid hepatic vein stenosis, in a hepatic vein large enough so that it will not develop thrombosis. Finally it must not be advanced to far into the portal vein so as not to hinder the possibility of liver transplantation. At the end of the procedure, a control portography is performed (Fig. 15.2). Some authors recommend embolization if large collaterals continue to be visualized after TIPS. However, on one hand, the efficacy of this procedure has not been demonstrated and, on the other hand, embolization might prove deleterious inasmuch as it could lead to portal vein obstruction and/or remote complications such as lung or brain abscesses.

Budd-Chiari syndrome and portal vein thrombosis raise specific problems. Regarding Budd-Chiari syndrome, if a hepatic vein stump persists, the TIPS technique is basically the same as described above although it might be somewhat more difficult, even under US guidance. In a few patients, hepatic veins are completely obstructed and cannot be catheterized so that the puncture is made directly through the anterior wall of the inferior vena cava aiming to enter the left branch of the portal vein through the hypertrophic caudate liver lobe [37]. The puncture route must be embolized thereafter.

Portal vein thrombosis was initially considered a contraindication for TIPS. Nowadays, on the contrary, it should be considered an indication whenever it is partial since the reversal of

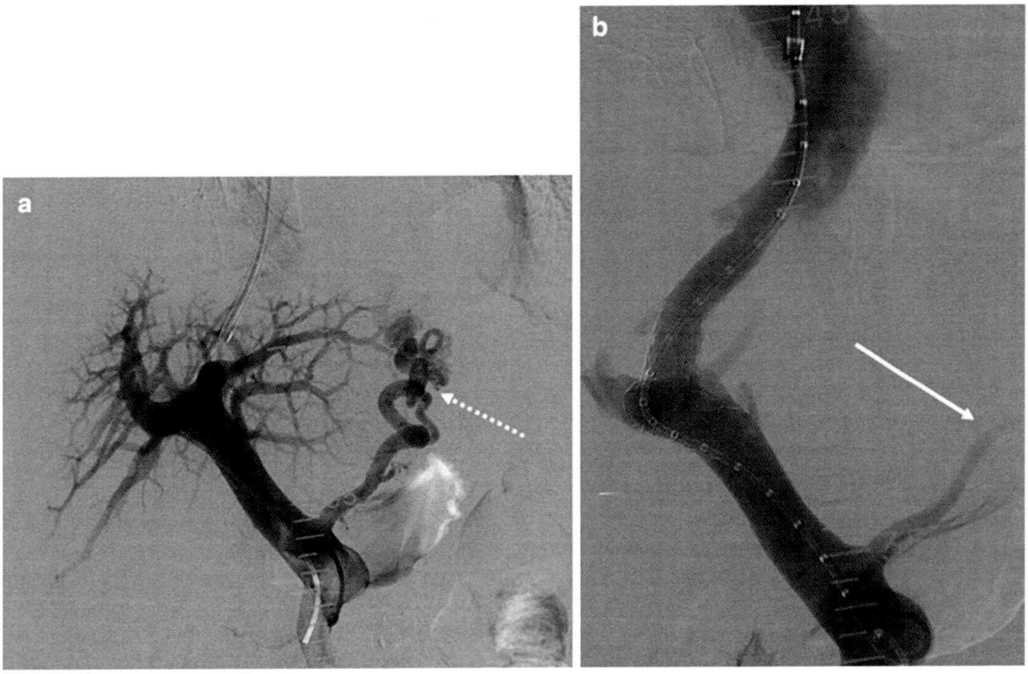

Fig. 15.2 (**a**) Pre-TIPS portography with large collaterals (*dashed arrow*). (**b**) Post-TIPS portography showing minimal opacification of collateral veins (*white arrow*)

blood flow from hepatofugal to hepatopetal may help dissolve the thrombus [38]. In patients with recent complete obstruction of the portal stem, TIPS can also be successfully performed without many difficulties. After the catheter is advanced upstream of the obstacle, the clot can be destroyed using different techniques (such as fragmentation, aspiration, or mechanical thrombectomy) or crushed by the expanded stent. The most difficult condition is portal vein cavernoma in which it may be extremely difficult, or even impossible, to identify a portal vessel large enough to release the prosthesis.

Indications

Among the indications of TIPS reported in the literature, only variceal hemorrhage and refractory ascites, which represent approximately 99% of the indications for TIPS worldwide, have been assessed in randomized controlled trials (RCTs).

Variceal Hemorrhage

Hemostasis

Multiple uncontrolled studies reported an average rate of hemostasis of 95% using TIPS as salvage therapy after the failure of drug and endoscopic therapies. TIPS was therefore considered a second line rescue procedure. In these settings, mortality was 20–30% higher than reported in elective conditions. This attitude has been challenged by two randomized controlled trials. Actually, early TIPS treatment in high-risk patients was found more effective than medical therapy by Monescillo et al. [39]. Among 116 consecutive patients with cirrhosis in whom HVPG was measured within 24 h after admission for variceal bleeding, 52 were considered "high-risk" patients given a HVPG equal or greater than 20 mmHg. Twenty-six were randomized to TIPS placement within 24 h after admission and 26 to standard pharmacological and/or endoscopic therapy. Patients in the TIPS group had fewer treatments failures (12% vs. 50% – $p=0.001$), lower transfusion requirements (2.2 ± 2.3 vs. 3.7 ± 2.7 blood units – $p=0.002$) and lower rates of in-hospital (11% vs. 38% – $p=0.02$) and 1-year (31% vs. 65% – $p=0.01$) mortality, compared to those in the standard treatment group. However, measurement of HVPG in emergency conditions is impossible in most centers and is not a convenient way to select candidates for early TIPS. In an international multicenter RCT, which found similar results, high-risk patients were defined as Child C patients or Child B patients with active bleeding at endoscopy. Early TIPS, using PTFE-covered stents, improved the control of the bleeding and overall survival without increasing the rate of hepatic encephalopathy (HE) [40]. Interestingly, seven patients from the standard treatment group had a salvage TIPS, of whom four (57%) died as compared to a mortality of 12.5% in the early TIPS group. This suggests that in high-risk patients with acute variceal hemorrhage, early treatment with TIPS should be considered as first line treatment, without waiting for the failure of endoscopic and drug therapies.

Recurrent Hemorrhage

Thirteen RCTs compare TIPS with bare stents to endoscopic therapy, sclerotherapy, or band ligation, with or without concomitant noncardioselective beta-blockers [41–53] (Table 15.2). Their results were pooled in three meta-analyses, which consistently found that TIPS was more effective than alternative treatment, though it did not improve survival and increased the rate of HE [54–56]. Similar results were found when comparing TIPS to the association of propranolol and isosorbide-5-mononitrate [57].

In a trial comparing surgical placement of small diameter prosthetic H-graft portocaval shunts with TIPS, the latter was found less effective ($p<0.02$) and had higher mortality and morbidity ($p<0.002$) [58]. However, the authors used a composite endpoint that included TIPS dysfunction and this was the endpoint that explained the efficacy difference between groups. In fact, in a 10-year follow-up study, survival in both groups was higher than predicted according to baseline MELD score and surgery was superior to TIPS only because it had fewer shunt failures [59].

Table 15.2 Randomized controlled trials of TIPS in the prevention of rebleeding

	Patients number			Rebleeding rate (%)		Mortality rate (%)		Encephalopathy (%)	
References	TIPS	Control group	Treatment in control group	TIPS	Control group	TIPS	Control group	TIPS	Control group
GEAIH [41]	32	33	EST + P	38[a]	68	50	42	NA	NA
Cabrera et al. [42]	31	32	EST	23[a]	52	7	18	33[a]	13
Rössle et al. [43]	61	65	EST/EVL + P	15[a]	41	13	12	36[a]	18
Sanyal et al. [44]	41	39	EST	22	21	29[a]	18	29	13
Cello et al. [45]	24	25	EST	13[a]	48	33	32	50	44
Sauer et al. [46]	42	41	EST + P	23[a]	57	31	33	29[a]	13
Jalan et al. [47]	31	27	EBL	10[a]	52	42	37	36	26
Merli et al. [48]	38	43	EST	24[a]	51	24	19	55[a]	26
Garcia-Villareal et al. [49]	22	24	EST	9[a]	50	15[a]	33	23	25
Pomier-Layrargues et al. [50]	41	39	EBL	18[a]	66	43	44	47	44
Narahara et al. [51]	38	40	EST	18[a]	33	29	18	34	15
Sauer et al. [52]	43	42	EBL	16[a]	43	26	29	37	21
Gülberg et al. [53]	28	26	EBL	25	27	14	15	7	19
Escorsell et al. [57]	47	44	P + IMN	13[a]	39	28	28	38[a]	14

EST endoscopic sclerotherapy; *EBL* endoscopic band ligation; *P* propranolol; *IMN* isosorbide-5-mononitrate
[a] Significantly different from control group

Henderson et al. [60] compared TIPS to distal splenorenal shunt and found no difference in rebleeding, de novo encephalopathy, 2- and 5-year survival, cost and quality of life. Thrombosis, stenosis and reintervention rates were higher in the TIPS group ($p<0.001$). The use of PTFE-covered prostheses dramatically decreases those complications [32], so that it is generally recommended that TIPS using these coated devices be preferred over surgery.

TIPS has also successfully been used in the treatment of hemorrhage from sources other than esophageal varices: gastric [61] or ectopic varices [62], or portal hypertensive gastropathy [63]. It was not effective for hemorrhages from gastric antral vascular ectasia [63], which could have been anticipated since these lesions are not a consequence of portal hypertension [64].

Refractory Ascites and Related Complications

The efficacy of TIPS with bare stents in the treatment of refractory ascites has been assessed in five RCTs [65–69] including a total of 330 patients (Table 15.3). As compared to large volume paracenteses with plasma volume expansion, TIPS significantly reduced the reaccumulation of ascites. In most studies survival was not improved and severe HE occurred significantly more often with TIPS [65–68]. However, a RCT by Salerno et al. reported a higher survival in patients treated with TIPS [69] and this result was confirmed in a meta-analysis of individual data from most of the published RCTs [70]. This meta-analysis analyzed 305 patients, 149 treated with TIPS and 156 with large volume paracentesis, and found less recurrence of ascites in the TIPS group (42% vs. 89% – $p<0.0001$), and a similar cumulative probability of developing the first episode of hepatic encephalopathy, although the average number of episodes of HE was higher ($p=0.06$) and there was better actuarial probability of transplant free survival ($p=0.035$) compared to treatment with large-volume paracentesis.

TIPS with bare stents has also been compared to peritoneovenous shunting and found to be more effective despite the need for multiple revisions to maintain shunt patency [71].

Uncontrolled series have also reported successful treatment of refractory hydrothorax [72], and type I and II hepatorenal syndrome [73, 74].

Miscellaneous Indications

In uncontrolled trials and case reports, TIPS has been successfully used in acute Budd-Chiari syndrome [75] (Chap. 13), immunosuppression-induced veno-occlusive disease [76], to facilitate abdominal surgery [77] and in patients awaiting liver transplantation [78].

The effects of TIPS on quality of life and on nutritional status are still controversial. Although both parameters were found to be improved after TIPS, it is not clear whether the improvement is greater than in long-term survivors receiving alternative treatments.

Complications

In a retrospective series that pooled 1,750 patients, the rate of lethal complications from TIPS was 1.7%, ranging from 3% in centers, where fewer

Table 15.3 Randomized controlled trials of TIPS vs. large volume paracenteses (LVP) in refractory ascites

	Number of patients		Control of ascites (%)		Encephalopathy (%)		Survival (%)	
References	TIPS	LVP	TIPS	LVP	TIPS	LVP	TIPS	LVP
Lebrec et al. [65]	13	12	69[a]	0	23[a]	0	29[a]	56
Rössle et al. [66]	29	31	61[a]	18	58	48	69	52
Gines et al. [67]	35	35	51[a]	17	77	66	41	35
Sanyal et al. [68]	52	57	58[a]	16	38	21	60	63
Salerno et al. [69]	33	33	61[a]	3	61	39	77[a]	52

[a] Significantly different from LVP group

than 150 procedures had been performed, to 1.4% in more experienced hands [79]. Procedural complications were reported at each step of the technique: hematoma of the neck after accidental puncture of the carotid artery and pneumothorax from puncture of the jugular vein, arrhythmia and tamponade while advancing the catheter through the right atrium, perforation of the inferior vena cava while trying to catheterize the hepatic vein, peritoneal bleeding from laceration of the liver capsule, or hemobilia from puncture of a bile duct when looking for a branch of the portal vein within the liver.

Four complications may be caused by stenting:

TIPS infection: the incidence of endotipsitis has been reported to be 1.2% in a series of 165 patients [80]. The most common presentation includes persistent bacteremia and fever together with either shunt occlusion, vegetation, or bacteremia in the presence of a patent shunt when other sources of bacteremia have been ruled out. Long-term antibiotic therapy is not always effective and liver transplantation may be indicated in a few patients.

Hemolysis: has been reported in up to 30% of patients. It is mostly asymptomatic, except for an increase in unconjugated bilirubin in serum. It is ascribed to erythrocyte damage on the metallic mesh of the stent and accordingly disappears with the development of a TIPS pseudo-intima [81].

Liver infarction: is a rare complication which can be caused by the laceration or acute thrombosis of a hepatic artery. Partial Budd-Chiari syndromes have also been reported after obliteration of a hepatic vein by the stent. The risk might be increased with covered prostheses [82].

Shunt dysfunction: may have two different origins: thrombosis or pseudo-intima overproliferation. Stent thrombosis usually occurs within the first 3 weeks after TIPS. Its incidence ranges from 10 to 15% [83]. It may be due to technical problems such as incomplete covering of the intraparenchymal tract or kinking of the prosthesis. Diagnosis is easily made by Doppler US. The shunt can be recanalized. Prophylactic anticoagulation has been proposed, but the efficacy of this treatment has not been proven and it may be harmful in patients with coagulation disorders and portal hypertension.

Within 3–4 weeks after insertion into the liver, the prosthesis is progressively covered by a smooth layer of fibrous tissue and a single layer of endothelial cells. This pseudo-intima offers adequate protection against thrombosis, but the process can be exaggerated and lead to a narrowing or even total obstruction of the shunt [84]. This pseudo-intimal overgrowth is the most common cause of shunt dysfunction and it has been reported to occur in 20–80% of cases within 1 year. Overproliferation of the intima may also involve the hepatic vein, where it is ascribed to an increased blood flow. Dysfunction from pseudo-intimal proliferation is very effectively prevented by using PTFE-covered stents [32, 85, 86], which completely inhibit its development.

Three types of complications can occur secondary to the shunting itself:

Cardiac failure: the sudden increase in cardiac preload by portosystemic shunting may decompensate cardiac function. Accordingly TIPS should not be performed in patients with an ejection fraction below 50%.

Liver failure: may be precipitated by shunting of portal blood flow. As a consequence, severe liver failure as assessed by a Child-Pugh score over 12 or a MELD score higher than 18 should be considered a contraindication for TIPS. The risk is increased in patients with hepatopetal blood flow and those with low arterial flow, conditions that should be ruled out by pre-TIPS Doppler US.

Hepatic encephalopathy: (HE): clinical studies consistently report an increased incidence of encephalopathy following TIPS. This complication is ascribed to shunting itself, so that a history of severe or recurrent HE is considered a contraindication for TIPS. Using bare stents, HE usually improves along with the narrowing of the shunt by pseudo-intimal proliferation. Therefore, the incidence and/or severity of this complication were expected to increase with the use of covered prostheses. However, this was not confirmed in clinical studies. On the contrary, the only published randomized trial reported a lower incidence of HE in patients treated with covered stents [32]. This was ascribed to a significantly less frequent need for hospitalizations, control angiographies and shunt revisions, and fewer rebleeding episodes or relapses of ascites. Should incapacitating HE occur after TIPS, the shunt could be reduced or even totally obstructed using specifically designed devices or a second coaxial stent [87].

Contraindications

These are summarized in Table 15.4. Most are relative contraindications and should be considered according to whether the complication to be treated is or is not life-threatening.

Cost-Effectiveness

Regarding prevention of recurrent variceal hemorrhage, TIPS has been found to be more cost-effective than endoscopic therapy [88] or surgical shunting [89]. In the trial from Escorsell et al., the direct costs were calculated and found to be roughly double in the TIPS group when compared to the drug therapy group [57]. Regarding refractory ascites, TIPS is 50% more expensive than large volume paracenteses [67]. All these studies were performed using bare stents. Although PTFE-covered prostheses are more expensive than bare ones, they should finally prove more cost-effective owing to a much lower need for shunt revisions and improved clinical outcome.

Table 15.4 Main contraindications for TIPS

Age >75
Child-Pugh score >12 or MELD score >18
Overt hepatic encephalopathy or history of severe and/or recurrent encephalopathy
Cardiac, respiratory or organic renal failure
Pulmonary arterial hypertension
Dilation of intrahepatic bile ducts
Hydatid cyst and polycystic liver
Hepatocellular carcinoma
Complete portal vein thrombosis

Conclusions

The efficacy of TIPS has been demonstrated by RCTs for severe acute, refractory and recurrent hemorrhage as well as in refractory ascites. Therefore, the technique has gained its place in the therapeutic armamentarium for portal hypertension. Initially, the main drawback of TIPS was shunt dysfunction. The use of PTFE-covered stents dramatically decreased this complication and improved clinical outcome. However, most published randomized controlled trials were performed with bare stents and their results should be challenged using these newer, more competitive devices. Furthermore, the experience accumulated over the last 20 years should allow a better selection of candidates, and therefore further improve the results obtained with TIPS.

References

1. Carbonell N, Pauwels A, Serfaty L, Fourdan O, Lévy VG, Poupon R. Improved survival after variceal bleeding in patients with cirrhosis over the past two decades. Hepatology. 2004;40:652–9.
2. Lunderquist A, Vang J. Transhepatic catheterization and obliteration of the coronary vein in patients with portal hypertension and esophageal varices. N Engl J Med. 1974;291:646–9.
3. Vinel JP, Scotto JM, Levade M, Teisseire R, Cassigneul J, Cales P, et al. Embolization of esophageal varices by the transjugular route in severe digestive hemorrhage in cirrhotic patients. Prospective study of 83 patients. Gastroenterol Clin Biol. 1985;9:814–8.
4. Smith-Laing G, Scott J, Long RG, Dick R, Sherlock S. Role of percutaneous transhepatic obliteration of varices in the management of hemorrhage from gastroesophageal varices. Gastroenterology. 1981;80:1031–6.
5. Terabayashi H, Ohnishi K, Tsunoda T, Nakata H, Saito M, Tanaka H, et al. Prospective controlled trial of elective endoscopic sclerotherapy in comparison with percutaneous transhepatic obliteration of esophageal varices in patients with nonalcoholic cirrhosis. Gastroenterology. 1987;93:1205–9.

6. Zhang CQ, Liu FL, Liang B, Sun ZQ, Xu HW, Xu L, et al. A modified percutaneous transhepatic variceal embolization with 2-octyl cyanoacrylate versus endoscopic ligation in esophageal variceal bleeding management: randomized controlled trial. Dig Dis Sci. 2008;53:2258–67.
7. Bonnière P, Henry-Amar M, Lescut D, Mathieu-Chandelier C, Colombel JF, Delhoustal L, et al. Transhepatic embolization and endoscopic sclerosing in digestive hemorrhage caused by rupture of esophageal varices in patients with Child's stage C cirrhosis. Gastroenterol Clin Biol. 1990;14:46B–51B.
8. Bengmark S, Börjesson B, Hoevels J, Joelsson B, Lunderquist A, Owman T. Obliteration of esophageal varices by PTP: a follow-up of 43 patients. Ann Surg. 1979;190:549–54.
9. Viamonte M, Pereiras R, Russell E, Le Page J, Hutson D. Transhepatic obliteration of gastroesophageal varices: results in acute and nonacute bleeders. AJR Am J Roentgenol. 1977;129:237–41.
10. Zamora CA, Sugimoto K, Tsurusaki M, Izaki K, Fukuda T, Matsumoto S, et al. Endovascular obliteration of bleeding duodenal varices in patients with liver cirrhosis. Eur Radiol. 2006;16:73–9.
11. Okazaki H, Higuchi K, Shiba M, Nakamura S, Wada T, Yamamori K, et al. Successful treatment of giant rectal varices by modified percutaneous transhepatic obliteration with sclerosant: report of a case. World J Gastroenterol. 2006;12:5408–11.
12. Chikamori F, Shibuya S, Takase Y. Percutaneous transhepatic obliteration for esophagojejunal varices after total gastrectomy. Abdom Imaging. 1998;23:560–2.
13. Ohnishi K, Nakata H, Terabayashi H, Tanaka H, Tsunoda T, Iida S, et al. The effects of endoscopic sclerotherapy combined with transhepatic variceal obliteration on portal hemodynamics. Am J Gastroenterol. 1987;82:1138–42.
14. Kanagawa H, Mima S, Kouyama H, Gotoh K, Uchida T, Okuda K. Treatment of gastric fundal varices by balloon-occluded retrograde transvenous obliteration. J Gastroenterol Hepatol. 1996;11:51–8.
15. Hirota S, Matsumoto S, Tomita M, Sako M, Kono M. Retrograde transvenous obliteration of gastric varices. Radiology. 1999;211:349–56.
16. Ninoi T, Nishida N, Kaminou T, Sakai Y, Kitayama T, Hamuro M, et al. Balloon-occluded retrograde transvenous obliteration of gastric varices with gastrorenal shunt: long-term follow-up in 78 patients. AJR Am J Roentgenol. 2005;184:1340–6.
17. Cho SK, Shin SW, Lee IH, Do YS, Choo SW, Park KB, et al. Balloon-occluded retrograde transvenous obliteration of gastric varices: outcomes and complications in 49 patients. Am J Roentgenol. 2007;189: W365–72.
18. Tanihata H, Minamiguchi H, Sato M, Kawai N, Sonomura T, Takasaka I, et al. Changes in portal systemic pressure gradient after balloon-occluded retrograde transvenous obliteration of gastric varices and aggravation of esophageal varices. Cardiovasc Intervent Radiol. 2009;32:1209–16.
19. Koconis KG, Singh H, Soares G. Partial splenic embolization in the treatment of patients with portal hypertension: a review of the English language literature. J Vasc Interv Radiol. 2007;18:463–81.
20. Ohmoto K, Yamamoto S. Prevention of variceal recurrence, bleeding, and death in cirrhosis patients with hypersplenism, especially those with severe thrombocytopenia. Hepatogastroenterology. 2003;50:1766–9.
21. Murata K, Shiraki K, Takase K, Nakano T, Tameda Y. Long term follow-up for patients with liver cirrhosis after partial splenic embolization. Hepatogastroenterology. 1996;43:1212–7.
22. Sakata K, Hirai K, Tanikawa K. A long-term investigation of transcatheter splenic arterial embolization for hypersplenism. Hepatogastroenterology. 1996;43:309–18.
23. Shah R, Mahour GH, Ford EG, Stanley P. Partial splenic embolization. An effective alternative to splenectomy for hypersplenism. Am Surg. 1990;56:774–7.
24. Sangro B, Bilbao I, Herrero I, Corella C, Longo J, Beloqui O, et al. Partial splenic embolization for the treatment of hypersplenism in cirrhosis. Hepatology. 1993;18:309–14.
25. Yoshida H, Mamada Y, Taniai N, Yamamoto K, Kaneko M, Kawano Y, et al. Long-term results of partial splenic artery embolization as supplemental treatment for portal-systemic encephalopathy. Am J Gastroenterol. 2005;100:43–7.
26. Harned II RK, Thompson HR, Kumpe DA, Narkewicz MR, Sokol RJ. Partial splenic embolization in five children with hypersplenism: effects of reduced-volume embolization on efficacy and morbidity. Radiology. 1998;209:803–6.
27. Vauthey JN, Tomczak RJ, Helmberger T, Gertsch P, Forsmark C, Caridi J, et al. The arterioportal fistula syndrome: clinicopathologic features, diagnosis, and therapy. Gastroenterology. 1997;113:1390–401.
28. Rosch J, Hanafee WN, Snow H. Transjugular portal venography and radiologic portacaval shunt: an experimental study. Radiology. 1969;92:1112–4.
29. Colapinto RF, Stronell RD, Gildiner M, Ritchie AC, Langer B, Taylor BR, et al. Formation of intrahepatic portosystemic shunts using a balloon dilatation catheter: preliminary clinical experience. AJR Am J Roentgenol. 1983;140:709–14.
30. Palmaz JC, Sibbitt RR, Reuter SR, Garcia F, Tio FO. Expandable intrahepatic portacaval shunt stents: early experience in the dog. AJR Am J Roentgenol. 1985;145:821–5.
31. Richter GM, Noeldge G, Palmaz JC, Roessle M, Slegerstetter V, Franke M, et al. Transjugular intrahepatic portacaval stent shunt: preliminary clinical results. Radiology. 1990;174:1027–30.
32. Bureau C, Garcia-pagan JC, Otal P, Pomier-layrargues G, Chabbert V, Cortez C, et al. Improved clinical outcome using polytetrafluoroethylene-coated stents for TIPS: results of a randomized study. Gastroenterology. 2004;126:469–75.
33. Teisseire R, Clanet J, Broussy P, Cassigneul J, Fourtanier G. Pascal JP.Transjugular approach to the

portal venous system. Applications to the diagnosis, prognosis and treatment of gastrointestinal bleeding in cirrhosis. Gastroenterol Clin Biol. 1979;3:425–32.
34. Darcy MD, Sterling KM. Comparison of portal vein anatomy and bony anatomic landmarks. Radiology. 1996;200:707–10.
35. Semba CP, Saperstein L, Nyman U, Dake MD. Hepatic laceration from wedged venography performed before transjugular intrahepatic portosystemic shunt placement. J Vasc Interv Radiol. 1996;7: 143–6.
36. Krajina A, Lojik M, Chovanec V, Raupach J, Hulek P. Wedged hepatic venography for targeting the portal vein during TIPS: comparison of carbon dioxide and iodinated contrast agents. Cardiovasc Intervent Radiol. 2002;25:171–5.
37. Soares GM, Murphy TP. Transcaval TIPS: indications and anatomic considerations. J Vasc Interv Radiol. 1999;10:1233–8.
38. Blum U, Haag K, Rössle M, Ochs A, Gabelmann A, Boos S, et al. Noncavernomatous portal vein thrombosis in hepatic cirrhosis: treatment with transjugular intrahepatic portosystemic shunt and local thrombolysis. Radiology. 1995;195:153–7.
39. Monescillo A, Martínez-Lagares F, Ruiz-del-Arbol L, Sierra A, Guevara C, Jiménez E, et al. Peña E.vInfluence of portal hypertension and its early decompression by TIPS placement on the outcome of variceal bleeding. Hepatology. 2004;40:793–801.
40. Garcia-Pagan JC, Caca K, Bureau C, Laleman W, Appenrodt B, Luca A, et al. Early TIPS (Transjugular Intrahepatic Portosystemic Shunt) Cooperative Study Group. Early use of TIPS in patients with cirrhosis and variceal bleeding. N Engl J Med. 2010 Jun 24;362(25):2370–9.
41. Groupe d'Etude des Anastomoses Intra-Hépatiques. TIPS vs. sclerotherapy + propranolol in the prevention of variceal rebleeding: preliminary results of a multicenter randomized trial (abstract). Hepatology 1995;22:A297.
42. Cabrera J, Maynar M, Granados R, Gorriz E, Reyes R, Pulido-Duque JM, et al. Transjugular intrahepatic portosystemic shunt versus sclerotherapy in the elective treatment of variceal hemorrhage. Gastroenterology. 1996;110:832–9.
43. Rössle M, Deibert P, Haag K, Ochs A, Olschweski M, Siegerstetter V, et al. Randomised trial of transjugular-intrahepatic-portosystemic shunt versus endoscopy plus propranolol for prevention of variceal rebleeding. Lancet. 1997;249:1043–9.
44. Sanyal AJ, Freedman AM, Velimir A, Purdum 3rd PP, Shiffman ML, Cole PE, et al. Transjugular intrahepatic portosystemic shunt compared with endoscopic sclerotherapy for the prevention of recurrent variceal hemorrhage: a randomized controlled trial. Ann Intern Med. 1997;126:849–57.
45. Cello JP, Ring EJ, Olcott EW, Koch J, Gordon E, Sandhu J, et al. Endoscopic sclerotherapy compared with percutaneous transjugular intrahepatic portosystemic shunt after initial sclerotherapy in patients with acute variceal hemorrhage: a randomized controlled trial. Ann Intern Med. 1997;126:858–65.
46. Sauer P, Theilmann L, Stremmel W, Benz C, Richter GM, Stiehl A. Transjugular intrahepatic portosystemic stent shunt versus sclerotherapy plus propranolol for rebleeding. Gastroenterology. 1997;113: 1623–31.
47. Jalan R, Forrest EH, Stanley AJ, Redhead DN, Forbes J, Dillon JF, et al. A randomized trial comparing transjugular intrahepatic portosystemic stent-shunt with variceal band ligation in the prevention of rebleeding from esophageal varices. Hepatology. 1997;26: 1115–22.
48. Merli M, Salerno F, Riggio O, de Franchis R, Fiaccadori F, Meddi P, et al. Transjugular intrahepatic portosystemic shunt versus endoscopic sclerotherapy for the prevention of variceal bleeding in cirrhosis: a randomized multicenter trial. Hepatology. 1998;27:40–5.
49. Garcia-Villareal L, Martinez-Lagares F, Sierra A, Guevara C, Marrero JM, Jimenez E, et al. Transjugular intrahepatic portosystemic shunt versus endoscopic sclerotherapy for the prevention od variceal rebleeding after recent variceal hemorrhage. Hepatology. 1999;29:27–32.
50. Pomier-Layrargues G, Villeneuve JP, Deschenes M, Bui B, Perreault P, Fenyves D, et al. Transjugular intrahepatic portosystemic shunt (TIPS) versus endoscopic variceal ligation in the prevention of variceal rebleeding in patients with cirrhosis: a randomised trial. Gut. 2001;48:390–6.
51. Narahara Y, Kanazawa H, Kawamata H, Tada N, Saitoh H, Matsuzaka S, et al. A randomized clinical trial comparing transjugular intrahepatic portosystemic shunt with endoscopic sclerotherapy in the long-term management of patients with cirrhosis after recent variceal hemorrhage. Hepatol Res. 2001;21: 189–98.
52. Sauer P, Hansmann J, Richter GM, Stremmel W, Stiehl A. Endoscopic variceal ligation plus propranolol vs transjugular intrahepatic portosystemic stent shunt: a long-term randomized trial. Endoscopy. 2002;34:690–7.
53. Gülberg V, Schepke M, Geigenberger G, Holl J, Brensing KA, Waggershauser T, et al. Transjugular intrahepatic portosystemic shunting is not superior to endoscopic variceal band ligation for prevention of variceal rebleeding in cirrhotic patients: a randomized controlled trial. Scand J Gastroenterol. 2002;37: 338–43.
54. Papatheodoridis GV, Goulis J, Leandro G, Patch D, Burroughs AK. Transjugular intrahepatic portosystemic shunt compared with endoscopic treatment for prevention of variceal rebleeding: a meta-analysis. Hepatology. 1999;30:612–22.
55. Luca A, D'Amico G, La Galla R, Midiri M, Morabito A, Pagliaro L. TIPS for prevention of recurrent bleeding in patients with cirrhosis: meta-analysis of randomized clinical trials. Radiology. 1999;212: 411–21.

56. Burroughs AK, Vangeli M. Transjugular intrahepatic portosystemic shunt versus endoscopic therapy: randomized trials for secondary prophylaxis of variceal bleeding: an updated meta-analysis. Scand J Gastroenterol. 2002;37:249–52.
57. Escorsell A, Banares R, Garcia-Pagan JC, Gilabert R, Mointinho E, Piqueras B, et al. TIPS versus drug therapy in preventing variceal rebleeding in advanced cirrhosis: a randomized controlled trial. Hepatology. 2002;35:385–92.
58. Rosemurgy AS, Goode SE, Zwiebel BR, Black TJ, Brady PG. A prospective trial of transjugular intrahepatic portosystemic stent shunts versus small-diameter prosthetic H-graft portacaval shunts in the treatment of bleeding varices. Ann Surg. 1996;224:378–84.
59. Rosemurgy AS, Bloomston M, Clark WC, Thometz DP, Zervos EE. H-graft portacaval shunts versus TIPS: ten-year follow-up of a randomized trial with comparison to predicted survivals. Ann Surg. 2005;241:238–46.
60. Henderson JM, Boyer TD, Kutner MH, Galloway JR, Rikkers LF, Jeffers LJ, et al. DIVERT Study Group. Distal splenorenal shunt versus transjugular intrahepatic portal systematic shunt for variceal bleeding: a randomized trial. Gastroenterology. 2006;130:1643–51.
61. Barange K, Péron JM, Imani K, Otal P, Payen JL, Rousseau H, et al. Transjugular intrahepatic portosystemic shunt in the treatment of refractory bleeding from ruptured gastric varices. Hepatology. 1999;30:1139–43.
62. Shibata D, Brophy DP, Gordon FD, Anastopoulos HT, Sentovich SM, Bleday R. Transjugular intrahepatic portosystemic shunt for treatment of bleeding ectopic varices with portal hypertension. Dis Colon Rectum. 1999;42:1581–5.
63. Kamath PS, Lacerda M, Ahlquist DA, McKusick MA, Andrews JC, Nagorney DA. Gastric mucosal responses to intrahepatic portosystemic shunting in patients with cirrhosis. Gastroenterology. 2000;118:905–11.
64. Payen JL, Calès P, Voigt JJ, Barbe S, Pilette C, Dubuisson L, et al. Severe portal hypertensive gastropathy and antral vascular ectasia are distinct entities in patients with cirrhosis. Gastroenterology. 1995;108:138–44.
65. Lebrec D, Giuily N, Hadengue A, Vilgrain V, Moreau R, Poynard T, et al. Transjugular intrahepatic portosystemic shunts: comparison with paracentesis in patients with cirrhosis and refractory ascites: a randomized trial. French Group of Clinicians and a Group of Biologists. J Hepatol. 1996;25:135–44.
66. Rössle M, Ochs A, Gülberg V, Siegerstetter V, Holl J, Deibert P, et al. A comparison of paracentesis and transjugular intrahepatic portosystemic shunting in patients with ascites. N Engl J Med. 2000;342:1701–7.
67. Ginès P, Uriz J, Calahorra B, Garcia-Tsao G, Kamath PS, Del Arbol LR, et al. Transjugular intrahepatic portosystemic shunting versus paracentesis plus albumin for refractory ascites in cirrhosis. Gastroenterology. 2002;123:1839–47.
68. Sanyal AJ, Genning C, Reddy KR, Wong F, Kowdley KV, Benner K. North American Study for the Treatment of Refractory Ascites Group. The North American Study for the Treatment of Refractory Ascites. Gastroenterology. 2003;124:634–41.
69. Salerno F, Merli M, Riggio O, Cazzaniga M, Valeriano V, Pozzi M, et al. Randomized controlled study of TIPS versus paracentesis plus albumin in cirrhosis with severe ascites. Hepatology. 2004;40:629–35.
70. Salerno F, Cammà C, Enea M, Rössle M, Wong F. Transjugular intrahepatic portosystemic shunt for refractory ascites: a meta-analysis of individual patient data. Gastroenterology. 2007;133:825–34.
71. Rosemurgy AS, Zervos EE, Clark WC, Thometz DP, Black TJ, Zwiebel BR, et al. TIPS versus peritoneovenous shunt in the treatment of medically intractable ascites: a prospective randomized trial. Ann Surg. 2004;239:883–9.
72. Strauss RM, Martin LG, Kaufman SL, Boyer TD. Transjugular intrahepatic portal systemic shunt for the management of symptomatic cirrhotic hydrothorax. Am J Gastroenterol. 1994;89:1520–2.
73. Guevara M, Ginès P, Bandi JC, Gilabert R, Sort P, Jiménez W, et al. Transjugular intrahepatic portosystemic shunt in hepatorenal syndrome: effects on renal function and vasoactive systems. Hepatology. 1998; 28:416–22.
74. LBrensing KA, Textor J, Perz J, Schiedermaier P, Raab P, Strunk H, et al. Long term outcome after transjugular intrahepatic portosystemic stent-shunt in non-transplant cirrhotics with hepatorenal syndrome: a phase II study. Gut. 2000;47:288–95.
75. Perelló A, García-Pagán JC, Gilabert R, Suárez Y, Moitinho E, Cervantes F, et al. TIPS is a useful long-term derivative therapy for patients with Budd-Chiari syndrome uncontrolled by medical therapy. Hepatology. 2002;35:132–9.
76. Azoulay D, Castaing D, Lemoine A, Samuel D, Majno P, Reynes M, et al. Successful treatment of severe azathioprine-induced hepatic veno-occlusive disease in a kidney-transplanted patient with transjugular intrahepatic portosystemic shunt. Clin Nephrol. 1998; 50:118–22.
77. Kim JJ, Dasika NL, Yu E, Fontana RJ. Cirrhotic patients with a transjugular intrahepatic portosystemic shunt undergoing major extrahepatic surgery. J Clin Gastroenterol. 2009;43:574–9.
78. Freeman Jr RB, FitzMaurice SE, Greenfield AE, Halin N, Haug CE, Rohrer RJ. Is the transjugular intrahepatic portocaval shunt procedure beneficial for liver transplant recipients? Transplantation. 1994;58:297–300.
79. Barton RE, Saxon RR, Lakin PC, Petersen BD, Keller FS. TIPS: short- and long-term results: a survey of 1750 patients. Sem Interv Radiol. 364;12:364–7.
80. Sanyal AJ, Reddy KR. Vegetative infection of transjugular intrahepatic portosystemic shunts. Gastroenterology. 1998;115:110–5.
81. Sanyal AJ, Freedman AM, Purdum III PP. TIPS-associated hemolysis and encephalopathy. Ann Intern Med. 1992;117:443–4.

82. Bureau C, Otal P, Chabbert V, Péron JM, Rousseau H, Vinel JP. Segmental liver ischemia after TIPS procedure using a new PTFE-covered stent. Hepatology. 2002;36:1554.
83. Rössle M, Siegerstetter V, Huber M, Ochs A. The first decade of the transjugular intrahepatic portosystemic shunt (TIPS): state of the art. Liver. 1998;18: 73–89.
84. Ducoin H, El-Khoury J, Rousseau H, Barange K, Peron JM, Pierragi MT, et al. Histopathologic analysis of transjugular intrahepatic portosystemic shunts. Hepatology. 1997;25:1064–9.
85. Otal P, Smayra T, Bureau C, Peron JM, Chabbert V, Chemla P, et al. Preliminary results of a new expanded-polytetrafluoroethylene-covered stent-graft for transjugular intrahepatic portosystemic shunt procedures. AJR Am J Roentgenol. 2002;178:141–7.
86. Bureau C, Pagan JC, Layrargues GP, Metivier S, Bellot P, Perreault P, et al. Patency of stents covered with polytetrafluoroethylene in patients treated by transjugular intrahepatic portosystemic shunts: long-term results of a randomized multicentre study. Liver Int. 2007;27:742–7.
87. Maleux G, Verslype C, Heye S, Wilms G, Marchal G, Nevens F. Endovascular shunt reduction in the management of transjugular portosystemic shunt-induced hepatic encephalopathy: preliminary experience with reduction stents and stent-grafts. AJR Am J Roentgenol. 2007;188:659–64.
88. Russo MW, Zacks SL, Sandler RS, Brown RS. Cost-effectiveness analysis of transjugular intrahepatic portosystemic shunt (TIPS) versus endoscopic therapy for the prevention of recurrent esophageal variceal bleeding. Hepatology. 2000;31:358–63.
89. D'Amico G, Luca A. TIPS is a cost effective alternative to surgical shunt as a rescue therapy for prevention of recurrent bleeding from esophageal varices. J Hepatol. 2008;48:387–90.

Surgical Intervention for Portal Hypertension

16

J. Michael Henderson

Abstract

In 2010, surgery for complications of portal hypertension is largely limited to liver transplantation. The use of surgical shunts and devascularization procedures for variceal bleeding is now limited to unusual patients who have bleeding refractory to medical management, cannot be managed by TIPS, and have sufficiently preserved liver function so that they do not need a liver transplant. This chapter gives an outline of the different types of surgical shunts available to decompress varices and of the approach devascularization procedures take in managing patients with refractory bleeding, and summarizes the most current outcome data for these treatments.

Keywords

Surgical shunts • Devascularization procedures • Surgical outcomes for variceal bleeding

The surgical management of patients with portal hypertension has changed dramatically in the last decade, with the only significant use of surgical treatment being liver transplantation. This is a significant change from the major role that surgical shunts and gastroesophageal devascularizations played in treating patients in the 1970–1990s. This has occurred because of significant improvement in overall management of patients with portal hypertension brought about by the advent of pharmacologic therapy, the increasing sophistication and expertise with endoscopic management, and the introduction of transjugular intrahepatic portal systemic shunt (TIPS) as a less invasive way of decompressing portal hypertension [1]. Liver transplantation has emerged as the most widely used option for patients with end stage liver disease and portal hypertension, and is the only treatment used in portal hypertension that has improved long-term survival.

Management of patients with portal hypertension depends on an overall team approach. This team comprises hepatologists, surgeons, endoscopists, radiologists, pathologists, and intensivists. To bring maximum benefit to patients, this team should have all treatment options available and be aware of the current evidence supporting each of these options. This

J.M. Henderson (✉)
Department of General Surgery, The Cleveland Clinic Foundation, 9500 Euclid Avenue/E32, Cleveland, OH 44195-000, USA
e-mail: henderm@ccf.org

L.D. DeLeve and G. Garcia-Tsao (eds.), *Vascular Liver Disease: Mechanisms and Management*,
DOI 10.1007/978-1-4419-8327-5_16,

requires standardization of practices, with protocols to evaluate, and manage patients with varices that have not bled, are acutely bleeding, and to prevent recurrent bleeding. In addition, the repertoire of complications of portal hypertension that this team needs to evaluate and treat has broadened to include ascites, hepatoma, portopulmonary syndromes, and end stage liver disease.

This chapter will review the surgical options that are available to this team and the indications for their use in context of overall management of patients with portal hypertension.

Patient Evaluation

The evaluation is the same no matter what a patient's management path will be. This includes:
1. Assessment of underlying liver disease.
2. Imaging studies of the liver and its vasculature.
3. Endoscopic assessment for varices and portal gastropathy.

The liver disease is evaluated by (1) a complete history and clinical findings, such as jaundice, ascites, muscle wasting, (2) appropriate laboratory tests, and (3) when indicated, liver biopsy and other specialized tests of liver function. This evaluation allows staging of the severity of liver disease as in a Child's Pugh score or a MELD score that will help guide treatment decisions.

Imaging studies in portal hypertension focus on liver morphology and vasculature. Liver ultrasound is the mainstay of imaging assessment, but may need to be augmented by CT scan or MRI for better definition of the liver or vessels. The morphologic assessment focuses on the overall size of the liver and evidence of any focal lesions that are suspicious for hepatocellular carcinoma. If focal lesions are identified, they may require further evaluation including biopsy. Hepatic and portal venous and arterial anatomy should be assessed with an emphasis on patency of the portal vein and its main tributaries. If surgical intervention is being considered, more detail may be required than can be achieved with ultrasound: this is when a CT scan and/or MRI may be required.

Endoscopic evaluation is for the presence, size, extent, and risk factors of varices and for the presence of portal hypertensive gastropathy. In patients with portal hypertension, endoscopic management is also a key component of treating such patients and may have a role in following their response to both pharmacologic and endoscopic management.

Gastroesophageal Varices

Time Points for Treatment of Varices

Table 16.1 summarizes treatment options for prophylaxis, acute variceal bleeding, and prevention of recurrent bleed bleeding, and ranks one approach to the value of pharmacologic, endoscopic, radiologic, surgical shunts, and liver transplant at the different time points.

Prophylaxis

Pharmacologic therapy with a beta blocker is the mainstay for preventing an initial bleed as discussed in Chap. 11. Occasionally endoscopic banding may be indicated for large varices of patients intolerant to beta blockers. There is no indication for TIPS or surgical shunt in preventing an initial

Table 16.1 Role of therapy options and different time points in managing variceal bleeding

	Pharmacotherapy	Endoscopic therapy	TIPS	Surgical shunt	Liver transplant
Prophylaxis	+++	+	−	−	+
Acute variceal bleed	+++	+++	++	−	−
Prevention of recurrent bleed	+++	+++	++	+	++

+++ = Primary therapy; + = occasional
++ = Secondary; − = not indicated

bleed. The only time a liver transplant is indicated in patients with portal hypertension, varices, and no bleeding, is when there is advanced end stage liver disease or hepatocellular carcinoma.

Acute Variceal Bleeding

The primary management for acute variceal bleeding is pharmacologic therapy and endoscopic banding as discussed in Chap. 11. In the 10% of patients in whom acute bleeding is not controlled with these therapies, TIPS may be indicated. There is no role for surgical shunt or liver transplant to manage patients with acute variceal bleeding.

Prevention of Recurrent Variceal Bleeding

Figure 16.1 shows an algorithm for managing patients with recurrent variceal bleeding.

Pharmacologic therapy with beta blockers and a course of endoscopic banding to obliterate varices are the primary management of patients to prevent recurrent bleeding after they are stabilized from an acute bleed. This is discussed in detail in Chap. 11. These two treatments will control variceal bleeding in 80% of patients. In patients who either rebleed through this primary treatment or have recurrent high risk varices, other treatments may be indicated. In patients with well-preserved liver function and recurrent bleeding, TIPS is the next treatment option. Surgical decompression with selective shunt has been shown to be as effective as TIPS, but is not as widely available and therefore remains an option rather than recommended treatment. In patients with extensive splanchnic venous thrombosis, recurrent bleeding, and adequate liver function to tolerate surgery, a gastroesophageal devascularization may be indicated. In patients with progressive and advanced liver disease with recurrent bleeding, liver transplant becomes the treatment of choice.

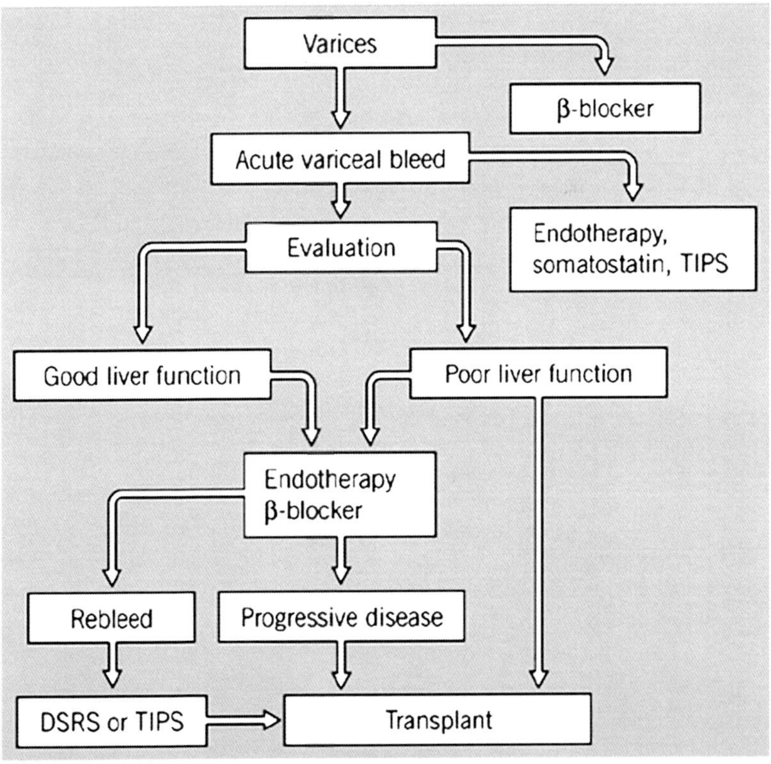

Fig. 16.1 Algorithm for prevention of variceal bleeding. Outside of liver transplant for end stage liver disease, surgery is not indicated for prophylaxis or management of acute bleeding. Selective shunt (DSRS) – or devascularization – may be indicated in some patients with preserved liver function and bleeding through primary therapy. Liver transplant is the most commonly used surgical treatment

The above recommendations are for patients with cirrhosis as the cause of portal hypertension. In considering the current role of surgical management in portal hypertension, other populations of patients need to be considered, as do geographic differences in diseases and available treatments. For example, patients with portal hypertension secondary to extrahepatic causes, such as portal vein thrombosis, who have well preserved liver function, may be excellent candidates for a surgical shunt if they have recurrent variceal bleeding despite pharmacologic and endoscopic therapy. Similarly, patients in India with noncirrhotic portal fibrosis have well preserved liver function, may not have good access for treatment requiring repeated visits such as endoscopic therapy or TIPS and may be good candidates for a selective surgical shunt. Other populations that may benefit from surgical management are (1) patients in remote locations who only get one chance at control of variceal bleeding, or (2) patients with schistosomiasis, and (3) patients with acute Budd–Chiari syndrome. In this latter population, the need may be for sinusoidal decompression, which can be achieved with a side-to-side portacaval shunt. While all of these patients can have decompression achieved with TIPS, long-term durability is less sure than management with a vein-to-vein surgical shunt. At the present time, it is incumbent upon the overall team managing such patients to have full working knowledge of all of these options and to have a defined management algorithm for patients with portal hypertension of all etiologies.

Surgical Procedures for Portal Hypertension

The main categories of surgical procedures for portal hypertension are:

1. Surgical shunts.
2. Surgical devascularization procedures.
3. Liver transplantation.

The surgical techniques for these are well described in a recent *Atlas of Upper Abdominal Surgery* [2]. Liver transplantation is dealt with elsewhere in this text and will not be discussed further. The following sections will briefly discuss the different types of surgical shunts and devascularization procedures and indicate where there may be roles for such management at the present time.

Surgical Shunt Procedures

These fall into three broad categories of total decompressive shunts, partial shunts, and selective shunts. These are illustrated in Figs. 16.2–16.4. In general terms, the difference with these options lies in the degree of maintenance of portal perfusion. All options provide decompression of gastroesophageal varices with a greater than 90% control of variceal bleeding. When a surgical shunt is indicated, the choice depends on the surgeon's familiarity with the given procedure and on the importance of maintaining some portal flow to lower the risk of encephalopathy.

Total Portal Systemic Shunts

These can be done either as a side-to-side portocaval shunt or an interposition mesocaval shunt that is more than 10 mm in diameter [2–5]. These shunts all divert portal flow away from the liver and are thus excellent in controlling bleeding. Since they also decompress the liver sinusoids they are also excellent in controlling ascites.

Figure 16.2 illustrates the side-to-side portocaval shunt. The main technical components are as follows:

1. Adequate exposure of the portal vein and subhepatic inferior vena cava.
2. Mobilization of sufficient length of the portal vein and inferior vena cava to allow approximation for direct anastomosis or safe placement of an interposition graft.
3. Completion of the anastomosis with running Prolene, ensuring no purse-stringing of the anastomosis which should be greater than 10 mm in diameter to provide total decompression.

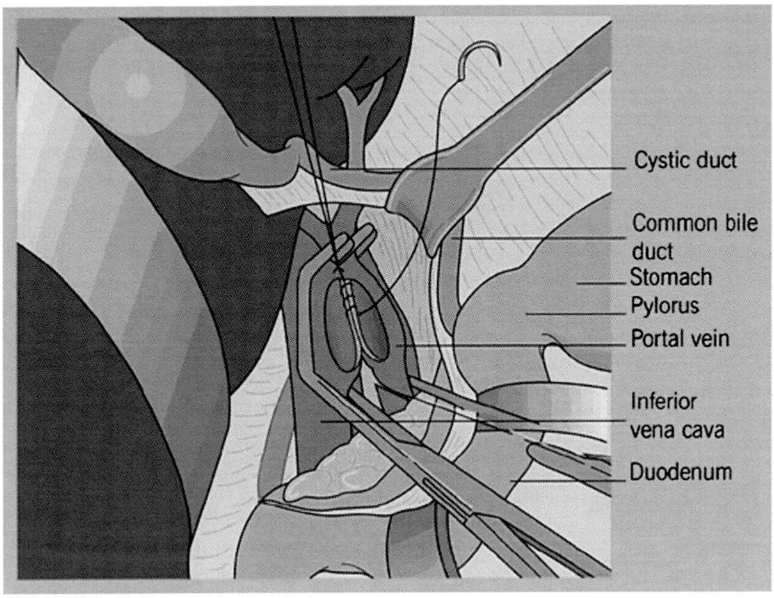

Fig. 16.2 Side-to-side portacaval shunt with direct anastomosis of the portal vein and inferior vena cava. To totally decompress portal hypertension, the anastomosis should be >10 mm

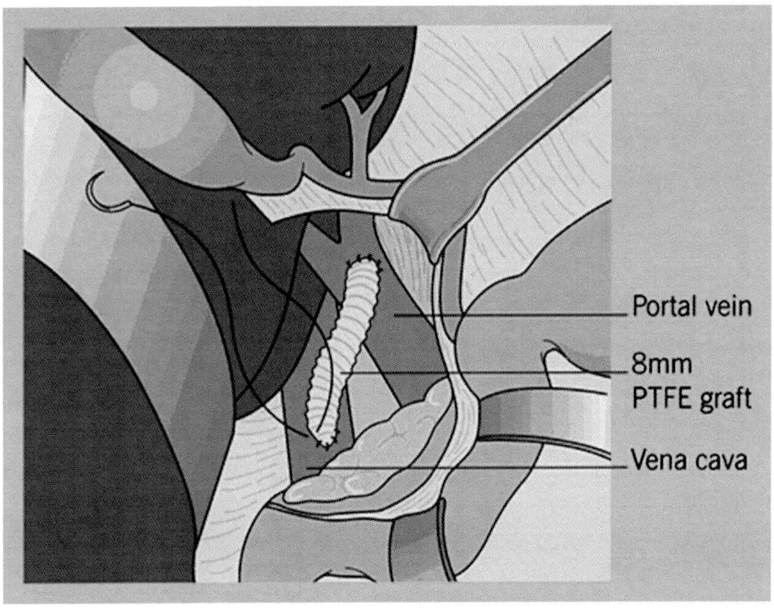

Fig. 16.3 Partial portacaval shunt with an 8 mm PTFE graft between the portal vein and inferior vena cava. This shunt will decompress varices and maintain some portal flow to the liver

Partial Portal Systemic Shunt

This shunt is achieved with an 8 mm graft between the portal vein and the inferior vena cava [2, 6]. The operative exposure and technique is similar to that for a side-to-side portocaval shunt, but the difference lies in the careful positioning of an 8 mm reinforced polytetrafluoroethylene (PTFE) graft between the IVC and the portal vein as shown in Fig. 16.3. The ends of the graft are

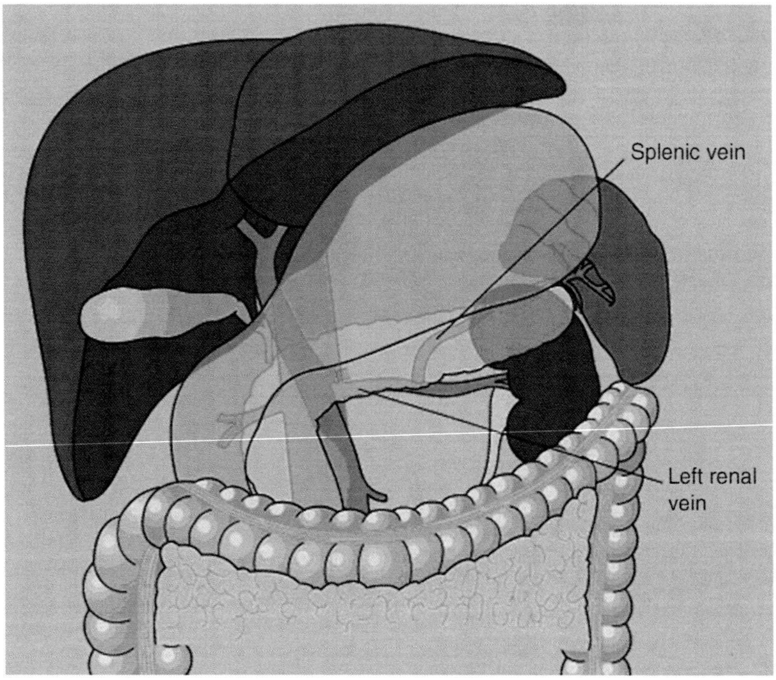

Fig. 16.4 Distal splenorenal shunt, which selectively decompresses varices through the spleen, while maintaining portal hypertension and hepatopedal flow in the portal vein

beveled to double the size of the anastomosis relative to the graft diameter and positioned at right angles to each other on the graft to avoid kinking of the graft when it sits in its correct position.

A small diameter shunt can also be used between the superior mesenteric vein and vena cava [7], but is considerably longer, so at greater risk of thrombosis.

Selective Surgical Shunt

Selective variceal decompression is most commonly done as the distal splenorenal shunt (DSRS) which has a different concept to those above – Fig. 16.4 [2, 8]. Varices are decompressed selectively from the spleen through the short gastric veins, the splenic vein, to the left renal vein, while portal hypertension is maintained in the superior mesenteric and portal veins to keep portal flow to the liver. The key steps to this shunt are:

1. Accessing the splenic vein on the back of the pancreas.
2. Dissecting the vein out of the posterior surface of the pancreas.
3. Dividing the splenic vein at its junction with the superior mesenteric vein.
4. The splenic vein is anastomosed to the left renal vein.
5. The operation is completed by ligating the coronary vein and other collaterals from the portal vein to isolate the portal and splenic systems.

Devascularization Procedures

Devascularization procedures have the overall goal of reducing inflow to varices, and have the components of splenectomy, gastric esophageal devascularization, and esophageal transection [2, 9]. Their success depends upon the extent of devascularization. The more extensive the devascularization, the lower the subsequent rebleeding rate. The operative approach for devascularization requires:

1. Sufficient exposure of the upper abdomen and left upper quadrant.

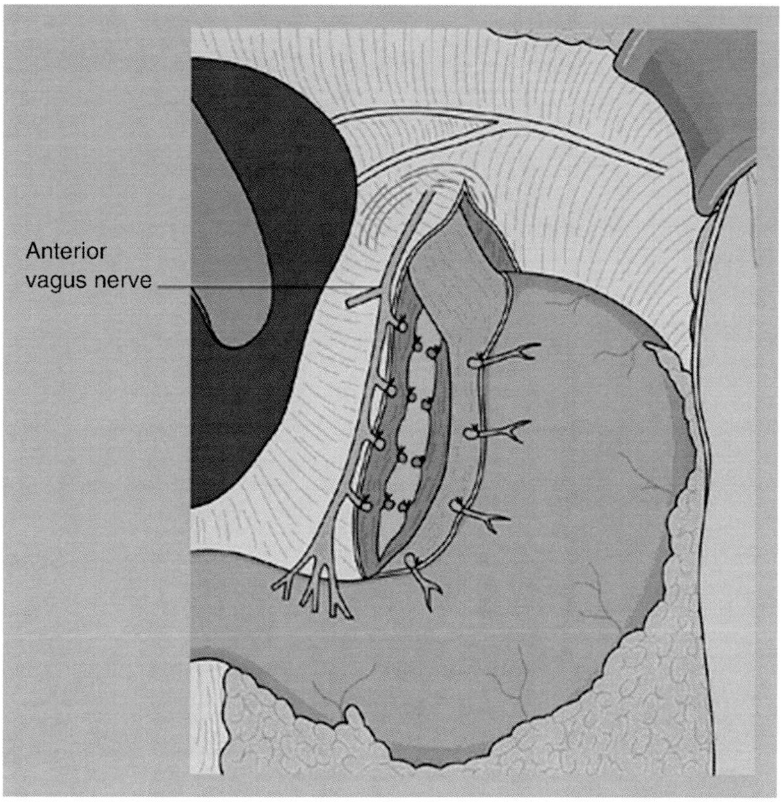

Fig. 16.5 Gastroesophageal devascularization of the distal 7 cm of esophagus, all of the greater curve and two-thirds of lesser curve of the stomach

2. Splenectomy.
3. Devascularization of the upper two-thirds of the lesser and all of the greater curvature of the stomach and at least 7 cm of the distal esophagus (Fig. 16.5).
4. Particular attention needs to be paid to the posterior aspect of the distal esophagus, where there are large penetrating veins from large paraesophageal venous plexuses.
5. Esophageal transection is controversial, because most patients have had extensive sclerotherapy and a thickened esophagus does not lend itself to a stapled transection. Most surgeons omit this component of devascularization procedures.

Various modifications have been made to devascularization. The initial approach to devascularization combined a transthoracic and transabdominal approach. This is now rarely done. Most patients only need a transabdominal approach to devascularization. Others have modified the transabdominal approach to avoid splenectomy and made a simpler procedure. Results from this appear to be satisfactory.

Perioperative Patient Management

When patients with portal hypertension are considered a candidate for surgical intervention, it is important that the whole team managing these patients is involved. This includes both careful preoperative assessment to make sure there are no contraindications to surgery in general terms, as well as being certain these are good risk patients from their liver disease perspective. Only Child's class A patients or patients without underlying liver disease and portal hypertension should be considered for surgical intervention. In the perioperative period, careful management from both the surgical and anesthesia team is essential. These patients should be managed somewhat differently than general surgical patients because of their risk of developing ascites. Perioperative fluids should be restricted to the minimum required to maintain an adequate intravascular volume. Similarly, in the postoperative period, fluid and electrolyte management is important with limiting sodium intake to reduce the risk of ascites. Similarly, caution with the use of narcotics and sedatives is important in patients with underlying liver disease. The risks in the perioperative period are deterioration of liver function, development of ascites, and the risk of infection. Attention to detail in managing these patients can minimize these risks.

Current Data

The data on surgical outcomes for patients with variceal bleeding is sparse over the past decade, and will be briefly reviewed for surgical shunts and devascularization.

Surgical Shunts

Two randomized trials have compared surgical shunts to TIPS in the last decade [10–13]. One compared TIPS and DSRS in Child's Class A and B patients [10]. The trial ran over 7 years, with a median follow-up of 42 months. The rebleeding rate in the DSRS group was 5.5% and in the TIPS group 10.5%, which were not significantly different ($p=0.29$). Encephalopathy rates were not significantly different, with 50% of patients in each group having at least one clinical encephalopathy event by 5 years. The survival rates were not significantly different, with 2 and 5 year survival rates of 81 and 62% in the DSRS patients and 88 and 61% in the TIPS patients ($P=0.87$). What was significantly different was the reintervention rate, which was 82% in the TIPS group and 11% in the DSRS group ($P<0.001$). It was the careful surveillance, protocol recatheterizations of TIPS at annual intervals, and completeness of follow-up that contributed to the low rebleeding rate in the TIPS group. This trial was conducted with uncovered stents. A European multicenter trial, compared covered and uncovered TIPS and the reintervention rate with covered stents was reduced to 15% at 1 year [14].

A cost effectiveness analysis of the DSRS versus TIPS trial [12] showed the average yearly costs of managing patients after TIPS and DSRS over 5 years were similar, $16,363 and 13,492, respectively. Cost of TIPS in surviving patients exceeded the cost of DSRS at years 3 and 5, but not significantly. Incremental Cost Effectiveness Ratios per life saved favored TIPS at year 5. Finally, an analysis of the effect of drinking on outcome in this trial showed that only those with alcoholic liver disease returned to drinking, and heavy drinking (>4 drinks/day) was associated with higher mortality and rebleeding rates [15].

The second trial compared TIPS to the 8-mm H-graft interposition portacaval shunt in an "all-comers" population [11]. In this trial 50% of patients entered were Child's C and 63% had alcoholic cirrhosis. At late follow-up [13], the rebleeding rate was significantly lower ($P<0.01$) in the surgical shunt group (3%) compared to the TIPS group (17%), and fewer patients in the surgical shunt group came to transplant ($P<0.01$). Mortality was not significantly different. Other variables were not different or not assessed.

A recently published randomized trial of emergency endoscopic sclerotherapy versus emergency portacaval shunt for acutely bleeding esophageal varices was performed by the San Diego Study Group [16]. This study entered all patients referred with acute bleeding with >80% having alcoholic liver disease and 27% being Child class C. They achieved 100% control of bleeding in the portacaval shunt group, but only 20% control in the sclerotherapy group. The 1, 5, and 10-year survivals in the two groups were: portacaval shunt 81, 73, and 46% and sclerotherapy 72, 21, and 9%, which were significantly ($P<0.001$) different. Of note, the rate of encephalopathy was significantly ($P<0.001$) lower in the portacaval shunt group at 15% compared to the sclerotherapy group at 35%. The authors conclude that early and complete control of bleeding in this population is the reason they achieved these remarkable results.

A review of the literature over the past 10 years shows only 22 cited papers on surgical shunts. These papers fall into the categories of the randomized studies cited above (7 reports), large series [17–21], or patients being shunted for specific circumstances. This paucity of recent publications on surgical shunts speaks to there being few indications for their use in 2009.

Devascularization Procedures

The use of these operations is limited to patients with extensive thrombosis of the portal venous system who have persistent bleeding through maximal pharmacologic and endoscopic therapy. There are no randomized trial evaluating devascularization procedures and the literature of the past 10 years includes a few small series of patients from across the world [22–26]. Rebleeding rates up to 20% are reported, but most series have poor follow-up. Again it bears emphasis that the control of bleeding with this procedure is primarily a function of the extent of devascularization, with best results being obtained in centers with experience. For individual patients, this may sometimes be the only option available.

Conclusions

A fitting way to conclude this chapter is to quote from a paper by one of the thoughtful stalwarts of surgery for portal hypertension, Dr Hector Orozco, publisher in the Archives of Surgery in 2007. This paper, "Rise and Downfall of the Empire of Portal Hypertension Surgery" [27] opens with the following paragraph:

> Frequently in life, there are things that appear in a coincidental way that tend to completely modify the environment of the human being. In the same way in other occasions, forces that had taken many years to show their utility for human beings tend to disappear without a clear explanation.

He goes on to outline the major phases, and successes of surgery in managing patients with portal hypertension. While there may indeed be great value in some of these options for some patients, "many new actors appeared on the scene", and the surgeons who performed these operations disappeared. He concludes with the following paragraph:

> What a pity. There have been many ideas to resolve a problem, many years of work, many patients treated, and 1 surgical solution that was approaching the ideal: low morbidity, low mortality, low recurrence of the hemorrhagic episodes, and long survival. Despite all of this, we threw it away because we did not know how, when, and to whom we might give it.

This epitaph for surgery for portal hypertension – other than liver transplant – is most fitting.

References

1. D'Amico G, Criscuoli V, Fili D, Pagliano L. Meta-analysis of trials for variceal bleeding. Hepatology. 2002;36:1023–4.
2. Henderson JM. Portal hypertension. In: Clavien PA, Sarr MG, Fong Y, editors. Atlas of upper gastrointestinal and hepatic-pancreato-biliary surgery. Berlin: Springer; 2007. p. 649–724.
3. Orloff MJ, Orloff MS, Orloff SL, et al. Three decades of experience with emergency portacaval shunt for acutely bleeding esophageal varices in 400 unselected patients with cirrhosis of the liver. J Am Coll Surg. 1995;180:257–72.
4. Stipa S, Balducci G, Ziparo V, et al. Total shunting and elective management of variceal bleeding. World J Surg. 1994;18:200–4.
5. Drapanas T. Interposition mesocaval shunt for treatment of portal hypertension. Ann Surg. 1972;176:435–48.
6. Sarfeh IJ, Rypins EB, Mason GR. A systematic appraisal of portocaval H-graft diameters. Clinical and hemodynamic perspectives. Ann Surg. 1986;204:356–63.
7. Mercado MA, Orozco H, Guillen-Navarro E, et al. Small-diameter mesocaval shunts: a 10-year evaluation. J Gastrointest Surg. 2000;4:453–7.
8. Warren WD, Zeppa R, Fomon JJ. Selective trans-splenic decompression of gastroesophageal varices by distal splenorenal shunt. Ann Surg. 1967;166:437–55.
9. Sugiura M, Futagawa S. Esophageal transaction with paraesophagogastric devascularizations (the Sugiura procedure) in the treatment of esophageal varices. World J Surg. 1984;8:673–9.
10. Henderson JM, Boyer TD, Kutner MH, Galloway JR, Rikkers LF, Jeffers LJ, et al. Distal splenorenal shunt versus transjugular intrahepatic portal systematic shunt for variceal bleeding: a randomized trial. Gastroenterology. 2006;130:1643–51.
11. Rosemurgy AS, Serofini FM, Zweibal BR, et al. TIPS versus small diameter prosthetic H-graft portacaval shunt: extended follow-up of an expanded randomized prospective trial. J Gastrointest Surg. 2000;4:589–97.

12. Boyer TD, Henderson JM, Heerey AM, Arrigain S, Konig V, Connor J, et al. Cost of preventing variceal rebleeding with transjugular intrahepatic portal systemic shunt and distal splenorenal shunt. J Hepatol. 2008;48:407–14.
13. Rosemurgy AS, Bloomston M, Clark WC, Thometz DP, Zervos EE. H-graft portacaval shunts versus TIPS: ten-year follow-up of a randomized trial with comparison to predicted survivals. Ann Surg. 2005;241: 238–46.
14. Bureau C, Garcia-Pagan JC, Otal P, et al. Improved clinical outcome using polytetrafluoroethylene-coated stents for TIPS: results of a randomized study. Gastroenterology. 2004;126:469–75.
15. Lucey MR, Connor JT, Boyer TD, Henderson JM, DIVERT Study Group. Alcohol consumption by cirrhotic subjects: patterns of use and effects on liver function. Am J Gastroenterol. 2008;103:1698–706.
16. Orloff MJ, Isenberg JI, Wheeler HO, et al. Randomized trial of emergency endoscopic sclerotherapy versus emergency portacaval shunt for acutely bleeding esophageal varices in cirrhosis. J Am Coll Surg. 2009;209:25–40.
17. Livingstone AS, Koniaris LG, Perez EA, Alvarez N, Levi JU, Hutson DG. 507 Warren-Seppa distal splenorenal shunts: a 34-year experience. Ann Surg. 2006;243:884–92.
18. Elwood DR, Pomposelli JJ, Pomfret EA, Lewis WD, Jenkins RL. Distal splenorenal shunt: preferred treatment for recurrent variceal hemorrhage in the patient with well-compensated cirrhosis. Arch Surg. 2006;141:385–8.
19. Orozco H, Mercado MA, Garcia JG, et al. Selective shunts for portal hypertension current role of a 21 year experience. Liver Transplant Surg. 1997;3: 475–80.
20. Rikkers LF, Jin G, Langnas AN, et al. Shunt surgery during the era of liver transplantation. Ann Surg. 1997;226:51–7.
21. Orozco H, Mercado MA. The evolution of portal hypertension surgery: lessons from 1000 operations and 50 years' experience. Arch Surg. 2000;135:1389–93.
22. Mercado MA, Chan C, Zenteno-Guichard G, et al. Results of surgical treatment (modified Sugiura-Futagawa operation) of portal hypertension associated to complete splenomesoportal thrombosis and cirrhosis. HPB Surg. 1999;11:157–62.
23. Qazi SA, Khalid K, Hameed AM, et al. Transabdominal gastro-esophageal devascularization and esophageal transaction for bleeding esophageal varices after failed injection sclerotherapy: long-term follow-up report. World J Surg. 2006;30:1329–37.
24. Rao KL, Goyal A, Menon P, et al. Extrahepatic portal hypertension in children: observations on three surgical procedures. Pediatr Surg Int. 2004;20:679–84.
25. Selzner M, Tuttle-Newhall JE, Dahm F, et al. Current indication of a modified Sugiura procedure in the management of variceal bleeding. J Am Coll Surg. 2001;193:166–73.
26. Orozco H, Mercado MA. Devascularizations in portal hypertension. J Am Coll Surg. 2002;194:247–9.
27. Orozco H, Mercado MA. Rise and downfall of the empire of portal hypertension surgery. Arch Surg. 2007;142:219–21.

Liver Transplantation and Vascular Disorders

17

Jan P. Lerut, Eliano Bonaccorsi-Riani, and Pierre Goffette

Abstract

One of the main advantages of liver transplantation (LT) has been to concentrate particular and rare liver diseases in a restricted number of centers. This policy has led to a much better understanding, diagnosis, and treatment of these, many times, difficult conditions.

This chapter gives a comprehensive and updated review in relation to vascular liver diseases. It is without any doubt that hemangioma, angiosarcoma (AS), infantile hemangioendothelioma (IHE), epithelioid hemangioendothelioma (EHE), hemorrhagic hereditary telangiectasia (HHT), Budd-Chiari syndrome (BCS), and nodular regenerative hyperplasia (NRH) took really profit of the latest developments in the field of LT. Based on the worldwide transplant experience, diagnostic and therapeutic algorithm of these diseases very much improved. We now know that LT is absolutely contraindicated in case of AS; that LT is of great value in the treatment of EHE and HHT and that indications of LT for IHE, BCS, and NRH must be highly individualized.

The second part of this chapter deals with particular features of hepatic and splanchnic vessels, which are of importance as well in the pre-LT as post-LT periods. These vascular modifications are important to know as well for the transplant physician and surgeon in order to make the transplant procedure successful.

Keywords

Vascular tumors – epithelioid hemangioendothelioma – infantile hemangioendothelioma • Hemangiosarcoma – nodular regenerative hyperplasia • Budd-Chiari syndrome • Hereditary hemorrhagic telangiectasia • Splanchnic venous thrombosis • Portal vein thrombosis • Caval thrombosis – cavoportal transposition – TIPSS – thrombectomy • Arterial thrombosis – coagulation – liver transplantation

J.P. Lerut (✉)
Department of Abdominal and Transplantation Surgery, Starzl Abdominal Transplant Unit, St. Luc Université Hospitals, Universite catholique de Louvain (UCL), Avenue Hippocrates 10, Brussels, Belgium
e-mail: jan.lerut@uclouvain.be

Introduction

Vascular hepatic disorders are rare indications for liver transplantation (LT). Indeed, vascular tumors, Budd-Chiari syndrome (BCS), hereditary

L.D. DeLeve and G. Garcia-Tsao (eds.), *Vascular Liver Disease: Mechanisms and Management*,
DOI 10.1007/978-1-4419-8327-5_17, © Springer Science+Business Media, LLC 2011

hemorrhagic telangiectasia (HHT), and nodular regenerative hyperplasia (NRH), respectively, represent 0.023, 1, 0.1, and 0.05% of 72,275 LT reported to the European Liver Transplant Registry (ELTR) between May 1968 and June 2008. Due to their rarity and variable clinical presentation, the role of LT in the therapeutic algorithm of most of these liver disorders is as yet unclear.

Many patients with cirrhosis present with localized or extensive splanchnic venous thrombosis at the time of LT. These conditions need a specific surgical strategy in order to allow a safe transplant procedure. Vascular complications after LT are rare events needing specific procedures, usually by interventional radiology.

Liver-based inherited thrombophilic or hemophilic diseases can be cured by LT, although exceptionally one may encounter transmission of such disorders by the liver allograft itself.

This chapter aims to give an overview regarding the role of LT in vascular and hemostatic liver disorders as well as surgical and radiological management of intra- and postoperative venous complications.

Vascular Hepatic Tumors

Vascular hepatic tumors form a continuum ranging from the completely benign hemangioma (HA) to the very aggressive hemangiosarcoma (HAS) [1].

Giant Hemangioma and Hemangiomatosis

Giant (>4 cm) hemangiomas represent an unusual indication for LT as these lesions, even if enormous, can be dealt with safely by liver resection. Most can be enucleated safely under (intermittent) occlusion of the hepatic vascular inflow. Rarely, a patient can present with a hepatic hemangiomatosis, a condition which can lead to the development of severe cardiac decompensation, a life-threatening condition that can only be cured by LT. Only a handful of patients reported to the ELTR were transplanted for this condition.

Hepatic Epithelioid Hemangioendothelioma (HEHE)

The HEHE is a rare (<1 per million population), low-grade malignancy, which has a behavior intermediate between HA and HAS [2]. This vascular tumor was first recognized in 1982 by Weiss and Enzinger in soft tissues, later on in the head and neck region, bones, lungs, and bronchi. Liver involvement occurs most often as a primary tumor. HEHE is more frequent in young adult women with a peak incidence during the fourth decade. HEHE has rarely been reported in children less than 15 years old. No definitive etiological factor has been clearly identified.

Ishak was the first to draw the attention of the hepatology community to this disease [2]. Macroscopically, HEHE appears as multifocal fibrous masses. Microscopically, it is characterized by medium- and large-sized pleiomorphic cells that are epithelioid in appearance and that spread within sinusoids and small veins at the periphery of the lesion, whereas the center is fibrous, studded with elongated tumor cells and sometimes with intracellular vascular lumina containing red blood cells. In contrast to HAS, the hepatic acinar landmarks are preserved. HEHE originates from endothelial cells, which explains the positive immunohistochemistry for factor VIII-related antigen and for the endothelial markers CD31 and CD34. Ultrastructural examination shows characteristic features of endothelial cells [2, 3].

Reviews derived from HEHE experiences by the European ELITA-ELTR (European Liver Intestine Transplant Association-European Liver Transplant Registry) and the American UNOS (United Network for Organ Sharing) have been pivotal in their early identification and, more importantly, in the refinement of their therapeutic algorithm [1, 4]. The clinical manifestations of HEHE are nonspecific, varying from an asymptomatic state to hepatic failure. More commonly, there is nonspecific upper abdominal or epigastric discomfort or pain, weakness, impaired general condition, and jaundice. About 20% of patients are asymptomatic and 10% present with pulmonary symptoms. Hepatosplenomegaly (50%) and weight loss (20%) are the most frequent clinical signs. Portal hypertension may be caused by tumor compression or venous infiltration. Anicteric cholestasis and cytolytic activity are present in 60 and 40%, respectively. Serum tumor markers are always normal in the absence of accompanying liver disease. The malignant potential of HEHE is unclear.

Radiological investigation identifies two different patterns of HEHE: the early peripheral and nodular, usually bilobar, type ("peripheral pattern") and the later confluent type ("diffuse pattern") with eventual invasion of the greater vessels (Fig. 17.1a and b). Focal calcifications are present in 20% of tumors. Angiography reveals only moderate vascularization with displacement of marginal vessels. Scintigraphy and FDG-PET imaging play an important role in the staging of the disease and of the early detection of recurrent disease after LT. Complete assessment is mandatory to exclude other, especially thoracic, organ involvement. If there is reason for concern, thoracoscopy with lung and/or pleural

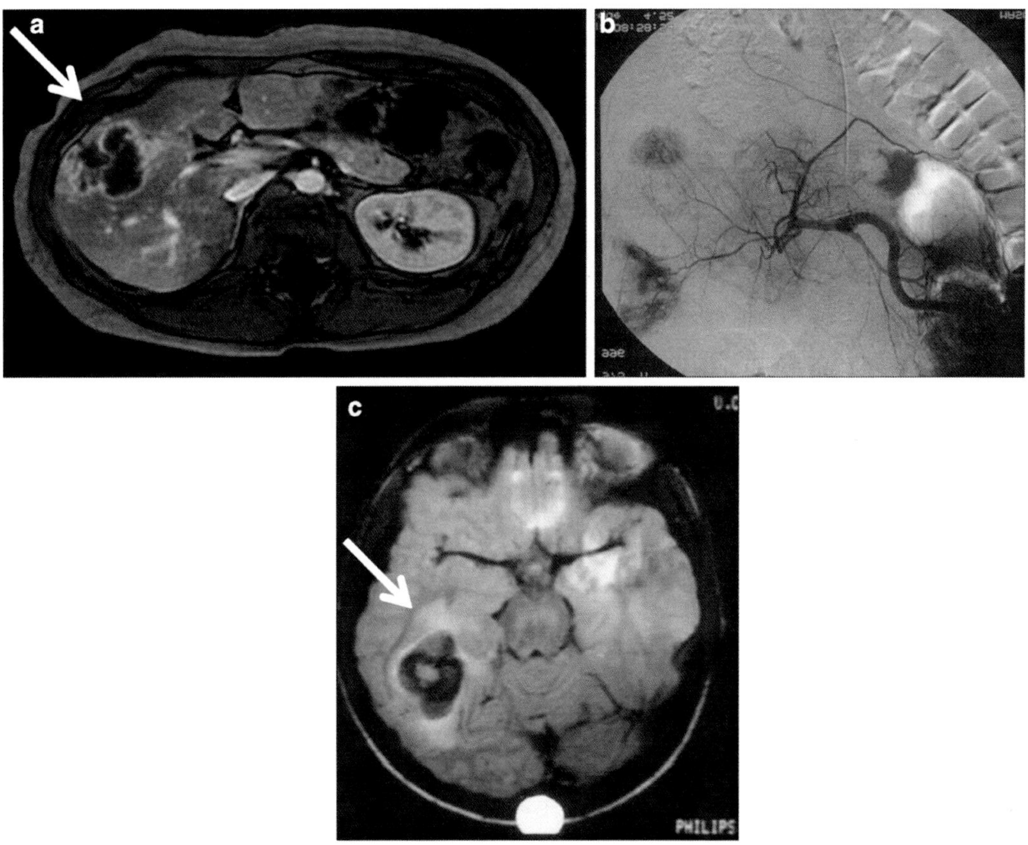

Fig. 17.1 (**a**) Nuclear magnetic resonance (NMR) shows typical peripheral lesions of hepatic epithelioid hemangioendothelioma (HEHE); (**b**) angiography confirms bilobar liver involvement; (**c**) cerebral NMR shows HEHE in the right cerebellum; this lesion was treated by neurosurgery and radiotherapy. The patient had a liver transplant 2 years later. He is alive and free of disease 14 years after liver transplant, off immunosuppression

biopsy is recommended in order to exclude frequent thoracic involvement. The definitive diagnosis of HEHE is based on a high degree of suspicion made by the combination of clinical and radiological features such as presentation in a young adult (female) with a good general status and a long-standing history despite the presence of numerous intrahepatic (often calcified) tumors [1, 2]. The diagnosis can only be confirmed by histology.

Until recently, the treatment algorithm for HEHE was far from standardized. Review of the literature reveals 13 small series (including 5 or more patients) and three reviews, all lacking detailed analysis, long-term follow-up, and comparisons between untreated and medically or surgically treated patients. Moreover, the role of LT has been questioned given the well-documented long-term survival, the high incidence (up to 45%) of extra-hepatic disease, the lack of predictive clinical or histological criteria, and the high incidence (up to 33%) of recurrent allograft disease [1, 2, 5]. The Pittsburgh group published the largest transplant series, which included 16 patients; 5-year patient and disease-free survival rates were 71 and 60%, respectively [7]. The presumed value of the radical transplant approach was confirmed in Mehrabi's literature review. In this review, the 5-year survival rates of LT, local or systemic chemo- and radiotherapy, and no treatment were 55, 30, and 0%, respectively [8]. Although partial resection has been reported as being successful in rare cases, this approach is illogical because the disease is nearly always multinodular and bilobar. Indeed, analysis of explants in the ELITA-ELTR study showed bilobar disease in 96% and presence of at least 15 tumor nodules in 86% of the cases. These observations go along with several case reports that document disease recurrence or need for LT after partial resection because of recurrent HEHE. Fortunately, pretransplant surgery does not impact patient survival after LT. The efficacy of nonsurgical treatments such as radiotherapy, local tumor ablation, hormone therapy, systemic or locoregional chemotherapy, transarterial embolization, and chemoembolization is impossible to assess, because of the lack of uniform treatment modalities and of long-term follow-up [1, 8].

The ELITA-ELTR study is the largest published detailed long-term study of HEHE and includes 59 patients [1]. The follow-up from diagnosis is 104 ± 72 months (median of 93 months) and from LT 83 ± 55 months (median of 79 months). This study validated the role of LT in the treatment of this disease, with 5- and 10-year posttransplant survival rates of 83 and 74%, respectively, and 5- and 10-year recurrence free survival rates of 82 and 64%, respectively. Medical and/or surgical pre-LT treatment (present in 30% of patients), invasion of regional lymph nodes (present in 33% of patients), and of (limited) extrahepatic disease (present in 17% of patients) were not formal contraindications to LT (Fig. 17.1c). Combined micro- and macrovascular invasion (present in 49% of patients) was the only parameter that significantly influenced post-LT outcome. Mitotic index and cellular pleiomorphism, criteria known to reflect a more aggressive tumor could not be analyzed because of the lack of central pathology reading [5, 6]. The recent UNOS data regarding 128 HEHE patients with a shorter median follow-up (24 months) are in line with the European experience, with 1- and 5-year survival rates of 80 and 64%, respectively [4].

There may even be a place for sequential or combined hepato-pulmonary transplantation in this disease (personal communication D. van Raemdonck, Lung Transplant Program, University Hospitals Leuven, B).

Recurrent disease after LT should be treated aggressively as prolonged, sometimes even disease-free, survival can be obtained [1]. The role of re-LT in the treatment of recurrent allograft disease is unclear as only one case has been reported [5].

In view of the high incidence of extrahepatic disease and of recurrence inside and outside the allograft (22% in the ELITA-ELTR study), a more radical approach combining total hepatectomy and antiangiogenic therapy, using of anti-VEGF-antibodies, α-interferon, and/or rapamycin could be of value in the treatment of HEHE [9]. Rapamycin is of particular interest in this context, as this immunosuppressive drug is regularly used not only as a renal sparing, but also as an antitumor drug in liver recipients. This approach, combined with a better study of molecular and genetic markers of tumor biology, may lead to improved outcomes, to determine efficacy of emerging neo- and adjuvant treatments, and to recognize the aggressive subtypes of HEHE.

Hepatic Infantile Hemangioendothelioma (HIHE)

The HIHE can be easily distinguished from HEHE as both have different, age-related, clinical and pathological features [2, 10]. HIHE, the most common mesenchymal tumor of the liver in infants (<3 years), is nearly always diagnosed during the first 6 months of life. This tumor is also more frequent in females and presents with symptomatic hepatosplenomegaly, failure to thrive, congestive cardiac failure (15%) due to intratumor arteriovenous shunting, cutaneous hemangiomas (20–40%), coagulopathy due to Kasabach–Merritt syndrome, and resistant hypothyroidism. HIHE may regress spontaneously in 5–10% of cases. The outcome is, however, poor because of associated anomalies or tumor complications that lead to a mortality as high as 90% [10, 11]. The main difficulty with HIHE lies in the difficult differential diagnosis with hemangiosarcoma. All diagnostic procedures, including large surgical biopsies, should be in order to exclude HAS.

The HIHE occurs either as a single or a multifocal tumor. The lesions are soft, spongy, red-tan nodules, sometimes more firm and gray-white or brown with areas of necrosis and hemorrhage. Histology identifies two types of HIHE. The most frequent, type 1, consists of intercommunicating small vascular channels lined by a single layer of regular endothelial cells. The more pleiomorphic type 2, containing nuclear atypia, multilayering and papillary projections, is now considered a form of HAS. Immunohistochemistry is of importance to differentiate HIHE from hepatic vascular malformations associated with capillary proliferation; immunoreactivity for GLUT-1 favors a diagnosis of HIHE [13]. The main problem is that these tumors may harbor foci of HAS. Data from the ELITA-ELTR showed that features of HAS were present in all children with HIHE with rapid deterioration due to acute liver failure or BCS. They all died of rapid recurrence.

Treatment of HIHE includes intensive medical therapies (using diuretics, digoxin, high-dose steroids, interferon, chemotherapy or radiotherapy, antiangiogenic drugs) and/or interventional radiology and/or surgery [10–12]. Symptomatic treatment may increase survival up to 40%. With specific therapy (such as liver resection), survival rate can be even higher. Liver resection series are sparse and usually include a few patients [18–20]. Five-year survival of 61% following LT has been described. The Boston algorithm for the treatment of this pediatric condition advocates partial hepatectomy if lesions are confined to one liver lobe and LT if the disease is diffuse or resistant to steroid therapy [14].

Hepatic Hemangiosarcoma (HAS)

The HAS is the most common primary liver sarcoma, accounting for up to 2% of all primary liver tumors [15–17]. Peak age incidence is in the sixth and seventh decades of life with a male-to-female ratio of 3/1. It has been rarely reported in children and, if so, is regarded as a distinct entity. Much attention has been given to this disease during the last decade because of the frequent association with several environmental carcinogens such as thorotrast, vinyl chloride monomer, radium, pesticides, cyclophosphamide, arsenical compounds, use of androgenic/anabolic steroids, iron overload such as seen in hemochromatosis, and external radiation. However, an etiological cause is not found in 70% of HAS [15].

The diagnosis, especially that of diffuse HAS, can be very difficult even if liver biopsy is available. Macroscopically, HAS appears as ill-defined spongy hemorrhagic nodules involving the whole liver. Four patterns of tumor growth are described: multiple nodular, large dominant mass, mixed patterns of multiple nodules and dominant mass, and, more rarely, diffusely infiltrating macronodular tumor. Extra-hepatic metastases seen in 20–40% of patients at the time of diagnosis are mostly located in lung, spleen, bone, and adrenals. Despite the introduction of nuclear magnetic resonance (NMR), the diagnosis of HAS is still difficult.

The most characteristic histological pattern is sinusoidal growth of malignant endothelial spindle cells on the surface of liver cell plates, leading to their atrophy and to formation of larger vascular channels and cavernous spaces with papillary projections into their lumen. Tumor cells have bizarre and hyperchromatic nuclei with numerous mitoses and they exhibit immunohistochemical positivity for endothelial markers F VIII, CD31, and CD 34. HAS differs from HEHE by its content of more atypical cells and its destruction of the liver architecture. Histological diagnosis on adequate tissue sampling is of utmost importance in order to avoid futile surgery. The difficulty of making a correct diagnosis is exemplified in the ELITA-ELTR study comprising 16 adults and 6 children [18]. A correct pre-LT histological diagnosis of HAS was made in only one third of 16 biopsied patients, so half of the patients were erroneously transplanted because of "HIHE or HEHE." At the time of LT, 15% of patients had metastatic disease. All four cases of HAS presenting as acute BCS were seen in children with a presumed diagnosis of HIHE. Biochemical expression of HAS is also nonspecific; with increased alkaline phosphatase in 70% of patients and negative tumor markers. In the early stages, HAS may present with hepatosplenomegaly, ascites, jaundice, signs of portal hypertension, weight loss, and muscle wasting; later on, pain, peripheral edema, acute BCS, acute abdomen due to tumor rupture, and thrombocytopenia may follow. In contrast to HEHE and HIHE, the course of these patients is much more rapid.

All patients died due to tumor recurrence after a median follow-up of only 6 months. Similar catastrophic results were recently reported by the Cincinnati Transplant Tumor and the Memorial Sloan Kettering group [16, 17]. Both European and American experiences confirm that HAS is an absolute contraindication to LT. In case of difficult differential diagnosis between HIHE or HEHE and HAS, a waiting period of 6 months (corresponding to the mean survival of HAS) on the waiting list should be advocated in order to document the course of the tumor, thereby avoiding the misuse of a scarce organ resource. The outcome of patients with HAS will only be improved by the development of a more effective interdisciplinary oncologic approach [1, 18].

Nodular Regenerative Hyperplasia (NRH)

The NRH of the liver is a rare condition, which most often presents with portal hypertension. Its prevalence is estimated to be between 0.7 and 2.6 % in autopsy series [19]. NRH is the major cause of noncirrhotic portal hypertension and is thought to be secondary to primary vasculopathy with alterations in blood flow. Portal venopathy, e.g., occlusion of terminal portal venules with or without accompanying hepatic arterial disorders, causes ischemia leading to atrophy with compensatory hyperplasia in adjacent unaffected areas. When a critical fraction of portal venules is affected, portal hypertension ensues. NRH is characterized by the formation of usually small, up to 1 cm, *nonfibrotic* parenchymal nodules. The absence of fibrosis distinguishes it from micronodular cirrhosis. Microscopically, these regenerative nodules are composed of large hyperplastic hepatocytes. They compress adjacent liver cell plates that become atrophic, a feature nicely underlined by reticulin stain. Hemodynamic investigation shows presinusoidal portal hypertension in association with a patent portal vein. Various systemic diseases are known to occur in association with NRH, such as primary biliary cirrhosis, BCS, HHT, lympho- and myeloproliferative disorders, collagen vascular diseases, congenital and acquired hepatic macrovascular abnormalities, as well as exposure to toxins such as azathioprine and some chemotherapeutic agents. Familial cases of NRH occurring without underlying or associated systemic disease have been described. These forms have a poor course and are often associated with progressive renal failure [20].

After LT, NRH has been reported to recur in the allograft, to develop de novo in the context of long-term azathioprine use and in living donor LT using small-for-size grafts. NRH and obliterative portal venopathy have also been documented in recipients transplanted for biliary tract disease complicated with severe noncirrhotic portal hypertension [21–23].

Four relatively large series and some case reports about successful LT for NRH have been reported [24]. Six patients with NRH were reported to the ELITA-ELTR. One patient had a previous kidney transplantation. Four patients had a favorable outcome and two died 20 and 42 months posttransplantation due to cardiac failure [18].

Hereditary Hemorrhagic Telangiectasia (HHT)

The HHT or Rendu–Osler–Weber disease is a rare, autosomal dominant disease which affects mainly skin and mucosa but can also be present in brain, lungs, and digestive tract (Chap. 14). Using modern imaging techniques, liver involvement has been shown to be present in up to 73% of patients (Fig. 17.2a). Fortunately, less than 15% of HHT patients are symptomatic [25–28]. According to shunt type and size, Garcia-Tsao et al. have classified patients into three groups presenting with either cardiac failure, biliary disease, or portal hypertension [29]. The clinical manifestations of hepatic involvement may overlap and fluctuate over time, sometimes even showing partial spontaneous remissions. Type 1 (arteriovenous) shunt can cause a cardiac and/or biliary-type clinical pattern. Cholestasis is the most frequent biochemical marker, indicating bile duct ischemia due to arterial stealing. Cardiac output is nearly always increased in HHT patients. Type 2 (arterioportal) shunts may cause portal hypertension, whereas the clinical impact of type 3 (portovenous) shunts has not been well defined.

The therapeutic algorithm of hepatic-based HHT, which should take into consideration the Garcia-Tsao classification, has again been refined recently [29, 30]. Indeed conservative management has been used mainly for first-line treatment followed by interventions to the hepatic arterial bed. Arterial ligation, banding, and embolization are not recommended given the high risk of biliary necrosis and sepsis, carrying a 20% mortality risk [30–32]. Moreover, these procedures may damage the liver vasculature leading to the development of new shunts. Arterial interventions are particularly hazardous when both hepatic artery–hepatic vein and portal vein–hepatic vein shunts are present because the intervention will cause interruption of any blood supply to the liver with resultant hepatic and biliary necrosis [33]. In very well-selected patients, arterial embolization can have a lasting clinical effect, even up to 50 months, due to the significant decrease of cardiac output immediately after the procedure [31].

The final therapeutic goal of hepatic involvement by HHT should be to eliminate hepatic arterio-venous malformations (AVM) and therefore it is logical to consider LT in the cure of this disorder [30, 32]. The first patient with HHT and LT, performed by the Hannover group in 1985, is still alive and in good condition. Unfortunately the two subsequent patients, transplanted in 1987 and 1989, died after LT due to intraoperative bleeding and primary graft nonfunction, underscoring the technical difficulties of transplant surgery in these patients. This negative experience was responsible for a guarded attitude of the transplant community in relation to this disease. The first case of LT for HHT reported in the English literature was published 10 years later. The reported world experience actually comprises 44 cases, four of whom were transplanted in the United States and the remaining 40 cases reported in the ELITA-ELTR study [30]. This was the first large study that focused on the role of LT in this setting, based on a detailed analysis of all transplanted patients. The results confirm that LT indeed represents a valuable, and most of all definitive, therapy in case of hepatic HHT leading to major cardiac failure and/or liver failure and/or massive biliary necrosis and/or development of major portal hypertension (Fig. 17.2b). Excellent 1-, 5-, and 10-year survival rates of 82.5% were observed. These results were obtained despite enhanced surgical difficulties reflected by greater transfusion requirements, longer

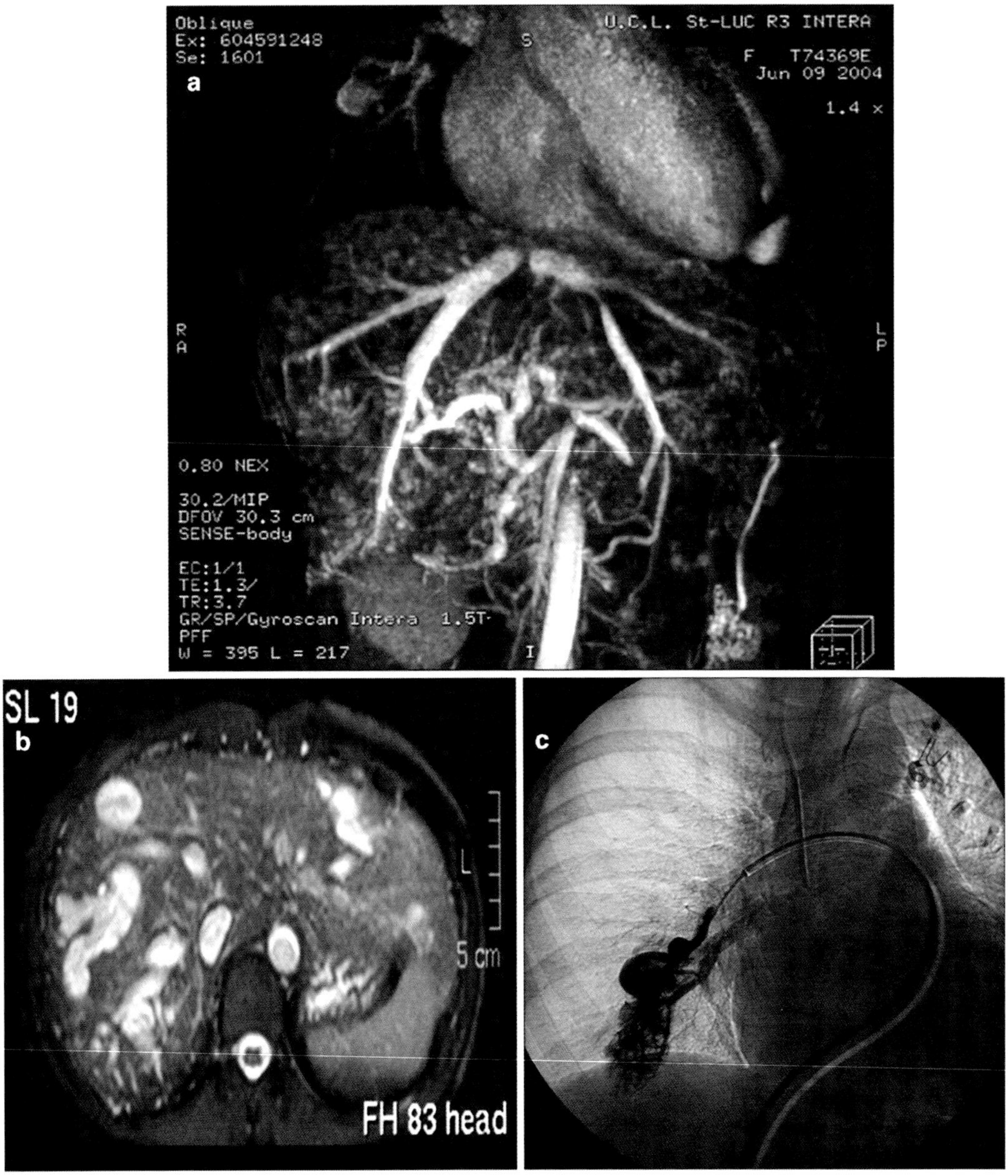

Fig. 17.2 (**a**) Angio-NMR of HHT patient showing simultaneous filling of intrahepatic arteries and veins. (**b**) Cholangio-NMR shows diffuse necrotic cavities due to extensive bile duct necrosis (**c**) Pulmonary AVM treated before transplantation using interventional radiology

operating time, prolonged hospital stay, and high postoperative morbidity and mortality related to heart failure and bleeding (Fig. 17.3a and b).

The timing of LT is essential especially in the setting of biliary infection with sepsis, major cardiac failure, and secondary pulmonary arterial hypertension. Ascites, the most common clinical expression of sinusoidal hypertension and/or heart failure, cholestasis, the major index of disease severity, and/or biliary sepsis should all lead to evaluating the necessity for LT. The necessity for timely LT is very well exemplified by a report from Yale showing that 17 of 51 HHT patients presenting with hepatic involvement died after a

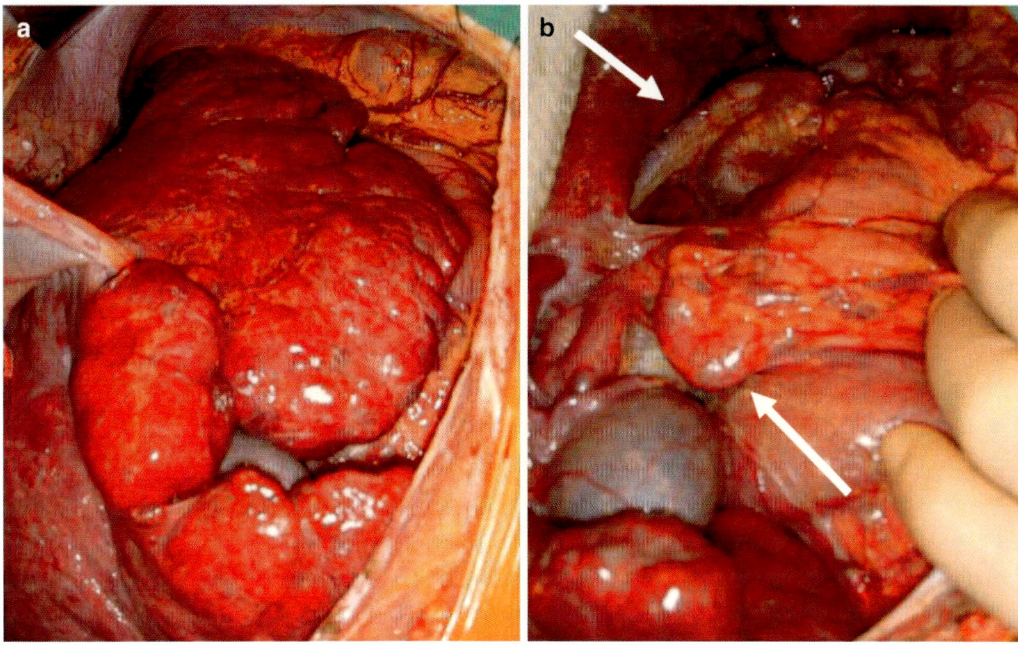

Fig. 17.3 (**a**) Intraoperative view of hepatic hereditary hemorrhagic telangiectasia showing a spongy enlarged liver. (**b**) Cystic, left and right hepatic arteries with a diameter of more than 1 cm

mean follow-up of 4.8 years; 14 (28%) of them died as a direct consequence of cardiopulmonary or biliary disease [34]. It can be easily understood that early LT permits complete recovery from these potentially lethal conditions by removing the source of ongoing (biliary) sepsis and cardiopulmonary failure. The Berlin, Paris, Cambridge, Lyon, and Besançon groups all provided evidence that right heart function, pulmonary pressure, cardiac output, and clinical symptoms normalize if LT can be done before fixed hypertension occurs [30, 31, 35, 36]. Treatment of major pulmonary and other splanchnic AVMs, using interventional radiology, should always be considered before LT, as these conditions can lead to severe or even lethal post-LT bleeding [30, 37] (Fig. 17.2c). The value of LT in symptomatic HHT is also exemplified by the dramatic improvement of Karnofsky scores, a very reliable and easy parameter to judge performance status of the transplant recipient [30]. The possible rare allograft recurrence recently described by Sabba in two female first-degree relatives remains intriguing [38]. These cases indicate that long-term follow-up and genetic HHT screening are both mandatory. Similar findings in other transplanted organs in HHT patients could provide more insight regarding the problem of disease recurrence. Unfortunately, such data are not available at present as only two cases of lung transplantation without follow-up have been reported [30, 39, 40]. A systematic registry of all hepatic HHT, including genetic counseling, will be the only way to further improve the outcome of symptomatic HHT patients allowing to further improve the therapeutic algorithm and better define the timing for LT [30, 40].

Budd-Chiari Syndrome (BCS)

Despite the fact that this syndrome was first described in 1845 by the British internist George Budd and that the histopathological features of the entity were documented by the Czech pathologist Hans Chiari exactly 100 years ago, the therapeutic algorithm of BCS has not yet been clearly established, again mainly due to the rarity and the protean clinical manifestations of this syndrome [41].

As discussed in Chap. 13, BCS is due to the obstruction of the hepatic venous outflow at any level from the small hepatic veins (HV) to the atriocaval junction. The main cause is thrombosis secondary to primary myeloproliferative diseases. Diagnosis of BCS is made by the combination of imaging studies (Doppler ultrasound, NMR, transjugular venography), liver biopsy, genetic and bone marrow examination. HVT has a protean clinical manifestation ranging from asymptomatic (incidental HVT) to acute [presenting the Budd-triad of abdominal pain, hepatomegaly, and ascites together with cytolysis (>5× elevation of AST/ALT), impaired coagulation and renal function] or chronic (presenting as a decompensated liver disease) liver failure. The treatment of BCS is based on supportive care (therapy for ascites and varices), treatment with anticoagulation and control of underlying thrombophilic disease and restoration of hepatic vein outflow (Chap. 13). This involves a stepwise, multidisciplinary approach over several weeks. Thrombolysis, surgical portosystemic shunting, and radiological angioplasty (except for partial or segmental stenosis) are nowadays abandoned in favor of the transjugular intrahepatic portosystemic shunt (TIPSS) [43–45]. Successful TIPSS, even when performed in high-risk patients, is associated with 1- and 5-year transplant free survival rates of 88 and 78%, respectively. If such treatment is unsuccessful or if BCS-TIPSS prognostic score is >7 [43, 44], LT should be considered [41, 44]. The ELITA-ELTR study includes 248 patients transplanted during the period 1988–1999 and showed 1- and 10-year actuarial survival rates of 76 and 68%. Pre-LT predictors of mortality in this study were impaired renal function (reflected nowadays as a high MELD score) and previous history of surgical shunt. Recurrent venous thrombosis and complications due to anticoagulation therapy were each seen in 11% of recipients [46]. These results remained almost identical in the 2008 ELTR update comprising 663 patients. The UNOS registry analysis, comprising 510 recipients, reports 3-year survival rates of 83% in the MELD era [47]. The Berlin group recently reported 5- and 10-year survival rates of 89 and 83%, respectively [48].

When considering LT, three particular problems deserve special attention from the transplant team: the technical aspect of the procedure, the higher incidence of vascular complications, and the modalities of antithrombotic treatment necessary to prevent recurrent disease [42, 49]. The transplant procedure is without any doubt more difficult due to liver congestion, the extensive (parietal and retroperitoneal) collateral venous network, and the often coexisting IVC and/or splanchnic venous thromboses (Fig. 17.4a and b). Early devascularization of the liver will facilitate total hepatectomy. In case of coexisting simple PVT, eversion thombectomy can easily solve the problem but in case of extensive splanchnic venous thrombosis, cavo-portal hemi-transposition may be the only way to revascularize the allograft [50, 51] (Fig. 17.5a and b). This technique directs blood flow from the IVC of the recipient to the portal vein of the allograft, either by performing an end-to-side or an end-to-end anastomosis. If coexisting thrombosis of the IVC exists, it is necessary to reconstruct or replace this vessel. In LDLT, partial or complete IVC reconstruction using free venous grafts is necessary [52]. Sometimes, extensive IVC involvement needs an anastomosis of the donor IVC with the right atrium.

As the posttransplant course may be complicated by recurrent thromboses and/or recurrent BCS, anticoagulation is necessary. During the first 4–7 days, IV heparin or low molecular weight heparin is administered followed by a switch to oral warfarin or fluindione. Long-term anticoagulation not only causes bleeding complications in about 10% of recipients, but also makes the follow-up more complicated especially if additional liver biopsy or surgical interventions are necessary. The Dallas group therefore proposed anticoagulation adapted to the thrombophilic status of the recipient [42, 49]. Patients with a hypercoagulable state such as protein C and S deficiencies completely corrected by LT do not need anticoagulation; recipients with "idiopathic" BCS need classical anticoagulation and/or therapy necessary to control their hypercoagulable state and finally patients with myeloproliferative diseases require antiplatelet therapy consisting of hydroxyurea (500–1,500 mg/day) and antiplatelet therapy (aspirin 325 mg/day) as a safe alternative to anticoagulation. Anagrelide may be preferred in case of thrombocytosis.

Splanchnic Venous Thrombosis and Portosystemic Shunt

Abnormalities of the portal vein and/or its tributaries were initially considered a contraindication to LT [50, 53]. As the incidence of PVT reaches 15–20% in patients with chronic liver disease and ranges from 6 to 21% in surgically treated cirrhotics, several technical modifications had to be developed in order to allow allograft implantation with reasonable morbidity and no mortality [54–56]. The prerequisites for successful LT in such cases are precise preoperative evaluation of the splanchnic vein and/or portosystemic shunt anatomy as well as extent of thrombosis [50, 53, 55]. The most used screening technique to investigate PVT is Doppler ultrasound. In case of previous surgery for portal hypertension and when there are pronounced portosystemic collaterals, selective angiography with or without NMR or CT angiography are required. The latter studies have the advantage that anatomic interrelationships are easier to evaluate, that less contrast medium is required, that PV can be visualized in the presence of reversed flow, and that phlebitis or perivascular inflammatory changes may be accurately recognized. The diagnosis of perivenous inflammation remains difficult and usually relies on indirect signs such as fatty perivascular infiltration. Angiography and angio-NMR should be done in order to get the maximal information about the modified vessel status and the extension of the thrombosis [57].

Appropriate choice and planning of pre-LT hepatobiliary or portal hypertension surgery is another means to avoid difficult intraoperative situations. If portal decompression is needed, mesocaval H-graft and distal splenorenal shunts are preferred as there is no liver hilum dissection. Pretransplant portocaval shunt is nowadays mostly replaced by TIPSS [58]. It should be noted that TIPSS may lead to technical difficulties related to stent dislocation into the suprahepatic vena cava,

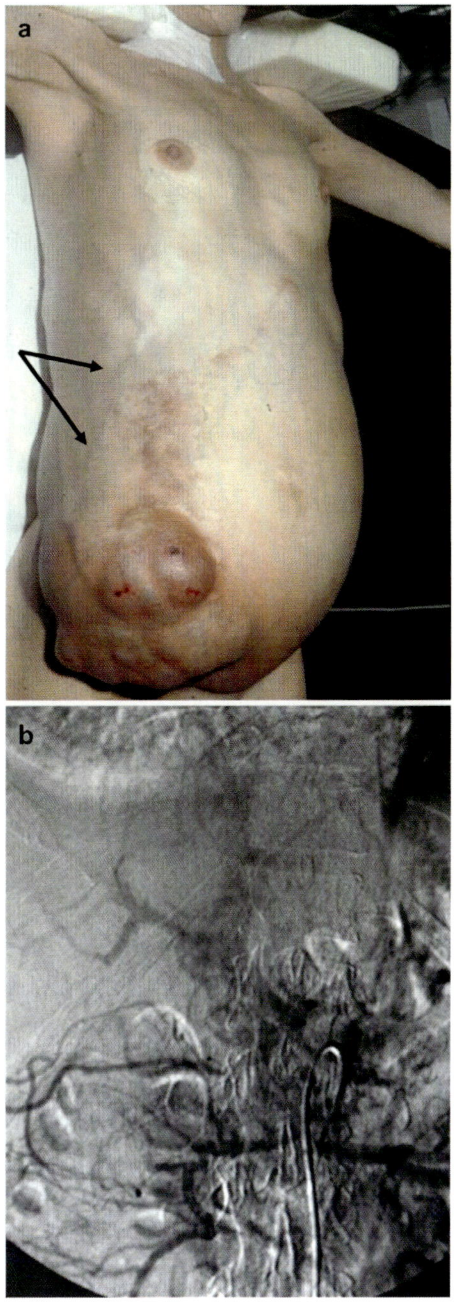

Fig. 17.4 (**a**) Budd-Chiari patient showing pronounced abdominal wall venous collaterals. (**b**) Splanchnic venography shows extensive splanchnic venous thrombosis

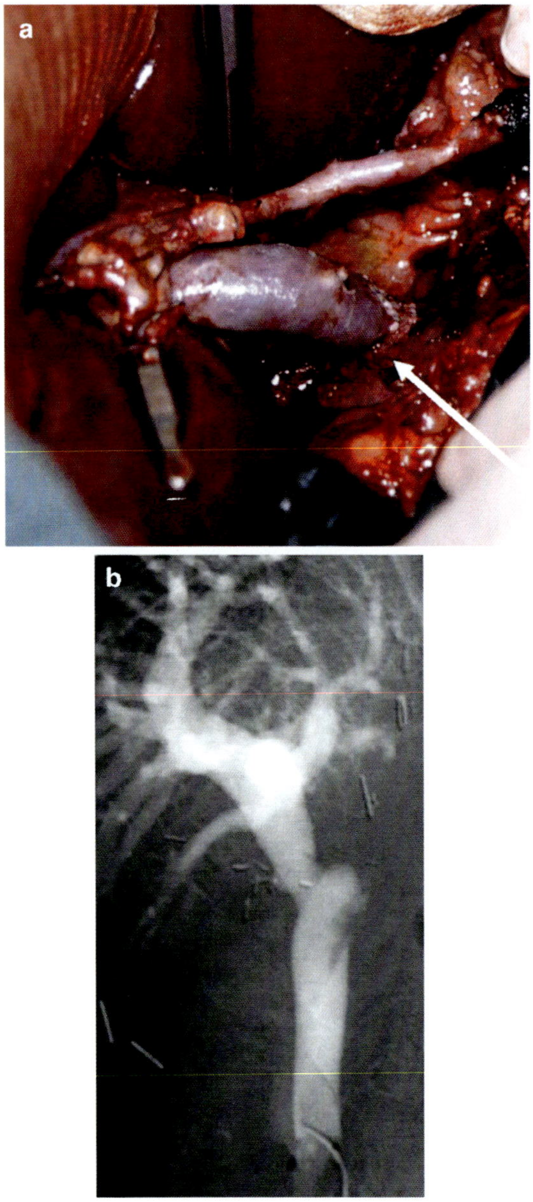

Fig. 17.5 (**a**) Intraoperative view of cavo-portal transposition showing the direct anastomosis between the portal vein and the infrahepatic IVC. (**b**) Posttransplant cavography confirms the adequate perfusion of the allograft

pericaval or portal inflammatory changes, and development of portal vein aneurysm (Fig. 17.6).

As splanchnic vein abnormalities are still responsible for enhanced morbidity and mortality due to possibly compromised allograft venous inflow, donor and recipient operations must be well scheduled in order to keep cold and warm ischemia times to a minimum and in order to plan the method of PV reconstruction *before* starting the implantation of the graft. In case of PV thrombosis, the surgical technique used *depends on the extent of thrombus and the quality of the vessel wall.* If the thrombosis is limited to the portal trunk or is present in a vessel which still has an adequate wall, a *hilar approach*, including dissection down to the splenomesenteric confluence in order to facilitate inflowing thrombectomy, is preferred. If the thrombus extends far into the superior mesenteric vein (SMV), if the PV is reduced to a fibrotic vessel remnant, or if inflammatory PV

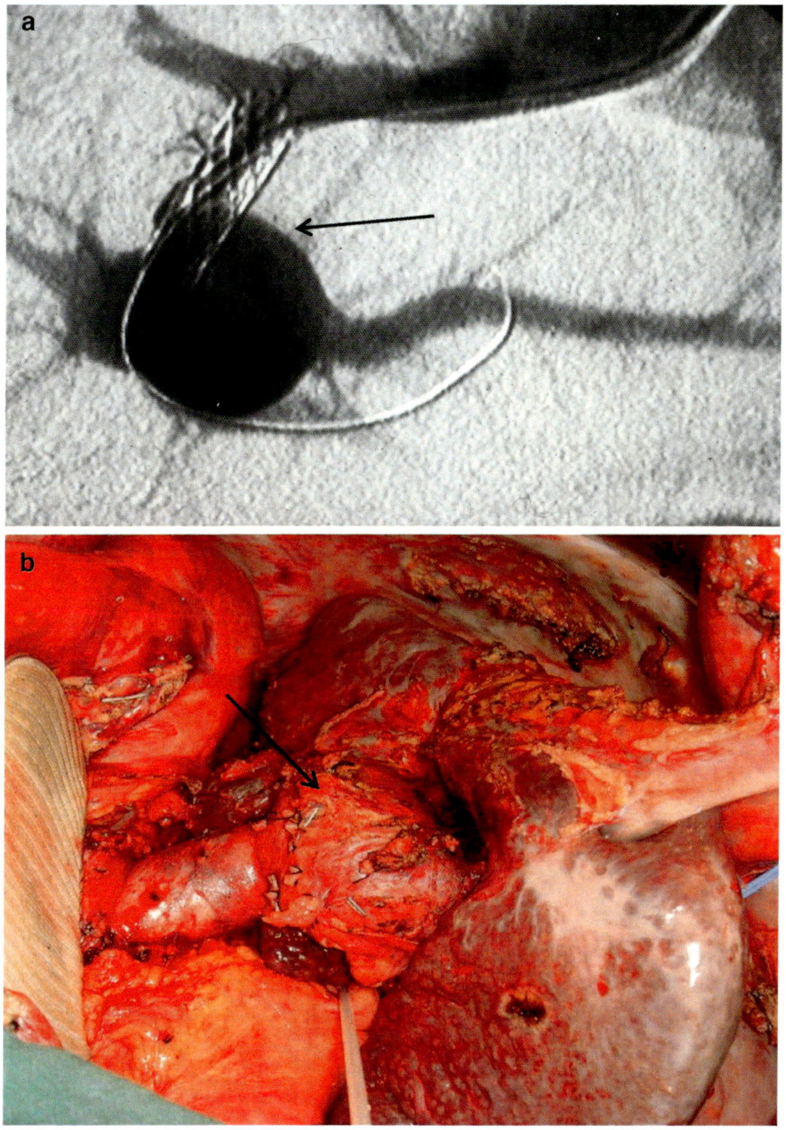

Fig. 17.6 Venography (**a**) and intraoperative view (**b**) of a portal vein aneurysm caused by the transjugular intrahepatic portosystemic shunt (TIPSS)

changes are present, an *infracolic approach* is performed [50, 53, 55, 57, 59]. Using the *hilar approach,* the PV is transected flush with the liver parenchyma once the liver is ready to be removed. Interruption of the collateral venous circulation such as very pronounced left gastric varices is rarely necessary to optimize portal perfusion. Eversion thrombectomy must be done under *complete visual control*. Using a carotid endarterectomy dissector, it is relatively easy to find the cleavage plane between thrombus and intima (Fig. 17.7). The thrombus is progressively freed by everting the venous wall, while the left index finger of the surgeon occludes the splenomesenteric confluence from behind. In contrast to blind thrombectomy, in which thrombotic material is grasped and pulled out, this maneuver allows complete thrombectomy under direct vision without major blood loss, with minimal risk of tearing out the vessel wall and with inspection of the intima of the thrombectomized vein. When severe inflammatory (peri)vascular changes are present, especially extending to the SMV and splenic veins, thrombectomy is too dangerous due to the

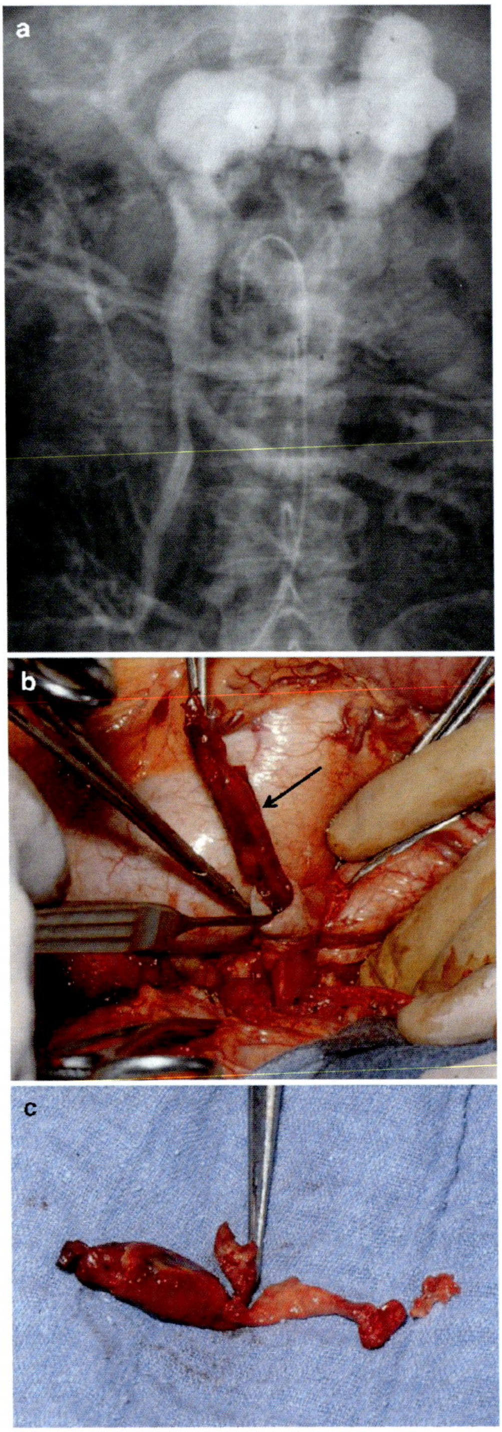

Fig. 17.7 (**a**) Venography showing a recanalized portal vein thrombosis. (**b**) Intraoperative view of hilar approach with porto-spleno-mesenteric eversion thrombectomy. (**c**) Porto-spleno-mesenteric fibrotic thrombus

high risk of venous wall tearing. In such cases, the SMV is prepared by an *infracolic* approach, to allow interposition of a free iliac vein homograft between donor PV and recipient SMV (Fig. 17.8). This graft is placed in a prepancreatic and retrogastric position. Extra PV length can be obtained during organ procurement by "en bloc" removal of the liver and pancreas, allowing retention of the portomesenteric venous axis [50, 53].

In some exceptional cases, anastomosis between donor PV and recipient splanchnic system is impossible. Intraoperative venography through the ileocolic or inferior mesenteric vein can help assess the venous anatomy. In such cases, successful restoration of portal allograft perfusion has been accomplished by anastomosing the donor PV to the left gastric vein, hepatoduodenal, bile duct, gastroepiploic, and ileocolonic varices and even by (partial) arterialization of the portal vein. If this is unfeasible, cavoportal transposition can be a "graft saving" procedure [51, 60]. One should be aware that this technique is usually unable to completely decompress the modified splanchnic venous system and frequently leads to post-LT gastro-intestinal bleeding. This complication can be managed by splenectomy or gastric devascularization. If diffuse thrombosis of the splanchnic veins is diagnosed, combined liver-intestinal transplantation may be the only therapeutic option [61].

If there are surgical portocaval shunts present, the surgical strategy also needs to be adapted [53, 62]. The shunt should be left intact until the end of the hepatectomy, as end-to-side portocaval and splenorenal shunts serve as an "internal" veno-venous bypass throughout the procedure. A distal splenorenal shunt only needs to be interrupted when intraoperative electromagnetic flow measurement reveals absent or low flow portal venous allograft perfusion.

Independent of the method used, portal allograft perfusion should be assessed by electromagnetic measurements. If inadequate, venous collaterals or surgical distal splenorenal shunt should be closed either surgically or by using intra- or peri-operative interventional radiology.

The safety of the transplant procedure in the presence of splanchnic vein anomalies can be further improved by performing a caval sparing

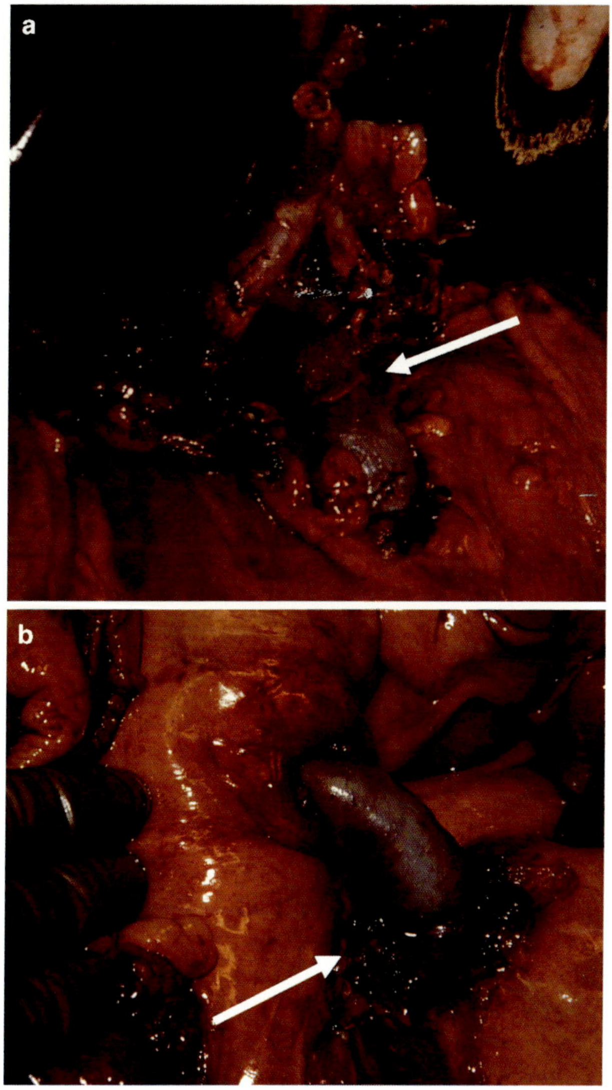

Fig. 17.8 Intraoperative views of free iliac vessel graft interposition between donor portal vein (**a**) and superior mesenteric (**b**) veins

transplant procedure. This technique involves dissection of the recipient liver from its own IVC without interrupting portal PV or dividing any portosystemic surgical shunt. The potentially most dangerous part of the recipient procedure, taking care of the thrombosed vessels or interruption of portosystemic shunt, can then be done immediately before completion of hepatectomy; a stage at which control of bleeding is usually easier to perform [63].

Venous Complications and LT

HV and IVC Thrombosis or Stenosis After Liver Transplantation

HV and IVC stenosis and thrombosis after LT are rare complications occurring in less than 1% of transplant procedures [53, 64]. Most of these problems can be successfully treated

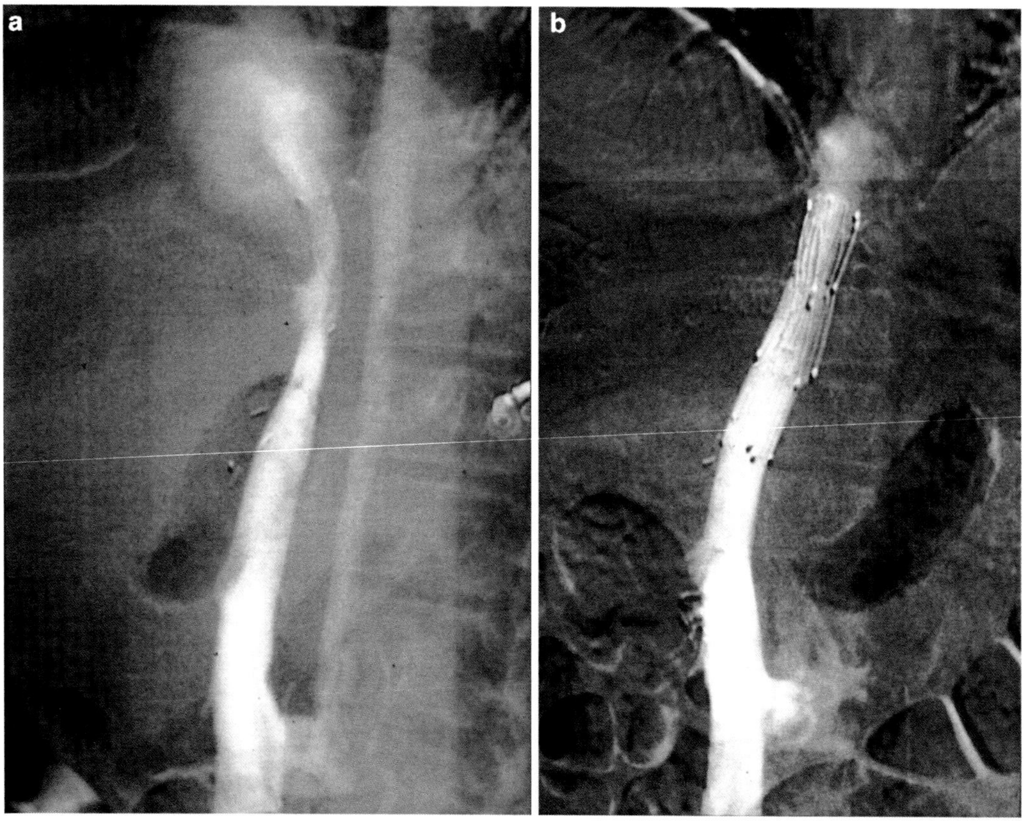

Fig. 17.9 Posttransplant retrohepatic IVC stenosis (**a**) responsible for refractory posttransplant ascites, resolved via stenting (**b**)

using interventional radiology (Fig. 17.9). Repermeabilization and angioplasty of the HV may need a combined transjugular and transhepatic venous approach [65, 66].

PV Thrombosis and Stenosis After Liver Transplantation

Early portal vein thrombosis after LT occurs in 1% of cases [50, 55]. This complication can be treated safely and successfully combining TIPSS and local thrombolysis [67, 68] (Fig. 17.10). This approach has several advantages such as performance under local anesthesia, avoidance of the more dangerous transcutaneous transhepatic approach, reduction of bleeding risk, creation of an adequate portal vein outflow, and finally repeated and easy accessibility to the PV for therapeutic as well as diagnostic purposes [69]. PV stenosis can easily be treated using balloon dilation and/or stenting [64, 65, 70] (Fig. 17.11).

TIPSS Before and After Liver Transplantation

Potential LT recipients presenting with refractory ascites and/or hepatic hydrothorax and/or gastrointestinal bleeding may have had TIPSS performed prior to transplantation. The indication for TIPSS must take into account the state of liver disease (Chap. 15). Patients having bilirubin levels of over 3 mg/dl are at risk of developing post-TIPSS liver failure [71].

The TIPSS may also be of interest in the treatment of recurrent allograft disease, redo-biliary

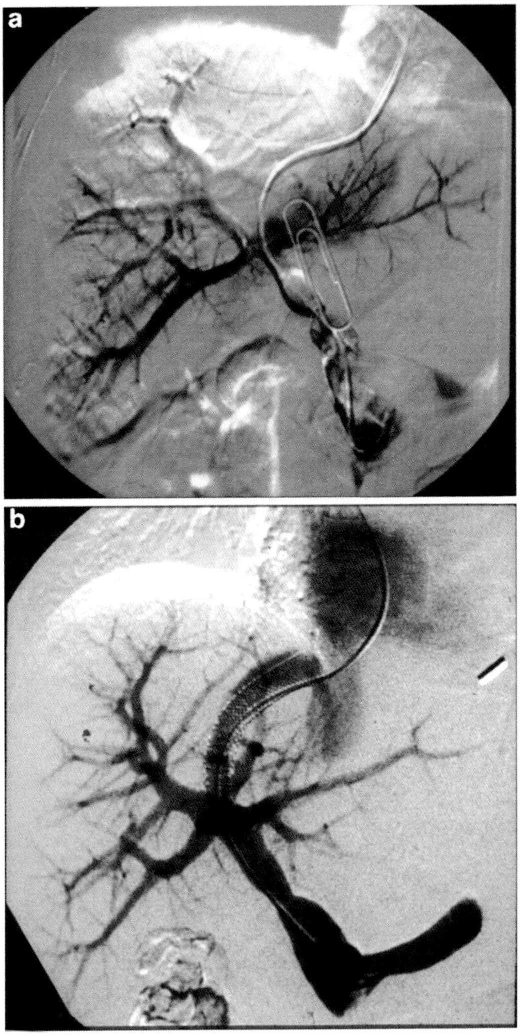

Fig. 17.10 Early recanalization of thrombosed PV using combination of TIPSS approach (**a**), thrombolysis and stenting (**b**). From Ciccarelli et al. [69]. Reprinted with kind permission from Wolters Kluwer Health

surgery, or re-LT in the presence of severe portal hypertension and also in case of veno-occlusive allograft disease refractory to medical treatment [72]. This procedure may be more difficult in the case of modified implantation techniques and when major atrophy/hypertrophy of the graft develops. An experienced interventional radiologist should be available to overcome all possible parenchymal and vascular modifications of the remodeled graft. It may be necessary to use a combined femoral and transjugular approach in order to position the TIPSS shunt correctly. The transplant surgeon should keep in mind possible posttransplant radiological interventions. When applying the cavo-caval anastomosis technique, the posterior cavotomy of the donor vena cava must therefore encompass the orifices of all HV in order to allow a later TIPSS procedure.

The TIPSS procedures in transplant recipients seem to have a higher incidence of encephalopathy, which may be explained by the combination of advanced stage of the liver disease and the use of neurotoxic drugs such as cyclosporine and tacrolimus. The portosystemic gradient should be reduced in such a way as to preserve hepatoportal perfusion. Immunosuppressive therapy needs to be monitored closely following TIPSS as cyclosporin and tacrolamus metabolism may be modified as a consequence of the elimination or reduction of their first-pass effect [72]. This condition may lead to neuro- and nephrotoxicity due to higher calcineurin inhibitor levels despite identical dosing.

Arterial Complications After Liver Transplantation

Hepatic artery thrombosis (HAT) is the most feared complications after LT because this complication usually needs to be treated by retransplantation. Its incidence varies from almost 0 to 15% in literature [53, 64, 73]. This complication has three different expressions: hepatic necrosis (Fig. 17.12), bile duct necrosis (Fig. 17.13), and infections. Different risk factors for HAT have been identified over the last years, such as inadequate technique, celiac trunk stenosis, arcuate ligament compression, aberrant donor or recipient anatomy, hepato-aortic conduits, periarterial arteritis due to locoregional chemotherapy, low recipient weight, difficult back-table reconstruction, hyperacute rejection, poor hepatic outflow due to severe ischemia–reperfusion injury, hypercoagulable state, and even high hematocrit levels. The fact that different Asian groups have reported an almost zero HAT rate in living donor LT suggests that this is a surgical complication [74]. Microscopic-assisted vascular technique, intraoperative flow measurement, and Doppler ultrasound are the best guarantee

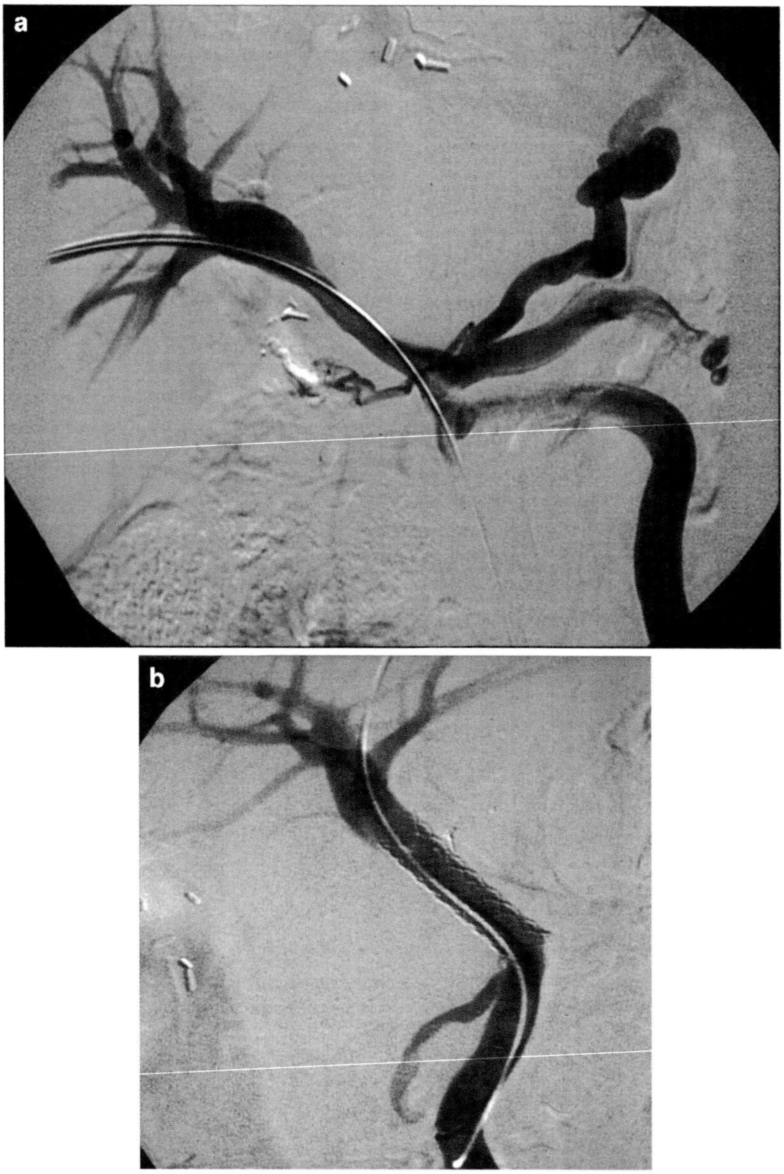

Fig. 17.11 Percutaneous portography (**a**) and stenting of a late posttransplant portal vein stenosis (**b**)

against early HAT. In contrast to HA stenosis, radiological intervention plays a minor role in HAT. Some rare grafts can be rescued by early surgical thrombectomy and thrombolysis.

Hepatic arterial steal syndrome can be observed in patients with severe portal hypertension; in such cases intraoperative ligation or early postoperative embolization of the proximal portion of the splenic artery can re-equilibrate the arterial splanchnic and hepatic flow.

Transmitted Hemostatic Disorders After LT

It has been well documented that LT cures several inherited hemostatic diseases, such as hemophilia, protein C and protein S deficiency [53, 75, 76]. Conversely, transmission by the allograft of factor VII, VIII, and XI, protein C and S deficiency, of dysfibrinogenemia, idiopathic thrombocytopenic

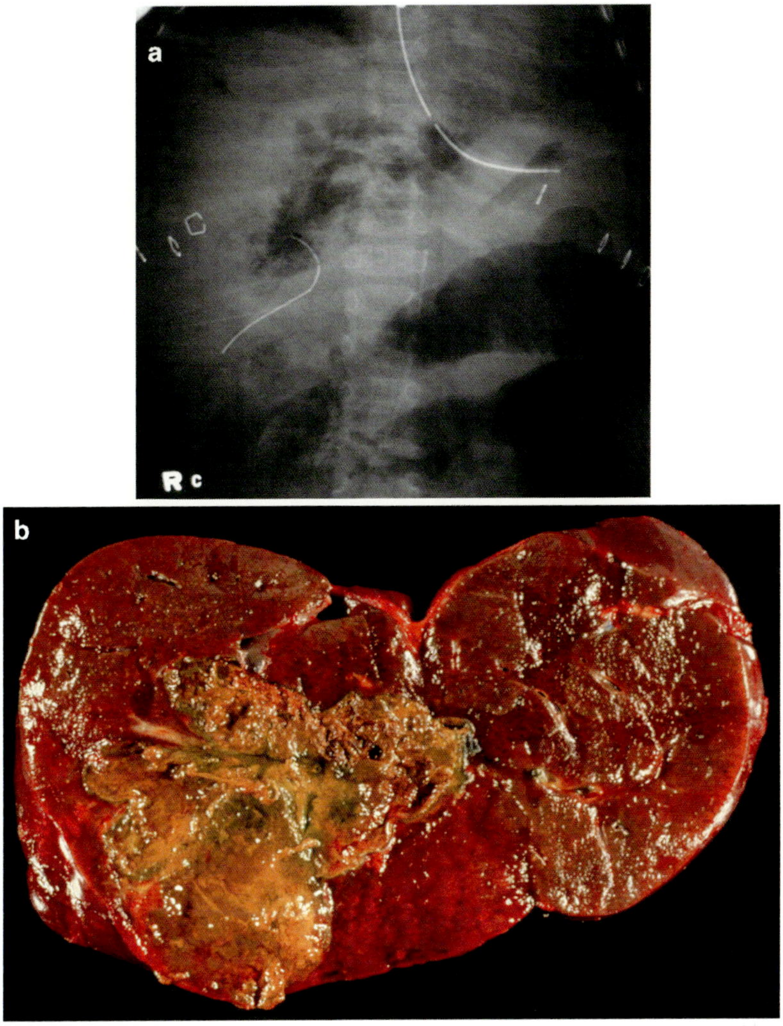

Fig. 17.12 Hepatic artery thrombosis causing massive allograft infarction visualized on plain abdominal X-ray (**a**) and macroscopic view of the liver (**b**)

disease, and von Willebrand disease (possibly) all have been reported [53, 76–81]. One should think about these acquired anomalies when confronted during the posttransplant period with unexplained hemostatic or thrombophilic disorders. Transmission of hemophilia needs to be treated by re-LT [81]. All these potential disease transmissions indicate the need to perform a complete hemostatic pretransplant workup in all potential liver recipients.

Conclusions

The transplant surgeon and internist can be faced with several vascular conditions before and after the transplant procedure. Except for frequent splanchnic venous thromboses, all vascular liver diseases are often difficult to diagnose and to treat due to their rarity and their protean clinical manifestation. More recent information, obtained trough a detailed analysis from larger, especially European, registry

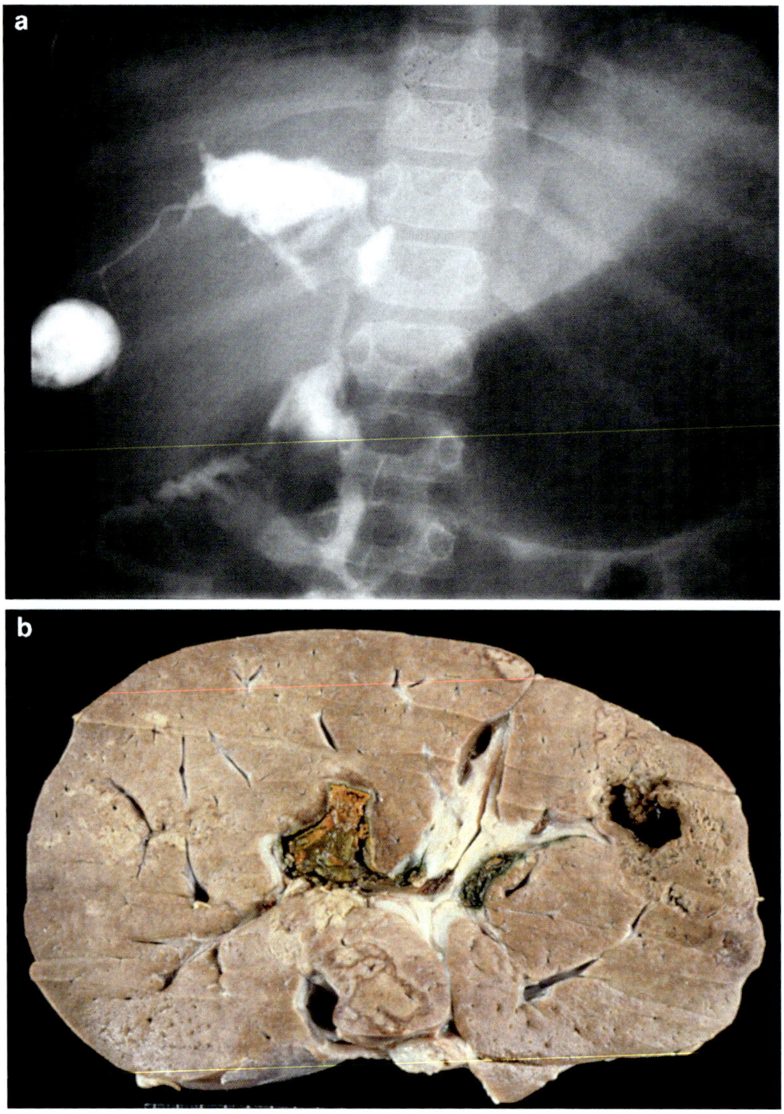

Fig. 17.13 Hepatic artery thrombosis causing bile duct necrosis (**a**); macroscopic view of the liver shows an infarcted zone impregnated with bile (**b**)

studies, has allowed to clarify therapeutic algorithms for these diseases. Of utmost importance is the fact that this knowledge has opened the door for these, often desperately ill, patients to a life-saving transplant procedure. One should have a high degree of suspicion in relationship to vascular liver diseases because they can have an extremely divergent clinical course. Aggressive diagnostic workup, adequate tissue sampling, and genetic analyses are mandatory in order to differentiate the potentially curable HEHE or HIHE from the incurable HAS. HEHE should be treated aggressively by total hepatectomy even in the presence of (limited) extrahepatic disease at the time of transplantation. The combination of LT and antiangiogenic drugs could be a way to further improve the outcome. HIHE has a variable disease expression that can lead to spontaneous regression as well as to fatal outcome. Diffuse HIHE resistant to steroid therapy should be treated using LT. The appearance of acute liver failure and/or BCS in these infants may indicate development of HAS. The outlook for HAS remains extremely dismal regardless of the therapy. LT is absolutely contraindicated due to very rapid disease recurrence and poor prognosis. In cases of unclear diagnosis, futile LT can be avoided when listing the patient for a minimal period of 6 months, a time span usually sufficient to observe the natural and fatal evolution of HAS.

Severe, symptomatic, noncirrhotic portal hypertension caused by NRH can be cured by LT if the available non-LT therapeutic armamentarium fails to control its severe complications.

The BCS must be treated using a multidisciplinary, stepwise approach going from anticoagulation to TIPSS to LT. Prognostic scores allow to better define the role and timing of LT in this disease. Posttransplant anticoagulation needs to be adapted to the thrombophilic state of the recipient.

Portal and splanchnic venous thrombosis, present in up to 20% of cirrhotic patients, initially were considered to be contraindications for LT. Adapted surgical techniques nowadays allow to perform the transplant procedure with minimal morbidity and mortality. Hepatic and caval venous complications are rare posttransplant complications, which can mostly be solved using different interventional radiology procedures. TIPSS of the allograft can be of help in overcoming complications of portal hypertension due to recurrent allograft disease.

Several hemostatic diseases can be transmitted by the allograft, indicating that a complete hematological workup should be done in every liver transplant candidate.

References

1. Lerut JP, Orlando G, Adam R, et al. The place of liver transplantation in the treatment of hepatic epitheloid hemangioendothelioma: report of the European liver transplant registry. Ann Surg. 2007;246:949–57.
2. Ishak K, Goodman Z, Stocker J. Tumors of the liver and intrahepatic bile ducts. Atlas of tumor pathology. Third series, fascicle 31. ed. Armed Forces Institute of Pathology. Washington, USA, 1999:282–307.
3. Makhlouf HR, Ishak KG, Goodman ZD. Epithelioid hemangioendothelioma of the liver: a clinicopathologic study of 137 cases. Cancer. 1999;85:562–82.
4. Rodriguez JA, Becker NS, O'Mahony CA, Goss JA, Aloia TA. Long-term outcomes following liver transplantation for hepatic hemangioendothelioma: the UNOS experience from 1987 to 2005. J Gastrointest Surg. 2008;12:110–6.
5. Demetris AJ, Minervini M, Raikow RB, Lee RG. Hepatic epithelioid haemangioendothelioma – biological questions based on pattern of recurrence in an allograft and tumor immunophenotype. Am J Surg Path. 1997;21:263–70.
6. Kelleher MB, Iwatsuki S, Iwatsuki S, Sheahan DG. Epithelioid haemangioendothelioma of the liver. Clinicopathological correlation of 10 cases treated by orthotopic liver transplantation. Am J Surg pathol. 1988;89:999–1008.
7. Madariaga JR, Marino IR, Karavia DD, et al. Long-term results after liver transplantation for primary hepatic epithelioid haemangioendothelioma. Ann Surg Oncol. 1995;2:483–7.
8. Mehrabi A, Kashfi A, Fonouni H, et al. Primary malignant hepatic epithelioid hemangioendothelioma: a comprehensive review of the literature with emphasis on the surgical therapy. Cancer. 2006;107:2108–21.
9. Miller MA, Sandler AD. Elevated plasma vascular endothelial growth factor levels in two patients with hemangioendothelioma. J Pediatr Surg. 2005; 40:17–9.
10. Lopez-Terrada DL, Finegold MJ. Liver tumors. In: Walker AW, Durie PR, Hamilton JR, Walker-Smith JA, Watkins J, editors. Pediatric gastrointestinal disease: pathophysiology, diagnosis, management. 5th ed. St. Louis, MO: CV Mosby; 2008. p. 911–26.
11. Selby DM, Stocker JT, Waclawiw MA, Hitchcock L, Ishak KG. Infantile hemangioendothelioma of the liver. Hepatology. 1994;20:39–45.
12. Daller JA, Bueno J, Gutierrez J, Dvorchik I, Towbin RB, Dickman PS, et al. Hepatic hemangioendothelioma: clinical experience and management strategy. J Pediatr Surg. 1999;34:98–106.
13. Mo JQ, Dimashkieh HH, Bove KE. GLUT1 endothelial reactivity distinguishes hepatic infantile hemangioma from congenital hepatic vascular malformation with associated capillary proliferation. Hum Pathol. 2004;35:200–9.
14. Christison-Lagay ER, Burrows PE, Alomari A, et al. Hepatic hemangiomas: subtype classification and development of a clinical practice algorithm and registry. J Pediatr Surg. 2007;42:62–8.
15. Maluf D, Cotterell A, Clark B, Stravitz T, Kauffman HM, Fisher RA. Hepatic angiosarcoma and liver transplantation: case report and literature review. Transplant Proc. 2005;37:2195–9.
16. Husted TL, Neff G, Thomas MJ, Gross TG, Woodle ES, Buell JF. Liver transplantation for primary or metastatic sarcoma to the liver. Am J Transplant. 2006;6:392–7.
17. Weitz J, Klimstra DS, Cymes K, et al. Management of primary liver sarcomas. Cancer. 2007;109:1391–6.
18. Lerut J, Weber M, Orlando G, Dutkowski P. Vascular and rare liver tumors: a good indication for liver transplantation? J Hepatol. 2007;47:466–75.

19. Wanless IR. Micronodular transformation (nodular regenerative hyperplasia) of the liver. A report of 64 cases among 2500 autopsies and a new classification of benign hepatocellular nodules. Hepatology. 1990;11:787–97.
20. Dumortier J, Boillot O, Chevallier M, et al. Familial occurrence of nodular regenerative hyperplasia of the liver: a report on three families. Gut. 1999;45:289–94.
21. Breen DP, Marinaki AM, Arenas M, Hayes PC. Pharmacogenetic association with adverse drug reactions to azathioprine immunosuppressive therapy following liver transplantation. Liver Transpl. 2005;11:826–33.
22. Gane E, Portmann B, Saxena R, Wong P, Ramage J, Williams R. Nodular regenerative hyperplasia of the liver graft after liver transplantation. Hepatology. 1994;20:88–94.
23. Demetris AJ, Kelly DM, Eghtesad B, et al. Pathophysiologic observations and histopathologic recognition of the portal hyperperfusion or small-for-size syndrome. Am J Surg Pathol. 2006;30:986–93.
24. Krasinskas AM, Eghtesad B, Kamath PS, Demetris AJ, Abraham SC. Liver transplantation for severe intrahepatic noncirrhotic portal hypertension. Liver Transpl. 2005;11:627–34.
25. Shovlin CL, Guttmacher AE, Buscarini E, et al. Diagnostic criteria for hereditary haemorrhagic telangiectasia (Rendu-Osler-Weber syndrome). Am J Med Genet. 2000;91:66–7.
26. Saurin JC, Dumortier J, Menard Y, et al. Les malformations vasculaires hépatiques de la maladie de Rendu-Osler. Gastroenterol Clin Biol. 2000;24:89–93.
27. Buscarini E, Buscarini L, Danesino C, et al. Hepatic vascular malformations in hereditary haemorrhagic telangiectasia: Doppler sonographic screening in a large family. J Hepatol. 1997;26:111–8.
28. Ianora AA, Memeo M, Sabba C, Cirulli A, Rotondo A, Angelelli G. Hereditary haemorrhagic telangiectasia: multi-detector row helical CT assessment of hepatic involvement. Radiology. 2004;230:250–9.
29. Garcia-Tsao G, Korzenik JR, Young L, et al. Liver disease in patients with hereditary haemorrhagic telangiectasia. N Eng J Med. 2000;343:931–6.
30. Lerut J, Orlando G, Sabba C, et al. Liver transplantation for hereditary haemorrhagic telangiectasia: report of the European Liver Transplant Registry. Ann Surg. 2006;244:854–64.
31. Neumann UP, Knoop M, Langrehr JM, et al. Effective therapy for hepatic Morbus Osler with systemic hypercirculation by ligation of the hepatic artery and subsequent liver transplantation. Transpl Int. 1998;11:323–6.
32. Odorico JS, Hakim MN, Becker YT, et al. Liver transplantation as definitive therapy for complications after arterial embolization for hepatic manifestations of hereditary haemorrhagic telangiectasia. Liver Transpl Surg. 1998;4:483–90.
33. Sawabe M, Arai T, Esaki Y, Tsuru M, Fukazawa T, Takubo K. Three-dimensional organization of the hepatic microvasculature in hereditary haemorrhagic telangiectasia. Arch Pathol Lab Med. 2001;125:1219–23.
34. Young L, Garcia-Tsao G, Henderson KJ, et al. Long-term outcomes in patients with symptomatic liver hereditary haemorrhagic telangiectasia. HHT Abstract 40, VI HHT-ROW Scientific Conference, Lyon, France; 2005.
35. Boillot O, Bianco F, Viale JP, et al. Liver transplantation resolves the hyperdynamic circulation in hereditary haemorrhagic telangiectasia with hepatic involvement. Gastroenterology. 1999;116:187–92.
36. Le Corre F, Golkar B, Tessier C, Kavafyan J, Marty J. Liver transplantation for hepatic arteriovenous malformation with high-output cardiac failure in hereditary haemorrhagic telangiectasia: hemodynamic study. J Clin Anesth. 2000;12:339–42.
37. Kjeldsen AD, Oxhoj H, Andersen PE, Green A, Vase P. Prevalence of pulmonary arteriovenous malformations and occurrence of neurological symptoms in patients with hereditary haemorrhagic telangiectasia. J Intern Med. 2000;248:255–62.
38. Sabba C, Gallitelli M, Longo A, Cariati M, Angelelli G. Orthotopic liver transplantation and hereditary haemorrhagic telangiectasia: do hepatic vascular malformations relapse? A long-term follow up study on two patients. J Hepatol. 2004;41:685–90.
39. Svetliza G, De la Canal A, Beveraggi E, et al. Lung transplantation in a patient with arteriovenous malformations. J Heart Lung Transplant. 2002;21:506–8.
40. Lesca G, Plauchu H, Coulet F, et al. Molecular screening of ALK / ACVRL1 and ENG genes in hereditary haemorrhagic telangiectasia in France. Hum Mutat. 2004;23:289–99.
41. Valla D-Ch. Primary Budd-Chiari syndrome. J Hepatol. 2009;50:195–203.
42. Stone MJ, Fulmer JM, Klintmalm GB. Transplantation for Budd-Chiari syndrome. In: Busuttil R, Klintmalm BG, editors. Transplantation of the liver. Philadelphia: Elsevier Saunders; 2005. p. 249–64.
43. Murad SD, Valla D-Ch, de Groen PC, et al. Determinants of survival and the effect of portosystemic shunting in patients with Budd-Chiari syndrome. Hepatology. 2004;39:500–508.
44. Garcia-Pagan JC, Heydtmann M, Raffa S, et al. TIPSS for Budd-Chiari syndrome: long-term results and prognostics factors in 124 patients. Gastroenterology. 2008;135:808–15.
45. Beckett D, Oliff S. Interventional radiology in the management of Budd-Chiari syndrome. Cardiovasc Intervent Radiol. 2008;31:839–47.
46. Mentha G, Giostra E, Majno PE, et al. Liver transplantation for Budd-Chiari syndrome: a European study on 248 patients from 51 centres. J Hepatol. 2006;44:520–8.
47. Segev DL, Nguyen GC, Locke JE, et al. Twenty years of liver transplantation for Budd-Chiari syndrome: a national registry analysis. Liver Transpl. 2007;13:1285–94.
48. Ulrich F, Pratschke J, Neumann U, et al. Eighteen years of liver transplantation experience in patients with advanced Budd-Chiari syndrome. Liver Transpl. 2008;14:144–50.

49. Melear JM, Goldstein RM, Levy MF, et al. Hematologic aspects of liver transplantation for Budd-Chiari syndrome with special reference to myeloproliferative disorders. Transplantation. 2002;74:1090–5.
50. Lerut J, Mazza D, Van Leeuw V, et al. Adult liver transplantation and abnormalities of splanchnic veins: experience in 53 patients. Transpl Int. 1997;10:125–32.
51. Borchert DH. Cavoportal hemitransposition for the simultaneous thrombosis of the caval and portal systems. A review of the literature. Ann Hepatol. 2008;7:200–11.
52. Yamada T, Tanaka K, Ogura Y, et al. Surgical techniques and long-term outcomes of living donor liver transplantation for Budd-Chiari syndrome. Am J Transplant. 2006;6:2463–9.
53. Starzl TE, Demetris J. Liver transplantation: a 21 years experience. Chicago: Year Book Medical Publishers; 1990.
54. Belli L, Sansalone CV, Aseni P, Romani F, Rondinara G. Portal thrombosis in cirrhotics: a retrospective analysis. Ann Surg. 1986;203:286–91.
55. Lerut J, Tzakis AG, Bron K, et al. Complications of venous reconstruction in human orthotopic liver transplantation. Ann Surg. 1987;205:404–14.
56. Francoz C, Belghiti J, Vilgrain V, et al. Splanchnic vein thrombosis in candidates for liver transplantation: usefulness of screening and anticoagulation. Gut. 2005;54:691–7.
57. Yerdel M, Gunson B, Mirza D, et al. Portal vein thrombosis in adults undergoing liver transplantation: risk factors, screening, management and outcome. Transplantation. 2000;69:1873–81.
58. Lerut JP, Laterre PF, Goffette P, et al. Transjugular intrahepatic portosystemic shunt and liver transplantation. Transpl Int. 1996;9:370–5.
59. Stieber AC, Zetti G, Todo S, et al. The spectrum of portal vein thrombosis in liver transplantation. Ann Surg. 1991;213:199–206.
60. Tzakis AG, Kirkegaard P, Pinna AD, et al. Liver transplantation with cavoportal hemitransposition in the presence of diffuse portal vein thrombosis. Transplantation. 1998;65:619–24.
61. Abu-Elmagd KM, Costa G, Bond GJ, et al. Five hundred intestinal and multivisceral transplantations at a single center: major advances with new challenges. 2009;250:567–581.
62. Mazzaferro V, Todo S, Tzakis AG, Stieber AC, Makowka L, Starzl TE. Liver transplantation in patients with previous portasystemic shunt. Am J Surg. 1990;160:111–6.
63. Lerut J, Molle G, Donataccio M, et al. Cavocaval liver transplantation without venovenous bypass and without temporary portocaval shunting: the ideal technique for adult liver grafting. Transpl Int. 1997;10:171–9.
64. Duffy JP, Hong JC, Farmer DG, et al. Vascular complications of orthotopic liver transplantation: experience in more than 4200 patients. J Am Coll Surg. 2009;208:896–905.
65. Miraglia R, Maruzzelli L, Caruso S, et al. Interventional radiology procedures in adult patients who underwent liver transplantation. World J Gastroenterol. 2009;15: 684–93.
66. Raby N, Karani J, Thomas S, O'Grady J, Williams R. Stenosis of vascular anastomoses after hepatic transplantation: treatment with balloon angioplasty. Am J Roentgenol. 1991;157:167–71.
67. Haskal ZJ, Naji A. Treatment of portal vein thrombosis with percutaneous thrombolysis and stent placement. J Vasc Interv Radiol. 1993;4:789–92.
68. Bhattacharjya T, Olliff SP, Bhattacharjya SH, Mirza DF, Mc Master PM. Percutaneous portal vein thrombosis and endovascular stent for management of posttransplant portal venous conduit thrombosis. Transplantation. 2000;69:2195–8.
69. Ciccarelli O, Goffette P, Laterre PF, Wittebolle V, Lerut J. Transjugular intrahepatic portosystemic shunt approach and local thrombolysis for treatment of early post-transplant portal vein thrombosis. Transplantation. 2001;72:159–61.
70. Calleja J, Echenagusia A, Banares R, et al. Portal stenosis in liver transplantation. Treatment by endoluminal prosthesis. Transpl Int. 1995;8:74–5.
71. Colombato L. The role of transjugular intrahepatic portosystemic shunt in the management of portal hypertension. J Clin Gastroenterol. 2007;41:S344–51.
72. Lerut J, Goffette P, Molle G, et al. Transjugular intrahepatic portosystemic shunt after adult liver transplant experience in eight patients. Transplantation. 1999;68: 379–84.
73. Gordon SA, Carmody IA. Arterial problems after liver transplantation. In: Busuttil R, Klintmalm BG, editors. Transplantation of the liver. Philadelphia: Elsevier Saunders; 2005. p. 953–61.
74. Lee SG, Hwang S, Kim KH, et al. Toward 300 liver transplants a year. Surg Today. 2009;39: 367–73.
75. Lerut J, Laterre PF, Lavenne-Pardonge E, et al. Liver transplantation and haemophilia A. J Hepatol. 1995;22:583–5.
76. Hunt BJ. Liver transplantation for severe von Willebrand's disease. Lancet. 1991;337:1553.
77. Friend PJ, McCarthy LJ, Filo RS, et al. Transmission of idiopathic (autoimmune) thrombocytopenic purpura by liver transplantation. N Engl J Med. 1990;323: 807–11.
78. Guy SR, Magliocca JF, Fruchtman S, et al. Transmission of factor VII deficiency through liver transplantation. Transpl Int. 1999;12:278–80.
79. de la Torre AN, Fisher A, Wilson DJ, Harrison J, Koneru B. A case report of donor to recipient transmission of severe thrombocytopenia purpura. Transplantation. 2004;77:1473–4.
80. Osborn NK, Ustundag Y, Zent CS, Wiesner RH, Rosen CB, Narayanan Menon KV. Factor XII deficiency acquired by orthotopic liver transplantation: case report and review of the literature. Am J Transplant. 2006;6:1743–5.
81. Hisatake GM, Chen TW, Renz JF, et al. Acquired hemophilia A after liver transplantation: a case report. Liver Transpl. 2003;9:523–6.

Index

L.D. DeLeve and G. Garcia-Tsao (eds.), *Vascular Liver Disease: Mechanisms and Management*, DOI 10.1007/978-1-4419-8327-5, © Springer Science+Business Media, LLC 2011

I

K

R